Life-Threatening Rashes

Emily Rose
Editor

Life-Threatening Rashes

An Illustrated, Practical Guide

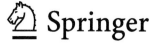 Springer

Editor
Emily Rose
Keck School of Medicine
University of Southern California
Los Angeles, CA
USA

ISBN 978-3-319-75622-6   ISBN 978-3-319-75623-3   (eBook)
https://doi.org/10.1007/978-3-319-75623-3

Library of Congress Control Number: 2018954623

This Springer imprint is published by the registered company Springer Nature Switzerland AG
The registered company address is: Gewerbestrasse 11, 6330 Cham, Switzerland

This book is dedicated to all providers who are entrusted with the care of patients. May you find wisdom, knowledge, and the ability to translate both compassionately to individuals who seek healing.

To my husband and our precious daughters— you are my home, my delight, and my joy in life.

And to my extended family—my parents (and parents-in-law), sisters, friends, and colleagues (who, gratefully, are too numerous to name)—thank you for your love, example, inspiration, and mentorship.

1 Peter 4:8

Preface

This book was inspired by a lecture given at the American College of Emergency Physicians' Scientific Assembly entitled "The Death Rash: Lethal Rashes You Can't Miss." This lecture has been one of the most attended lectures of the conference. Despite knowing these conditions, providers continue to fear missing the diagnosis and the resultant significant clinical consequences.

Many life-threatening conditions present with mucocutaneous findings. These diagnoses are essential to recognize, and clinicians must be able to accurately diagnose these conditions, even when subtle or atypical in presentation. Early recognition and intervention frequently can reverse the disease course. These life-threatening conditions are relatively rare, and clinicians are far more likely to see benign mimics of these encounters. For that reason, several typically benign conditions are also discussed with key features emphasized to help differentiate them from more serious underlying conditions.

This book has been written by a tremendous group of educators and giants in emergency medicine, each with significant expertise on their given topic. All authors were instructed to make the chapter a highly visual, pragmatic guide for the practicing clinician. Each topic was chosen based on its potential for lethal consequences or for the fact that it is a common mimic of a serious diagnosis. This book is not exhaustive but rather emphasizes several diagnoses that are important to exclude due to their potential lethality and other diagnoses that are fairly common benign mimics. The authors highlight key differentiating diagnostic features, detail atypical presentations, discuss differential diagnoses of each condition, and give clinically relevant, high-yield take-home points that can be applied at the bedside.

I would like to thank each author who worked tirelessly to help accomplish the vision of this book. Every chapter has tremendous practical, clinically relevant pearls. Your work is appreciated, and your dedication is admirable. And thank you to ACEP for the inspiration and opportunity to teach such a fun course. May this book enhance your clinical knowledge and help you save lives.

Los Angeles, CA, USA   Emily Rose

Contents

Contributors

Tiffany M. Abramson LAC+USC Medical Center, Department of Emergency Medicine, Keck School of Medicine, Los Angeles, CA, USA

Solomon Behar Pediatric Emergency Medicine, Long Beach Memorial/Miller Children's Hospital & Children's Hospital Los Angeles, Los Angeles, CA, USA

Julie C. Brown Division of Pediatric Emergency Medicine, Department of Pediatrics, University of Washington School of Medicine, Seattle, WA, USA

David Burbulys Health Sciences Clinical Professor of Emergency Medicine, David Geffen School of Medicine at UCLA, Los Angeles, CA, USA

Harbor-UCLA Medical Center, Department of Emergency Medicine, Torrance, CA, USA

Ilene Claudius Harbor-UCLA Medical Center,, Los Angeles, CA, USA

Elizabeth Crow Los Angeles County Medical Center, Department of Emergency Medicine, Los Angeles, CA, USA

Brittney K. DeClerck Keck School of Medicine, Los Angeles, CA, USA

Matthieu P. DeClerck Keck School of Medicine, LAC+USC Medical Center, Los Angeles, CA, USA

James Dill Emergency Medicine/Pediatrics, University of Arizona, Tucson, AZ, USA

Julie Furmick Department of Pediatrics, University of Arizona, Tucson, AZ, USA

Katrina Harper-Kirksey Department of Emergency Medicine, Department of Anesthesia Critical Care, NYU Langone Medical Centers, New York, NY, USA

Molly Hartrich Department of Emergency Medicine, University of Southern California, Los Angeles, CA, USA

Farhan Huq Department of Dermatology, University of Michigan, Ann Arbor, MI, USA

Paul Ishimine Departments of Emergency Medicine and Pediatrics, University of California, San Diego School of Medicine, San Diego, CA, USA

Nathaniel Johnson Emergency Medicine/Pediatrics, University of Arizona, Tucson, AZ, USA

John T. Kanegaye Department of Pediatrics, University of California, San Diego School of Medicine, San Diego, CA, USA

Alex Koyfman Department of Emergency Medicine, The University of Texas Southwestern Medical Center, Dallas, TX, USA

Brett Lee Department of Emergency Medicine, Los Angeles County + University of Southern California Medical Center, Los Angeles, CA, USA

Tracy LeGros Louisiana State University School of Medicine, Emergency Medicine Residency, New Orleans, LA, USA

Brit Long Department of Emergency Medicine, Brooke Army Medical Center, Fort Sam Houston, TX, USA

Louise Malburg Department of Pediatrics, University of Arizona, Tucson, AZ, USA

Mariana Martinez Department of Emergency Medicine, Los Angeles County + University of Southern California Medical Center, Los Angeles, CA, USA

Maureen McCollough David Geffen School of Medicine at UCLA, Department of Emergency Medicine, Los Angeles, CA, USA

Oliveview-UCLA Medical Center, Sylmar, CA, USA

Heather Murphy-Lavoie Louisiana State University School of Medicine, Emergency Medicine Residency, New Orleans, LA, USA

Talib Omer Department of Emergency Medicine, Keck School of Medicine, University of Southern California, Los Angeles, CA, USA

Garrett S. Pacheco Departments of Emergency Medicine & Pediatrics, University of Arizona, Tucson, AZ, USA

Patricia Padlipsky David Geffen School of Medicine at UCLA, Los Angeles, CA, USA

Harbor-UCLA Medical Center, Department of Emergency Medicine, Torrance, CA, USA

Emily Rose Division of Emergency Medicine, Keck School of Medicine of the University of Southern California, Los Angeles County + USC Medical Center, Los Angeles, CA, USA

Genevieve Santillanes Department of Emergency Medicine,, Keck School of Medicine of USC, Los Angeles, CA, USA

Ghazala Q. Sharieff University of California, San Diego, CA, USA
Scripps Health, San Diego, CA, USA

Jan M. Shoenberger Department of Emergency Medicine, Los Angeles County + USC Medical Center, Keck School of Medicine of the University of Southern California, Los Angeles, CA, USA

Elicia Skelton Emergency Medicine, Bellevue/NYU Emergency Department, New York, NY, USA

Stuart Swadron LAC+USC Medical Center, Department of Emergency Medicine, Keck School of Medicine, Los Angeles, CA, USA

Anand Swaminathan Emergency Medicine, St. Joseph's Regional Medical Center, New York, NY, USA

Taku Taira Department of Emergency Medicine, University of Southern California, Los Angeles, CA, USA

Danielle Wickman Department of Emergency Medicine, Los Angeles County + USC Medical Center, Keck School of Medicine of the University of Southern California, Los Angeles, CA, USA

Dale Woolridge Department of Emergency Medicine, University of Arizona, Tucson, AZ, USA

Loren Yamamoto University of Hawai'i John A. Burns School of Medicine, Honolulu, HI, USA
Kapi'olani Medical Center For Women & Children, Honolulu, HI, USA

Kelly D. Young Health Sciences Clinical Professor of Emergency Medicine, David Geffen School of Medicine at UCLA, Los Angeles, CA, USA
Harbor-UCLA Medical Center, Department of Emergency Medicine, Torrance, CA, USA

The Algorithmic Approach to the Unidentified Rash

Heather Murphy-Lavoie and Tracy LeGros

Background

Approximately 5% of emergency department visits are for dermatologic conditions, and there are more than 3000 dermatologic diagnoses. Therefore, it is important to have a systematic approach to a patient with a rash in order to identify the life-threatening and diagnose common conditions. For the purpose of organization and simplicity, this chapter will divide rashes into four basic categories: diffuse erythema, maculopapular rashes, vesiculobullous rashes, and petechial and purpuric rashes [1–7].

History and Physical Exam

When taking the history of a patient with a rash, it is important to gather the following information: age; duration; associated symptoms such as fever, itching, pain, sore throat, and eye irritation; travel history; sick contacts; past medical history; medication history; menstrual history; sexual history; and vaccination history?

The evaluation of a patient with a rash should begin with ascertaining patient acuity with particular attention to mental status and the presence or absence of fever. Then evaluate the rash morphology: is it diffusely erythematous, maculopapular (blanches by definition), vesiculobullous, or petechial/purpuric?

Then assess rash distribution: Is it central, peripheral, on flexural surfaces or extensor surfaces, intertriginous, or dermatomal? Eliciting the initial distribution and progression of the rash is essential. Does it involve the palms and soles? Is there mucous membrane involvement? Next describe the appearance: What color is it? Is it scaly/moist, crusting, umbilicated, palpable, or hyper-/hypopigmented?

H. Murphy-Lavoie (✉) · T. LeGros
Louisiana State University School of Medicine, Emergency Medicine Residency,
New Orleans, LA, USA

© Springer International Publishing AG, part of Springer Nature 2018
E. Rose (ed.), *Life-Threatening Rashes*, https://doi.org/10.1007/978-3-319-75623-3_1

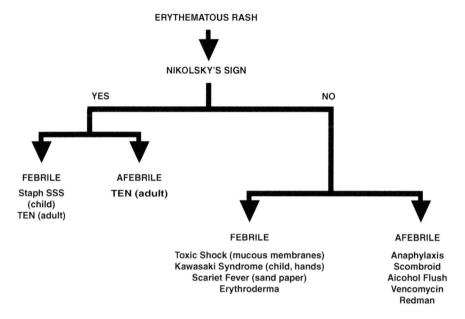

Fig. 1.1 Algorithm for diffuse erythematous rashes. (Reproduced with permission from Murphy-Lavoie and LeGros [1, 2])

Diffuse Erythema

These rashes are characterized by redness of the skin due to capillary congestion and are differentiated by the presence or absence of a Nikolsky sign or a fever (Fig. 1.1). A Nikolsky sign is positive when mild lateral pressure to the skin results in skin sloughing leaving an area of denuded pink tender skin. The presence of a Nikolsky sign indicates either toxic epidermal necrolysis (which is the most serious cutaneous drug reaction in adults; see Chap. 2) or staphylococcal scalded skin syndrome (an emergent infection in children; see Chap. 7). If fever is present without a Nikolsky sign, the differential includes toxic shock syndrome (Chap. 10), Kawasaki syndrome (Chap. 10), scarlet fever (Chap. 10), and erythroderma (Chap. 10). Patients with diffuse erythema and no fever or Nikolsky may be having an anaphylactic reaction (see Chap. 10), scombroid, or red man syndrome from drugs such as vancomycin or alcohol flushing [1–3].

Maculopapular Rashes

Maculopapular rashes are by definition a portmanteau of macules and papules, typically with pink to red hues. They are differentiated by the distribution and presence of systemic toxicity and target lesions (Fig. 1.2). Viral exanthems

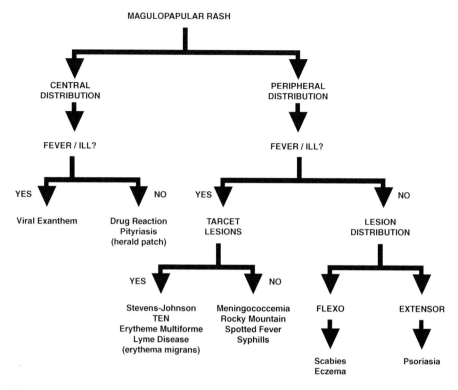

Fig. 1.2 Algorithm for maculopapular rashes. (Reproduced with permission from Murphy-Lavoie and LeGros [1, 2])

frequently have a central distribution initially and then spread centrifugally. Drug reactions also tend to start centrally but are not typically characterized by fever. Maculopapular rashes that start peripherally and are associated with fever include those with target lesions such as Stevens-Johnson syndrome/TEN and those without target lesions such as meningococcemia, syphilis, and Rocky Mountain spotted fever.

Vesiculobullous Rashes

The key factors for differentiating vesiculobullous rashes are degree of distribution (localized versus diffuse) and fever (Fig. 1.3). Febrile patients with diffuse vesiculobullous changes should be evaluated for varicella (Chap. 10), smallpox (Chap. 10), disseminated gonococcemia, and purpura fulminans (Chap. 10) depending on the color and stage of the blisters. Patients without fever and with diffuse blistering should be evaluated for autoimmune conditions such as pemphigus vulgaris and bullous pemphigoid (Chap. 10).

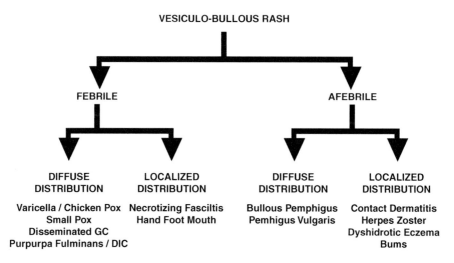

Fig. 1.3 Algorithm for vesiculobullous rashes. (Reproduced with permission from Murphy-Lavoie and LeGros [1, 2])

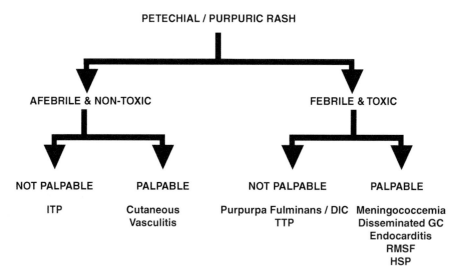

Fig. 1.4 Algorithm for petechial/purpuric rashes. (Reproduced with permission from Murphy-Lavoie and LeGros [1, 2])

Petechial and Purpuric Rashes

Petechial and purpuric rashes are associated with a devastating differential of deadly conditions (Fig. 1.4). Palpable petechiae are vasculitis, and many have an infectious cause such as meningococcemia or Rocky Mountain spotted fever. Notably, both of these conditions start as maculopapular and then become petechial over time. This rash is also present in the more benign conditions such as Henoch-Scholein purpura (see Chap. 10). Nonpalpable petechiae are associated with thrombocytopenia or platelet dysfunction. In the setting of fever and systemic toxicity, thrombocytopenic patients should be evaluated for DIC and thrombotic thrombocytopenic purpura.

Pearls and Take-Home Points
- Generate a differential diagnosis in the setting of fever with a rash to identify some of the more dangerous dermatologic conditions.
- A Nikolsky sign is a harbinger of an emergent condition.
- The presence of mucous membrane involvement should raise the suspicion of a life-threatening condition.
- Petechial rashes with palpable lesions are vasculitis and may have an infectious etiology.
- Nonpalpable petechiae are due to platelet dysfunction or thrombocytopenia.
- The involvement of the palms and soles is a characteristic of specific infectious and autoimmune conditions.
- Hemorrhagic bullae (can be seen in conditions such as necrotizing fasciitis and purpura fulminans) are especially ominous since they usually represent tissue necrosis but may also be present in HSP (see Chap. 10).

References

1. Murphy-Lavoie H, LeGros T. Emergent diagnosis of the unknown rash: the algorithmic approach. Em Med Mag. 2010;42(3):6–17.
2. Murphy-Lavoie H, LeGros T. Approach to the adult rash. In: Adams JG, editor. Emergency medicine: clinical essentials. 2nd ed. Philadelphia: Elsevier Publishing; 2013. p. 1598–608.
3. Ashton R, Leppard B. Differential diagnosis in dermatology. 3rd ed. United Kingdom: Radcliffe Publishing; 2005.
4. Fleischer A, Feldman S, et al. Emergency dermatology: a rapid guide to treatment. New York: McGraw Hill; 2002.
5. Ghatan H. Dermatologic differential diagnosis and pearls. 2nd ed. New York: Parthenon Publishing; 2002.
6. Sauer G, Hall J. Manual of skin diseases. 7th ed. Philadelphia: Lippincott-Raven; 1996.
7. Nguyen T, et al. Dermatologic emergencies: diagnosing and managing life-threatening rashes. Emergency medicine practice: an evidenced based approach to. Emerg Med. 2002.

Anaphylaxis

2

Genevieve Santillanes and Julie C. Brown

Background

Anaphylaxis is a potentially fatal disorder which can present suddenly in previously healthy patients. It is frequently under-recognized and inadequately treated, even in emergency departments [1–5]. Atypical and subtle forms of anaphylaxis are particularly challenging to diagnose. The rate of hospitalization for anaphylaxis has increased, driven mainly by an increase in food-related anaphylaxis [6]. In the outpatient setting, peanuts, tree nuts, fish, shellfish, cow's milk, soy, egg, and sesame are the most common triggers for anaphylaxis [7]. Other triggers include medications, insect venom, and latex.

Anaphylaxis is a systemic allergic reaction due to IgE produced by sensitized B cells. Allergen present in the body binds to IgE. This activates mast cells to release histamine, leukotrienes, prostaglandins, and other immune mediators, which act on end organs throughout the body, such as mucous glands, blood vessels, and smooth muscles, resulting in vasodilation, bronchoconstriction, and smooth muscle contraction. Anaphylactoid reactions circumvent the classic IgE-mediated pathway, and triggers directly activate mast cells. The pathophysiologic distinction is not clinically important in the acute setting, as the emergency management of anaphylactoid reactions is the same as the emergent management of anaphylactic reactions.

G. Santillanes (✉)
Department of Emergency Medicine, Keck School of Medicine of USC, Los Angeles, CA, USA
e-mail: Genevieve.santillanes@usc.edu

J. C. Brown
Division of Pediatric Emergency Medicine, Department of Pediatrics, University of Washington School of Medicine, Seattle, WA, USA
e-mail: Julie.brown@seattlechildrens.org

© Springer International Publishing AG, part of Springer Nature 2018
E. Rose (ed.), *Life-Threatening Rashes*, https://doi.org/10.1007/978-3-319-75623-3_2

Classic Clinical Case Presentation

Anaphylaxis generally presents as a constellation of signs and symptoms, all of which are also seen in other diseases common in acute care settings. No single finding is pathognomonic for anaphylaxis, and no single finding is invariably present in anaphylaxis. The National Institute of Allergy and Infectious Disease/Food Allergy and Anaphylaxis Network (NIAID/FAAN) developed clinical criteria for the diagnosis of anaphylaxis (Table 2.1) [5]. However, these criteria are complex and rely on history that may not be available at presentation. Furthermore, patients with known allergies or a history of anaphylaxis may present early in the course of illness with suggestive symptoms, but not yet meet the NIAID/FAAN clinical criteria for anaphylaxis. Strict adherence to these criteria could lead to unnecessary delay in treatment. A more clinically useful approach to anaphylaxis is that in the appropriate clinical context, patients with one major symptom (such as tight throat, respiratory distress, or fainting) or milder symptoms involving two systems (such as a lump in the throat and vomiting or rash and abdominal pain) warrant treatment with epinephrine [1, 8–10]. Table 2.2 lists signs and symptoms in the most commonly involved organ systems.

Over 90% patients with anaphylaxis have skin or mucosal changes at some point in the clinical course, usually accompanied by pruritus, but cutaneous involvement may not be initially present [3, 11–13]. Involvement of the superficial dermis produces diffuse urticaria and/or flushing as seen in Figs. 2.1, 2.2, 2.3, 2.4, 2.5, and 2.6. Involvement of the subcutaneous dermis produces angioedema which may be localized or diffuse and frequently involves the face as seen in Figs. 2.2, 2.3, 2.4, 2.5, and 2.6. Both angioedema and urticaria are vascular inflammatory reactions. Although angioedema is not necessarily indicative of a more severe reaction, angioedema of

Table 2.1 NIAID/FAAN clinical criteria for diagnosis of anaphylaxis. Anaphylaxis is highly likely if any of the following three criteria are fulfilled

Acute (minutes to several hours) onset of illness with skin or mucosal involvement (generalized hives, pruritus, flushing, swelling of the lips, tongue, or uvula)
PLUS
Respiratory compromise
(dyspnea, bronchospasm, stridor, hypoxemia)
OR
Reduced blood pressure or associated symptoms
(collapse, syncope, incontinence)

Two of the following within minutes to several hours after exposure to a likely allergen for that patient
1. Skin or mucosal involvement (generalized hives, pruritus, flushing, swelling of the lips, tongue, or uvula)
2. Respiratory compromise (dyspnea, bronchospasm, stridor, hypoxemia)
3. Reduced blood pressure or associated symptoms (collapse, syncope, incontinence)
4. Persistent gastrointestinal symptoms (crampy abdominal pain, vomiting)

Reduced blood pressure minutes to several hours after exposure to a known allergen for the patient

Adapted from Sampson et al. [47]

Table 2.2 Possible signs and symptoms of anaphylaxis

Organ system	Signs/symptoms
Skin and mucosa	Urticaria, erythema, angioedema, itching, itchy eyes, conjunctival injection, and edema
Respiratory	Wheezing, stridor, hypoxia, dyspnea, chest pain, cough, sneeze, profuse rhinorrhea
Cardiovascular	Hypotension, tachycardia, delayed capillary refill
Gastrointestinal	Nausea, vomiting, diarrhea, abdominal cramping
Genitourinary	Uterine cramping, urinary incontinence
Neurologic	Syncope or pre-syncope, dizziness, anxiety, altered level of consciousness, irritability in infants

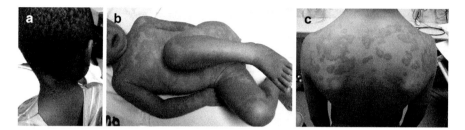

Fig. 2.1 (**a**) Urticaria. (**b**) Urticaria. (Photo credit: Professor Pete Smith). (**c**) Urticaria. (Photo credit: Professor Pete Smith)

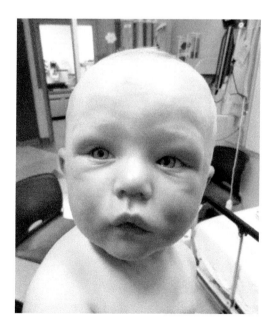

Fig. 2.2 Child with facial flushing and angioedema

Fig. 2.3 Child with angioedema of the lips and Urticaria. (Photo credit: Professor Pete Smith)

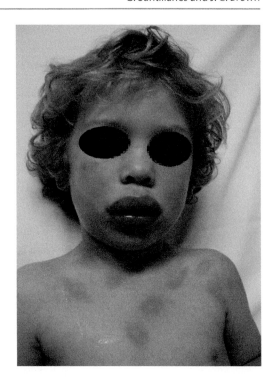

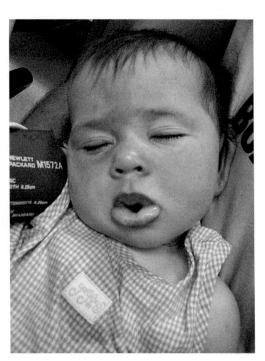

Fig. 2.4 Child with flushing and angioedema of the lips. Urticaria. (Photo credit: Professor Pete Smith)

Fig. 2.5 Child with flushing and angioedema of eyelids. Urticaria. (Photo credit: Professor Pete Smith)

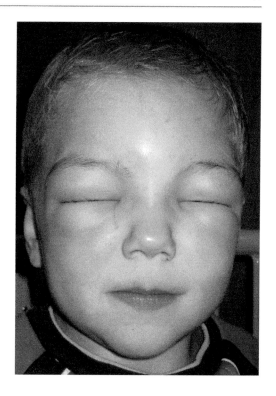

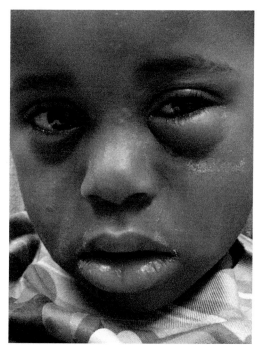

Fig. 2.6 Child with urticaria and angioedema of the eyelid

the oral or pharyngeal mucosa may result in difficulty securing the airway if that becomes necessary.

Anaphylaxis generally involves signs in more than one organ system. Other systems commonly involved in anaphylactic reactions are the respiratory system, the cardiovascular system, the gastrointestinal system, and the neurologic system. Upper respiratory findings include nasal congestion, hoarseness, and stridor. Lower respiratory findings include cough, dyspnea, wheezing, or other evidence of bronchospasm or hypoxia. Histamine release in the gastrointestinal tract may result in crampy abdominal pain, nausea, vomiting, and diarrhea. Vasodilation may manifest with vital sign changes including tachycardia and hypotension and symptoms including pallor, sweating, dizziness, and syncope. In severe cases, marked vasodilation can lead to cardiac arrest.

Atypical Presentation

The lack of unique signs and symptoms and the wide spectrum of possible presentations likely contribute to underdiagnosis of anaphylaxis. Lack of skin involvement can make the diagnosis particularly challenging. Patients and health-care providers must be aware that anaphylaxis can present without cutaneous findings. Cutaneous signs and symptoms are absent in 3–8% of cases of anaphylaxis [3, 11, 14] and are the initial finding in only 65% of cases [12]. Several recent studies found that urticaria is present in only 62–72% of cases [3, 11].

While most cases of anaphylaxis are identified when two or more organ systems are involved, severe symptoms in a single system should be treated without delay if anaphylaxis is suspected [5]. In addition, in the appropriate clinical context, such as the ingestion of a known allergen in a patient with a history of a severe reaction, even milder symptoms, such as widespread rash, warrant treatment for anaphylaxis [5].

Associated Systemic Symptoms

Anaphylaxis is a systemic reaction. Signs and symptoms of anaphylaxis in the respiratory, gastrointestinal, cardiovascular, and neurologic systems are detailed in Table 2.2. Respiratory involvement is seen in 80–97% of cases [3, 11]. Gastrointestinal, neurologic, and cardiovascular signs and symptoms are less common, with each of these systems involved in less than half of cases [3, 14].

Time Course of Disease

Most cases of anaphylaxis present within 1 h of exposure to the trigger. One study found that the mean time from exposure to first symptoms was 31 min with a median of 10 min [14], although symptoms can be delayed for 10 or more hours.

Common Mimics and Differential Diagnosis

As anaphylaxis has myriad presentations, the differential diagnosis varies based on the patient's presenting signs and symptoms. Table 2.3 presents the differential diagnosis based on presenting symptom.

Scombroid is a type of food poisoning that can be clinically indistinguishable from anaphylaxis. It is seen when histidine is broken down to histamine in poorly refrigerated fish resulting in ingestion of large amounts of histamine. Patients may present with oral tingling or burning, rash, pruritus, nausea, vomiting, abdominal cramping, diarrhea, tachycardia, and hypotension [15]. The diagnosis should be suspected if multiple people develop symptoms after eating fish or if a patient has an apparent anaphylactic reaction to a type of fish they have eaten many times previously.

Table 2.3 Differential diagnosis by predominant symptom

Predominant symptom	Differential diagnosis
Rash	Isolated urticaria
	Contact dermatitis
	Erythroderma (toxic shock syndrome or other etiology)
	Carcinoid syndrome
	Viral syndrome
	Henoch-Schonlein purpura
	Erythema multiforme
	Cutaneous drug reaction
	Mastocytosis
Dyspnea/wheeze/stridor/hypoxia	Asthma/chronic obstructive pulmonary disease
	Croup
	Choking event
	Foreign body aspiration
	Epiglottitis
	Pulmonary embolism
	Congestive heart failure
	Panic attack
	Psychogenic stridor
Angioedema (oral)	Angioedema due to ACE inhibitor
	Hereditary angioedema
Angioedema (eyes)	Simple allergic reaction
	Nephrotic syndrome
	Infection (blepharitis, periorbital cellulitis)
Dizziness/syncope/near-syncope	Seizure
	Postural orthostatic tachycardia syndrome
	Syncope (vasovagal, cardiogenic)
	Arrhythmia
	Vertebral basilar insufficiency
	Central vertigo
	Dehydration
	Breath-holding spell
Chest pain	Myocardial infarction
	Arrhythmia
	Aortic dissection

(continued)

Table 2.3 (continued)

Hypotension	Septic shock
	Myocarditis/other cardiogenic shock
	Hypovolemic shock
	Unrecognized trauma
Vomiting/diarrhea/abdominal cramping	Gastroenteritis
	Food poisoning
	Mastocytosis
	Carcinoid syndrome
Difficulty swallowing	Caustic ingestion
	Esophageal foreign body
Altered level of consciousness	Stroke
	Drug/alcohol ingestion
	Meningitis/encephalitis
	Postictal state
	Intracranial hemorrhage
	Cerebral contusion
	Hypoxia
	Psychogenic

Key Physical Exam Findings and Diagnostic Features

The key to making the diagnosis of anaphylaxis is an acute onset of symptoms in two or more organ systems in a patient with a suspected allergic reaction. No physical exam feature is uniformly present in anaphylaxis, and no single organ system is invariably involved in cases of anaphylaxis. There is no finding that is pathognomonic for anaphylaxis; all findings are also seen in other disease processes. Consequently, the clinician must consider symptoms and signs in the context of a carefully gathered history and have a low threshold for treating, even when the diagnosis is uncertain.

Findings of anaphylaxis are not always immediately obvious. Subtle signs of anaphylaxis include conjunctival injection and sudden, profuse rhinorrhea. Decreased breath sounds may be missed without a careful pulmonary examination. Mild facial swelling may not be easily appreciated; asking family members or viewing recent photos can be helpful. Cutaneous findings of anaphylaxis vary greatly and may be limited to erythema of the skin. Even when urticaria is present, there is great variability in the appearance as demonstrated in Fig. 2.1. Urticaria and erythema may be harder to appreciate in patients with dark skin tones.

Management

Epinephrine

Epinephrine is the only first-line therapy for anaphylaxis [1, 5, 7]. Epinephrine should be given immediately in all cases of anaphylaxis and in all cases in which anaphylaxis is the most likely diagnosis. Epinephrine treats all of the signs and symptoms of anaphylaxis and stabilizes mast cells, preventing further histamine

Table 2.4 Effects of epinephrine and antihistamines on signs of anaphylaxis

Effects of cytokines	Effects of epinephrine	Effects of antihistamines (H1 blockers)
	Stabilizes mast cells	
Vasodilation	Vasoconstriction	Block histamine H1 receptor-mediated vasodilation
Bronchoconstriction	Bronchodilation	Block histamine H1 receptor-mediated bronchoconstriction
Smooth muscle contraction	Smooth muscle relaxation	Block histamine H1 receptor-mediated muscle contraction
Increased or decreased pulse	Increased pulse	
Decreased blood pressure	Increased blood pressure	
Decreased coronary perfusion	Increased coronary perfusion[a]	
Onset of action	Almost immediate	15–60+ minutes

[a]Although epinephrine is a vasoconstrictor, in anaphylaxis, its other effects are postulated to result in improved coronary perfusion

release (see Table 2.4). Patients frequently improve dramatically within minutes of receiving intramuscular epinephrine (see Fig. 2.7). Intramuscular epinephrine is best administered in the lateral thigh and may be repeated every 5 min or even sooner if clinically warranted. The risk of complications from appropriately dosed intramuscular epinephrine is extremely low, and there are no absolute contraindications to epinephrine administration [1, 16–18].

Early use of epinephrine improves outcomes. Early use has been shown to decrease the odds of requiring multiple doses of epinephrine [19]. Early epinephrine administration is also associated with decreased emergency department length of stay and decreased risk of hospitalization [20]. Many anaphylaxis deaths are associated with delayed epinephrine use [21, 22]. Unfortunately, many patients treated in emergency departments for anaphylaxis do not receive epinephrine [2, 3, 23, 24]. Patients more frequently receive antihistamines which may be used as adjunctive treatment but have limited effects on the systemic findings of anaphylaxis as demonstrated in Table 2.4.

Other Resuscitative Measures

Supplemental oxygen is indicated for hypoxia, respiratory distress, or cardiovascular symptoms. In patients with evidence of airway edema such as stridor or a hoarse voice, preparations for airway management are necessary in the event that the patient does not improve with epinephrine administration. Patients with anaphylaxis should be presumed to have difficult airways. Intravascular volume can be rapidly depleted in anaphylaxis; bolus intravenous fluids are indicated for hypotension or poor perfusion. Unless patients must be upright due to respiratory distress, the supine position is preferred in nonpregnant patients, and left lateral decubitus positioning is recommended for patients late in pregnancy [1, 7, 25, 26]. The left lateral decubitus position is also preferred for patients who are vomiting.

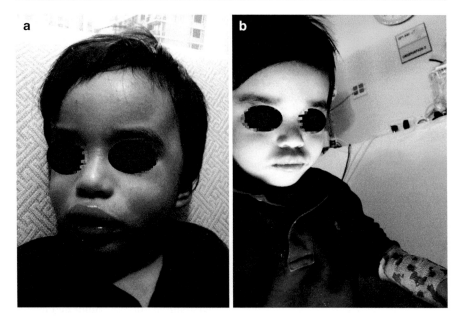

Fig. 2.7 A child with anaphylaxis prior to receiving treatment with epinephrine and minutes after administration of epinephrine

In patients with significant persistent symptoms despite multiple doses of intramuscular epinephrine, an intravenous epinephrine infusion is appropriate. Based on anecdotal experience and the use of nebulized epinephrine in croup, nebulized epinephrine is an option in patients with evidence of upper airway edema despite intramuscular epinephrine [1]. Beta-agonist bronchodilators may also be administered for bronchospasm that does not resolve with intramuscular epinephrine.

Patients taking beta-blocking medications are at risk of persistent bronchospasm and hypotension despite appropriate treatment with epinephrine. Although evidence is limited to case reports, a glucagon infusion may be used to treat patients with refractory anaphylaxis and beta-blocker exposure [27]. Glucagon theoretically improves hypotension and bronchospasm via increased cellular cyclic adenosine monophosphate and can be considered in patients with severe refractory anaphylaxis even in the absence of beta-blocker exposure [1]. Because the evidence is quite limited, a glucagon infusion should only be used as a supplemental treatment and should not delay epinephrine, fluids, and other resuscitative measures.

Delaying administration of epinephrine has been associated with increased reaction severity, increased morbidity, a greater likelihood of biphasic reactions, and an increased risk of fatality even in some cases in which the initial symptoms were mild. (Nowak et al. Customizing anaphylaxis guidelines for emergency medicine. *The Journal of Emergency Medicine.*)

Adjunctive Therapies

Adjunctive therapies include antihistamines and corticosteroids. Administration of adjunctive treatments should never delay the administration of epinephrine or other emergent resuscitative measures. Although there is no direct evidence that histamine blockers are beneficial in anaphylaxis [1, 28], H1 and H2 blockers may be used to treat cutaneous symptoms of anaphylaxis. There is some evidence that a combination of H1 and H2 blockers is superior to monotherapy with an H1 blocker in patients with allergic reactions [29]. Diphenhydramine is often administered, but use of nonsedating antihistamines such as cetirizine avoids sedation which may confuse the clinical picture [30].

Corticosteroids do not work quickly enough to treat the acute phase of anaphylaxis [4]. They are often given to decrease the risk of biphasic reactions; multiple published guidelines state that their use is optional as adjunctive treatment [1, 5]. While theoretically plausible, there is no compelling evidence that corticosteroids lower the risk of biphasic reactions [14, 31–35]. No randomized trials have been performed, but information from cohort studies suggests no benefit of corticosteroids in ED patients [31, 33, 34, 36]. In one retrospective study of patients requiring hospitalization for anaphylaxis, corticosteroid administration was associated with a shorter length of stay [37]. Based on this study, corticosteroid use should be strongly considered in hospitalized patients and those with symptoms that persist after initial treatment [37]. Doses for medications commonly used to treat anaphylaxis are listed in Table 2.5.

Table 2.5 Medications commonly used in the treatment of anaphylaxis

Medication	Pediatric dose	Adult dose
Epinephrine (1 mg/ml = 1:1000)	0.01 mg/kg IM	0.3–0.5 mg IM
H1 blocker		
Diphenhydramine	1.25 mg/kg PO/IV	25–50 mg PO/IV
Cetirizine	<2 years old: 0.25 mg/kg PO up to 2.5 mg 2–5 years old: 2.5 mg PO 6 years and up: 5 mg PO	10 mg PO
H2 blocker		
Ranitidine	2 mg/kg PO 1 mg/kg IV	150 mg PO 50 mg IV
Famotidine	0.5 mg/kg IV	20 mg IV
Corticosteroids		
Prednisone/prednisolone	1–2 mg/kg PO	30–60 mg PO
Methylprednisolone	1–2 mg/kg IV	125 mg IV

IM intramuscular, PO oral, IV intravenous

Disposition

Most patients with anaphylaxis can be discharged home after a period of observation in the emergency department. Due to the risk of biphasic reaction, guidelines recommend a period of observation of at least 4 h even in patients with complete resolution of symptoms [1, 5]. Admission or longer observation periods may be indicated in patients with severe or refractory symptoms (e.g., hypotension or pharyngeal edema) or risk factors for biphasic reactions or fatal anaphylaxis (e.g., history of asthma). Predictors for biphasic reaction in one recent study included a delay in presentation to the emergency department, need for more than one dose of epinephrine, need for inhaled beta-agonists in the emergency department, and a wide pulse pressure on arrival [32]. Delay in epinephrine administration has also been associated with an increase in biphasic reactions [14].

Patients with an episode of anaphylaxis must be prescribed epinephrine auto-injectors at discharge because they are at risk of biphasic reactions and repeated episodes of anaphylaxis. There are currently three different auto-injector designs on the market: Mylan products (EpiPen and generic, Mylan Specialty, L.P., Canonsburg, PA), Impax/Lineage epinephrine which is a generic for Adrenaclick (Impax Laboratories, Inc., Fort Washington, PA), and Auvi-Q (kaléo, Richmond, Virginia) (see Fig. 2.8). All devices are currently available in

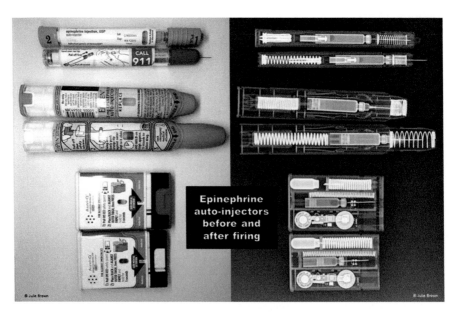

Fig. 2.8 Available epinephrine auto-injectors before and after firing. (© Julie Brown)

0.15 mg and 0.3 mg doses. The manufacturer instructions for the 0.15 mg auto-injectors suggest the use in patients weighing 15 kg up to 30 kg. The 0.3 mg auto-injector is suggested for patients weighing 30 kg or more. A 2017 American Academy of Pediatrics (AAP) clinical report states that it is appropriate to switch to the 0.3 ml auto-injector for children weighing 25–30 kg [38]. Until recently, epinephrine auto-injectors were not available in doses less than 0.15 mg. However, in 2018, the US FDA approved an Auvi-Q 0.1 mg epinephrine auto-injector (kaléo, Richmond, Virginia) with a shorter needle, designed for infants and children weighing less than 15 kg [39]. Ideally the new 0.1 mg auto-injector can be prescribed for all patients weighing less than 15 kg. If a 0.1 mg auto-injector is not available, alternatives for children weighing less than 15 kg include having caregivers draw up an appropriate dose of epinephrine from a 1 ml ampule, giving families syringes pre-filled with epinephrine or prescribing a 0.15 mg epinephrine auto-injector. These options are suboptimal as they risk delay of epinephrine administration, incorrect dosing, or degradation of medication.

The benefit of adjunctive treatments such as corticosteroids and antihistamines after discharge is less clear, but a prescription for a short course of adjunctive medications can be considered at discharge. All patients with a first presentation of anaphylaxis should be referred to an allergist for evaluation [1, 4].

Patient and family education is vital when discharging patients with their first diagnosis of anaphylaxis. Patients and families must understand the importance of early epinephrine administration. In one study of food-related anaphylaxis deaths, most patients had known food allergies, but did not have their epinephrine auto-injector available at the time of the reaction, demonstrating the importance of patient education [40]. Patients must also be instructed in allergen avoidance and signs and symptoms of biphasic or repeat anaphylactic reactions. The various brands of auto-injectors are operated differently, so patients must be instructed in the use of the auto-injector they will receive. This choice may sometimes be determined by cost rather than patient or provider preference, as costs of different auto-injectors may vary greatly based on insurance. Parents of young children diagnosed with anaphylaxis should be instructed to restrain the child appropriately and immobilize the leg before administering epinephrine, to prevent laceration injury [41]. Figure 2.9 demonstrates various restraint methods for a single adult administering an intramuscular injection to a child.

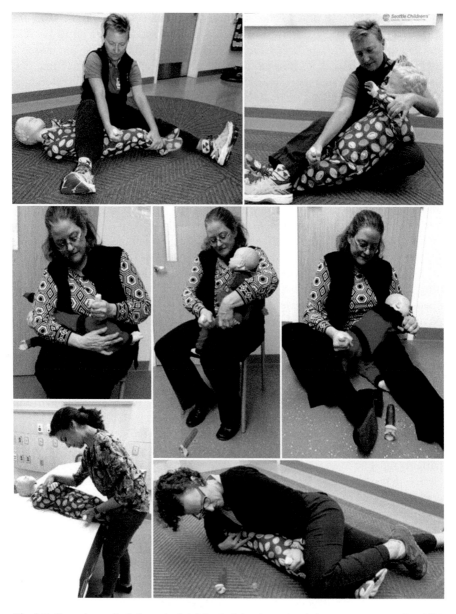

Fig. 2.9 Restraint methods for a single adult administering epinephrine to an uncooperative child. (© Julie Brown)

Complications

Anaphylaxis is a potentially fatal disease. Although fatality due to anaphylaxis is rare with less than one death per million population per year, many of these deaths are preventable deaths occurring in young, otherwise healthy patients [42–44]. Patients with asthma are at increased risk for fatal anaphylaxis [5].

Other less serious complications of anaphylaxis include digit injections, lacerations, and retained needles from epinephrine auto-injectors [45, 46]. Digit injections occur primarily from pen-shaped devices, which are easy to accidentally use upside down [46]. Instructions for use should include training that emphasizes the correct direction of use, such as the "blue to the sky, orange to the thigh" jingle for the Mylan devices. Laceration injuries can be minimized by restraining the thigh before injection if the patient is uncooperative and never reinserting a needle. The instructions for Mylan devices recently changed from a 10-s hold to a 3-s hold, which will hopefully decrease these injuries. The Lineage generic device, however, still has instructions to hold the device in place for 10 s. The Auvi-Q device has a needle that self-retracts in less than 2 s, allowing less time for laceration injury to occur [45].

Bottom Line: Anaphylaxis Clinical Pearls
- Consider the diagnosis of anaphylaxis in patients with a relatively acute onset of symptoms or signs in two or more organ systems, or severe symptoms in a single system, in the context of a suspected allergic reaction.
- Administer epinephrine intramuscularly immediately to any patient with an anaphylactic reaction.
- Antihistamines, corticosteroids, and inhaled beta-agonists are adjunctive therapies for anaphylaxis and should never delay or replace administration of epinephrine.
- Prescribe epinephrine auto-injectors at discharge. Patients also require teaching in auto-injector use, allergen avoidance, recognition of anaphylaxis, and when to treat with epinephrine.

References

1. Campbell RL, Li JT, Nicklas RA, Sadosty AT. Emergency department diagnosis and treatment of anaphylaxis: a practice parameter. Ann Allergy Asthma Immunol. 2014;113:599–608.
2. Clark S, Bock SA, Gaeta TJ, Brenna BE, Cydulka RK, Camargo CA Jr. Multicenter study of emergency department visits for food allergies. J Allergy Clin Immunol. 2004;113:347–52.
3. Grabenhenrich LB, Dolle S, Moneret-Vautrin A, et al. Anaphylaxis in children and adolescents: The European Anaphylaxis Registry. J Allergy Clin Immunol. 2016;137:1128–37.e1.
4. Nowakgerc R, Farrar JR, Brenner BE, Lewis L, Silverman RA, Emerman C, et al. Customizing anaphylaxis guidelines for emergency medicine. J Emerg Med. 2013;45:299.
5. Sampson HA, Munoz-Furlong A, Campbell RL, Adkinson NF, Bock SA, et al. Epidemiology of anaphylaxis: findings of the American College of Allergy, asthma and immunology epidemiology of anaphylaxis working group. Ann Allergy Asthma Immunol. 2006;97:596–602.
6. Lin RY, Anderson AS, Shah SN, Nurruzzaman F. Increasing anaphylaxis hospitalizations in the first 2 decades of life: New York State, 1990–2006. Ann Allergy Asthma Immunol. 2008;101:387–93.
7. Lieberman P, Nicklas R, Oppenheimer J, Kemp S, Lang D. The diagnosis and management of anaphylaxis practice parameter: 2010 update. J Allergy Clin Immunol [AnaphylaxisPracticeParameterAAAAI]. 2010;126:477–80.
8. Boyce JA, Assa'ad A, Burks AW, et al. Guidelines for the diagnosis and management of food allergy in the United States: summary of the NIAID-sponsored expert panel report. J Allergy Clin Immunol. 2010;126:1105–18.

 9. Wang J, Sicherer SH, Section on Allergy and Immunology. Guidance on completing a written allergy and anaphylaxis emergency plan. Pediatrics. 2017;139 https://doi.org/10.1542/peds.2016-4005. Epub 2017 Feb 13.
10. Food allergy & anaphylaxis emergency care plan. Available at: http://www.foodallergy.org/document.doc?id=234. Accessed 10 Aug 2014.
11. de Silva IL, Mehr SS, Tey D, Tang ML. Paediatric anaphylaxis: a 5 year retrospective review. Allergy. 2008;63:1071–6.
12. De Swert LF, Bullens D, Raes M, Dermaux AM. Anaphylaxis in referred pediatric patients: demographic and clinical features, triggers, and therapeutic approach. Eur J Pediatr. 2008;167:1251–61.
13. Rudders SA, Banerji A, Clark S, Camargo CA Jr. Age-related differences in the clinical presentation of food-induced anaphylaxis. J Pediatr. 2011;158:326–8.
14. Lee JM, Greenes DS. Biphasic anaphylactic reactions in pediatrics. Pediatrics. 2000;106:762–6.
15. Feng C, Teuber S, Gershwin ME. Histamine (scombroid) fish poisoning: a comprehensive review. Clin Rev Allergy Immunol. 2016;50:64–9.
16. Nowak RM, Macias CG. Anaphylaxis on the other front line: perspectives from the emergency department. Am J Med. 2014;127:S34–44.
17. Lieberman P, Simons FE. Anaphylaxis and cardiovascular disease: therapeutic dilemmas. Clin Exp Allergy. 2015;45:1288–95.
18. Wood JP, Traub SJ, Lipinski C. Safety of epinephrine for anaphylaxis in the emergency setting. World J Emerg Med. 2013;4:245–51.
19. Hochstadter E, Clarke A, De Schryver S, et al. Increasing visits for anaphylaxis and the benefits of early epinephrine administration: a 4-year study at a pediatric emergency department in Montreal, Canada. J Allergy Clin Immunol. 2016;137:1888–1890.e4.
20. Fleming JT, Clark S, Camargo CA Jr, Rudders SA. Early treatment of food-induced anaphylaxis with epinephrine is associated with a lower risk of hospitalization. J Allergy Clin Immunol Pract. 2015;3:57–62.
21. Pumphrey RS. Fatal anaphylaxis in the UK, 1992–2001. Novartis Found Symp. 2004;257:116–28. discussion 128–32, 157–60, 276–85
22. Pumphrey RS, Gowland MH. Further fatal allergic reactions to food in the United Kingdom, 1999-2006. J Allergy Clin Immunol. 2007;119:1018–9.
23. Clark S, Bock SA, Gaeta TJ, et al. Multicenter study of emergency department visits for food allergies. J Allergy Clin Immunol. 2004;113:347–52.
24. Russell S, Monroe K, Losek JD. Anaphylaxis management in the pediatric emergency department: opportunities for improvement. Pediatr Emerg Care. 2010;26:71–6.
25. Pumphrey RS. Fatal posture in anaphylactic shock. J Allergy Clin Immunol. 2003;112:451–2.
26. Simons FE, Ardusso LR, Bilo MB, et al. 2012 update: world allergy organization guidelines for the assessment and management of anaphylaxis. Curr Opin Allergy Clin Immunol. 2012;12:389–99.
27. Thomas M, Crawford I. Best evidence topic report. Glucagon infusion in refractory anaphylactic shock in patients on beta-blockers. Emerg Med J. 2005;22:272–3.
28. Nurmatov UB, Rhatigan E, Simons FE, Sheikh A. H2-antihistamines for the treatment of anaphylaxis with and without shock: a systematic review. Ann Allergy Asthma Immunol. 2014;112:126–31.
29. Lin RY, Curry A, Pesola GR, et al. Improved outcomes in patients with acute allergic syndromes who are treated with combined H1 and H2 antagonists. Ann Emerg Med. 2000;36:462–8.
30. Banerji A, Long AA, Camargo CA Jr. Diphenhydramine versus nonsedating antihistamines for acute allergic reactions: a literature review. Allergy Asthma Proc. 2007;28:418–26.
31. Lee S, Bellolio MF, Hess EP, Erwin P, Murad MH, Campbell RL. Time of onset and predictors of biphasic anaphylactic reactions: a systematic review and meta-analysis. J Allergy Clin Immunol Pract. 2015;3:408–16.e1–2.
32. Alqurashi W, Stiell I, Chan K, Neto G, Alsadoon A, Wells G. Epidemiology and clinical predictors of biphasic reactions in children with anaphylaxis. Ann Allergy Asthma Immunol. 2015;115:217–223.e2.

33. Choo KJ, Simons FE, Sheikh A. Glucocorticoids for the treatment of anaphylaxis. Cochrane Database Syst Rev. 2012;4:CD007596.
34. Grunau BE, Wiens MO, Rowe BH, et al. Emergency department corticosteroid use for allergy or anaphylaxis is not associated with decreased relapses. Ann Emerg Med. 2015;66:381–9.
35. Joint Task Force on Practice Parameters, American Academy of Allergy, Asthma and Immunology, American College of Allergy, Asthma and Immunology, Joint Council of Allergy, Asthma and Immunology. The diagnosis and management of anaphylaxis: an updated practice parameter. J Allergy Clin Immunol. 2005;115:S483–523.
36. Dhami S, Panesar SS, Roberts G, et al. Management of anaphylaxis: a systematic review. Allergy. 2014;69:168–75.
37. Michelson KA, Monuteaux MC, Neuman MI. Glucocorticoids and hospital length of stay for children with anaphylaxis: a retrospective study. J Pediatr. 2015;167:719–24.e1–3.
38. Sicherer SH, FER S, Section on Allergy and Immunology. Epinephrine for first-aid management of anaphylaxis. Pediatrics. 2017;139 https://doi.org/10.1542/peds.2016-4006. Epub 2017 Feb 13
39. In brief: Auvi-Q epinephrine auto-inejctor for infants and toddlers. The Medical Letter on Drugs and Theraputics. Issue 1547. May 21, 2018.
40. Bock SA, Munoz-Furlong A, Sampson HA. Fatalities due to anaphylactic reactions to foods. J Allergy Clin Immunol. 2001;107:191–3.
41. Brown JC, Tuuri RE, Akhter S, et al. Lacerations and embedded needles caused by epinephrine autoinjector use in children. Ann Emerg Med. 2016;67(3):307–315.e8.
42. Liew W, Williamson E, Tang ML. Anaphylaxis fatalities and admissions in Australia. J Allergy Clin Immunol [AnaphylaxisDeathsAustralia]. 2009;123(2):434–42.
43. Turner PJ, Gowland MH, Sharma V, et al. Increase in anaphylaxis-related hospitalizations but no increase in fatalities: an analysis of United Kingdom national anaphylaxis data, 1992–2012. J Allergy Clin Immunol. 2015;135:956–63.e1.
44. Ma L, Danoff TM, Borish L. Case fatality and population mortality associated with anaphylaxis in the United States. J Allergy Clin Immunol. 2014;133:1075–83.
45. Brown JC, Tuuri RE. Lacerations and embedded needles due to EpiPen use in children. J Allergy Clin Immunol Pract. 2016;4:549–51.
46. Cluck D, Odle B, Rikhye S. Therapeutic management of accidental epinephrine injection. J Pharm Technol [AccidentalEpi]. 2013;29:123–9.
47. Sampson HA, Muñoz-Furlong A, Campbell RL, et al. Second symposium on the definition and management of anaphylaxis: summary report—second National Institute of Allergy and Infectious Disease/Food Allergy and Anaphylaxis Network symposium. J Allergy Clin Immunol. 2006;117(2):391–7.

Pemphigus Vulgaris

3

Brit Long and Alex Koyfman

Background

Pemphigus is a group of life-threatening cutaneous disorders that also involves mucosal surfaces. There are four types of pemphigus including pemphigus vulgaris, pemphigus foliaceus, IgA pemphigus, and paraneoplastic pemphigus [1–7]. These forms differ in their clinical features and laboratory studies. The most common pemphigus disorder is pemphigus vulgaris [1, 3–5]. The incidence ranges from 0.1 to 0.5 per 100,000 people per year and is highest in descendants from India, Southeast Asia, and the Middle East [3, 4].

Pemphigus disorders possess several common features including mucosal involvement and blistering. Table 3.1 demonstrates the features of each disease [1, 3, 4].

The underlying cause of disease manifestation is loss of keratinocyte adhesion due to autoantibodies, specifically IgG in pemphigus vulgaris. These autoantibodies bind to epithelial cell surface antigens, resulting in the destruction of these cells. Desmoglein proteins are the predominant transmembrane glycoproteins targeted. Loss of these proteins leads to blister formation [1, 3–9].

B. Long (✉)
Department of Emergency Medicine, Brooke Army Medical Center, Fort Sam Houston, TX, USA

A. Koyfman
Department of Emergency Medicine, The University of Texas Southwestern Medical Center, Dallas, TX, USA

Table 3.1 Disease features of pemphigus subtypes (distinguishing features in bold)

Disease	Features
Pemphigus vulgaris	Painful mucosal or mucosal and skin involvement, autoantibodies against desmoglein 3 or desmoglein 3 and 1 *Oral mucosal lesions appear first, followed by cutaneous blister formation*
Pemphigus foliaceus	Skin involvement only, with autoantibodies against desmoglein 1 Often involves the scalp *No oral involvement*
IgA pemphigus	Subcorneal pustular dermatosis type IgA pemphigus, neutrophilic IgA dermatosis
Paraneoplastic pemphigus	Occurs with malignancy, often lymphoma *Extensive stomatitis*, pustules, erythema with plaques and crusts Often involves the lungs (bronchiolitis obliterans) and esophagus Subcorneal blisters Autoantibodies against desmoglein 1

There are several contributing factors associated with the autoimmune dysregulation that trigger the onset of disease. A genetic association has been suggested. Associated diseases include autoimmune thyroid disorders, insulin-dependent diabetes, lupus, myasthenia gravis, and rheumatoid arthritis [3, 4, 10]. Ultraviolet light, acidic foods, radiation, viral infection, penicillamine, captopril, rifampin, nonsteroidal anti-inflammatory drugs, penicillins, and cephalosporins may also contribute to disease occurrence [10–14].

Classic Clinical Presentation

This chapter will focus primarily on pemphigus vulgaris. The disease typically affects males and females equally between the ages of 40–60 years [15–17]. The disease is rare in children, except for pemphigus foliaceus, which occurs more commonly in children [18]. The vast majority of patients with pemphigus vulgaris develop mucosal involvement during the disease course. Oral cavity involvement is most common and is the initial site in 50–70% of patients, typically affecting the buccal and palatine mucosa [1, 3–5, 19]. Blisters erode quickly, leaving behind an erosion that may be the only sign found. Other sites include conjunctiva, nasal passages, esophagus, vulva, vagina, anus, and cervix. *Pain with the mucosal lesions is often severe* and worse with chewing or swallowing [1, 3, 4, 19–23].

Cutaneous development often follows, with flaccid blisters on normal skin or on skin with diffuse erythema (Figs. 3.1 and 3.2). These blisters can rupture easily, leaving bleeding erosions. Of note, patients normally do not experience pruritis [3–5]. Nikolsky sign is usually present with cutaneous blisters, in which skin pressure results in erosion and blister extension [5]. Table 3.2 demonstrates typical and classic findings.

Fig. 3.1 Arm blisters from
PV with erosions

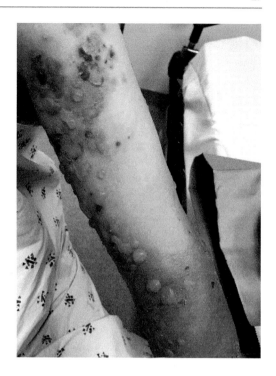

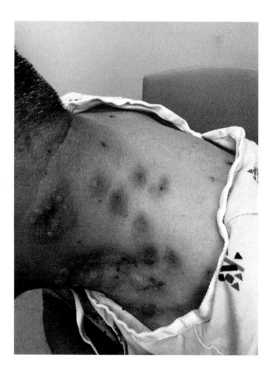

Fig. 3.2 Blisters with erosions and
erythema on the neck from PV

Table 3.2 Classic features of pemphigus vulgaris

Typical presentation
Painful oral mucosal lesions with blisters and erosions
Painful cutaneous blisters and bullae
Diffuse skin involvement includes flaccid blisters or bullae filled with clear fluid
Positive Nikolsky sign
Patient is afebrile and does not have pruritus
Patient is typically 40–60 years of age

Fig. 3.3 Blisters with eruption and bleeding

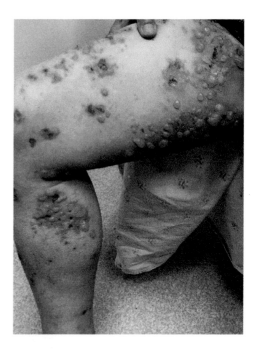

Atypical Presentation

Some forms of pemphigus do not display mucosal involvement, such as pemphigus foliaceus with autoantibodies to desmoglein 1 and 3 [23–25]. In children and young adults, pemphigus foliaceus is the most common form of pemphigus [18]. Pemphigus vegetans demonstrates plaques with granulation tissue and crusting on the scalp, face, axilla, groin, and flexor areas [24, 25]. Urticarial lesions with vesicles is referred to as pemphigus herpetiformis [26]. This form is associated with pruritis, as well as burning sensation.

Associated Systemic Symptoms

Patients are typically afebrile and without pruritis. However, the lesions are extremely painful and may bleed following blister rupture (Fig. 3.3) [3–5, 15, 16]. Other sites of involvement besides oral mucosa include nasal passages, esophagus, and vaginal area. If these areas are affected, patients can present with ocular symptoms, hoarseness, dysphagia, sore throat, dysuria, and dyspareunia. Patients usually do not present with myalgias. Nail involvement is common with dystrophies, subungual hematomas, and chronic paronychia [19–22]. Lung involvement can be seen in paraneoplastic pemphigus, resulting in bronchiolitis obliterans [1–5].

Disease Progression

The disease course varies in patients (Fig. 3.4). The typical sequence in pemphigus vulgaris is the development of oral blisters and erosions, followed by cutaneous flaccid blister formation. These blisters then rupture, resulting in erosions over the first several weeks. With prompt treatment, lesions usually stabilize within 2 weeks, followed by complete resolution by 6-8 weeks [3–5, 15, 16, 27–29].

Common Mimics and Differential Diagnosis

There are a significant number of mimics, with a large differential diagnosis. A key aspect is to differentiate whether the patient is febrile and the distribution of the rash (Table 3.3) [3–5].

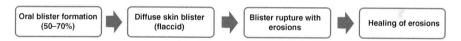

Fig. 3.4 Disease timeline

Table 3.3 Differential diagnosis of pemphigus vulgaris based on associated features

Location	Febrile	Afebrile
Diffuse	Varicella Smallpox Gonococcal disease (disseminated) DIC Purpura fulminans	Bullous pemphigoid Drug-induced bullous disease Pemphigus vulgaris Phytophotodermatitis Erythema multiforme major
Localized	Necrotizing fasciitis Hand-foot-mouth disease	Contact dermatitis Herpes zoster Dyshidrotic eczema Burns Dermatitis herpetiformis Erythema multiforme minor Poison oak, ivy, sumac dermatitis Impetigo

Key Physical Exam Findings

The vital signs may be normal with the absence of fever. Mild tachycardia induced by pain may be present. Hypovolemia-induced tachycardia with hypotension may rarely be present with fluid loss from diffuse blisters or erosions. Patients typically have mucosal blisters or erosions, most commonly in the mouth. Cutaneous involvement is usually diffuse, with flaccid blisters filled with clear fluid. These blisters rupture, resulting in erosions that bleed. Lesions are painful, with positive Nikolsky sign [3–5, 15, 16].

Management

Diagnosis

Diagnosis includes a combination of history, physical examination, and laboratory testing. As seen in Table 3.3, a variety of diseases may present with similar features. Definitive diagnosis of pemphigus requires biopsy of affected cutaneous areas, with histopathological examination demonstrating intraepithelial cleavage in the suprabasal regions, retention of basal keratinocytes within the basement membrane zone, and inflammatory eosinophilic infiltrates within the dermis [1, 4, 11]. Direct immunofluorescence is only completed on normal appearing skin or mucosa (Fig. 3.5). Intracellular IgG deposition will be seen. ELISA testing may also be completed to evaluate for circulating autoantibodies [1, 3–5, 11, 16]. An electrolyte panel is indicated if there is diffuse skin involvement and/or the patient is toxic appearing.

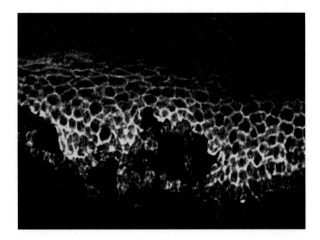

Fig. 3.5 Positive direct immunofluorescence. (From https://upload.wikimedia. org/wikipedia/commons/ thumb/3/3c/Pemphigus_ immunofluorescence. jpg/200px-Pemphigus_ immunofluorescence.jpg)

Treatment

Untreated pemphigus has a high mortality rate, which is typically a result of secondary infection. The goal of treatment is the remission of the disease while limiting side effects of medications. Systemic glucocorticoids are the primary treatment to achieve control of the disease, whether the presentation is early and mild or severe. Before corticosteroids, mortality ranged from 70% to 100% for pemphigus vulgaris [5, 7, 27–29]. With treatment including corticosteroids, mortality is often less than 10%. Corticosteroids include prednisone, prednisolone, or methylprednisolone [27–29]. Prednisone at 1–1.5 mg/kg by mouth or IV per day is often the initial treatment. Patients usually display rapid response to corticosteroid therapy, within 2 weeks commonly. Unfortunately, patients may require extended corticosteroid therapy, which increases the risk of side effects. To minimize this risk, adjunctive immunosuppressive agents may be utilized. These include IV gamma globulin, rituximab, azathioprine, mycophenolate mofetil, and cyclophosphamide [27–36]. The emergency physician can begin the steroid course, but the use of these other agents typically requires admission and further consultation (Table 3.4).

Local skin care is important for patient comfort and limiting infection risk. Blisters can be punctured in a sterile manner to facilitate fluid drainage, leaving the blister roof intact and covering the wound, but this practice is controversial. Erosions should be kept clean and covered with antibiotic ointment and bandage. A high potency topical corticosteroid may be used on erosions that do not improve with systemic glucocorticoid therapy [3–5, 30, 32–35].

Oral lesions produce significant discomfort. Patients must avoid acidic, abrasive, spicy, or hot foods. Topical anesthetics such as viscous lidocaine 2% may assist in numbing the oral mucosa. Oral hygiene is imperative [3–5, 30, 34–36].

For patients who are nontoxic appearing with localized blisters, discharge home with dermatology follow-up is possible. However, the patient with extensive blisters, toxic appearance, or abnormal hemodynamic status should be admitted for management and further monitoring. Fluid resuscitation and

Table 3.4 Treatment of pemphigus vulgaris

Treatment
Systemic glucocorticoids, prednisone 1–1.5 mg/kg per day
Keep skin lesions clean; may cover erosions with antibiotic ointment and bandage
Ttreat oral lesions with topical lidocaine or corticosteroids; avoid topically aggravating foods, and maintain good oral hygiene
Adjunctive treatments include gamma globulin, rituximab, azathioprine, mycophenolate mofetil, and cyclophosphamide

Table 3.5 Factors associated with clinical improvement of pemphigus vulgaris

Factors indicating effective treatment
Absence of new lesions
Limited blistering
Negative Nikolsky sign
Remission of active lesions

electrolyte management may be required for patients with diffuse involvement, and the patient may require transfer to a burn center for diffuse involvement [30, 33–35].

Superinfection of mucosal and skin lesions may occur with many organisms (see section "Complications" below). Targeted treatment to combat these infections should be administered including topical and/or oral antibiotics and antiviral and antifungal medications as indicated.

Patient improvement is monitored through several aspects (Table 3.5). With these factors present, medications should be tapered. Full resolution is often observed within 6–8 weeks [4, 5, 30, 33–35].

Complications

Due to the painful oral and cutaneous blisters, a variety of complications may develop. Poor intake with weight loss and malnutrition can occur. Electrolyte disorders, hypoalbuminemia, fluid loss/dehydration, local infections, and systemic infections may occur in the setting of diffuse involvement [3–5, 30, 32–35]. Ocular involvement may be extensive, requiring ophthalmology evaluation and management including debridement and topical steroids. Topical steroids should only be provided with ophthalmology consultation.

Patients must be monitored for signs of infection, a major cause of morbidity and mortality in patients with pemphigus vulgaris. Skin lesions and erosions may become secondarily infected with bacterial species (most commonly *Staphylococcus* or *Streptococcus*) or herpes simplex virus (Fig. 3.6) [35–37]. Mucosal lesions may become secondarily infected with *Candida* (Fig. 3.7), especially with glucocorticoid use [34–36].

The medications utilized for initial control and disease remission can have significant side effects. Glucocorticoids may cause hypertension, diabetes, hyperlipidemia, osteoporosis, gastrointestinal ulcers, and increase infection risk. Other immunomodulators may result in increased risk of infection, renal injury, liver dysfunction, nausea/vomiting, and bone marrow suppression [27–37].

Fig. 3.6 Herpes simplex
virus infection. (From
https://upload.wikimedia.
org/wikipedia/commons/d/
dc/Herpes_zoster_neck.png)

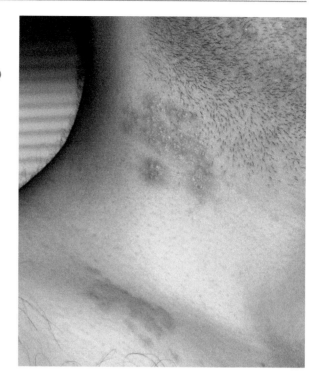

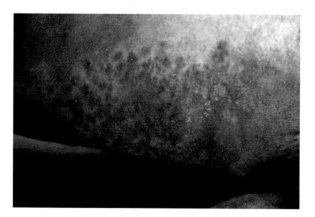

Fig. 3.7 Candidiasis of the
skin. (From https://en.
wikipedia.org/wiki/
Candidiasis#/media/
File:Derm-57.jpg)

Bottom Line: Pemphigus Vulgaris Clinical Pearls
- Pemphigus vulgaris has a high mortality rate without treatment.
- The classic clinical course is initial painful mucosal blisters and erosions.
- Mucosal lesions most commonly occur in the mouth, but any mucosal surface may be involved.
- Cutaneous blistering/bullae typically occur after mucosal lesions and are characterized by a positive Nikolsky sign.
- Pain, not pruritus, is the predominant symptom of lesions.
- Fever is not common but may indicate superinfection.
- The diagnosis is suspected clinically but confirmed by biopsy.
- Treatment includes systemic glucocorticoids, oral care, skin care, and adjunctive treatments as needed to facilitate resolution of lesions.
- Superinfection increases risk of morbidity and mortality and should be treated.
- Extensive lesions, severe superinfection, and toxic appearance require admission.
- Complications include electrolyte disorders, hypovolemia, secondary infection, and medication side effects.

Acknowledgments The view(s) expressed herein are those of the author(s) and do not reflect the official policy or position of Brooke Army Medical Center, the US Army Medical Department, the US Army Office of the Surgeon General, the US Department of the Air Force, the US Department of the Army or the Department of Defense, or the US Government.

References

1. Stanley JR, Amagai M. Pemphigus, bullous impetigo, and the staphylococcal scalded-skin syndrome. N Engl J Med. 2006;355:1800.
2. Mihai S, Sitaru C. Immunopathology and molecular diagnosis of autoimmune bullous diseases. J Cell Mol Med. 2007;11:462.
3. Kneisel A, Hertl M. Autoimmune bullous skin diseases. Part 1: clinical manifestations. J Dtsch Dermatol Ges. 2011;9:844.
4. Bystryn JC, Rudolph JL. Pemphigus. Lancet. 2005;366:61.
5. Venugopal SS, Murrell DF. Diagnosis and clinical features of pemphigus vulgaris. Dermatol Clin. 2011;29:373.
6. Sitaru C, Zillikens D. Mechanisms of blister induction by autoantibodies. Exp Dermatol. 2005;14:861.
7. Grando SA. Pemphigus autoimmunity: hypotheses and realities. Autoimmunity. 2012;45:7.
8. Amagai M, Tsunoda K, Zillikens D, et al. The clinical phenotype of pemphigus is defined by the anti-desmoglein autoantibody profile. J Am Acad Dermatol. 1999;40:167.
9. Ding X, Aoki V, Mascaro JM Jr, et al. Mucosal and mucocutaneous (generalized) pemphigus vulgaris show distinct autoantibody profiles. J Invest Dermatol. 1997;109:592.
10. Firooz A, Mazhar A, Ahmed AR. Prevalence of autoimmune diseases in the family members of patients with pemphigus vulgaris. J Am Acad Dermatol. 1994;31:434.
11. Brenner S, Goldberg I. Drug-induced pemphigus. Clin Dermatol. 2011;29:455.
12. Ruocco V, Pisani M. Induced pemphigus. Arch Dermatol Res. 1982;274:123.
13. Ruocco V, Ruocco E, Lo Schiavo A, et al. Pemphigus: etiology, pathogenesis, and inducing or triggering factors: facts and controversies. Clin Dermatol. 2013;31:374.

14. Brenner S, Tur E, Shapiro J, et al. Pemphigus vulgaris: environmental factors. Occupational, behavioral, medical, and qualitative food frequency questionnaire. Int J Dermatol. 2001;40:562.
15. Joly P, Litrowski N. Pemphigus group (vulgaris, vegetans, foliaceus, herpetiformis, brasiliensis). Clin Dermatol. 2011;29:432.
16. James KA, Culton DA, Diaz LA. Diagnosis and clinical features of pemphigus foliaceus. Dermatol Clin. 2011;29:405.
17. Brenner S, Wohl Y. A survey of sex differences in 249 pemphigus patients and possible explanations. Skinmed. 2007;6:163.
18. Diaz LA, Sampaio SA, Rivitti EA, et al. Endemic pemphigus foliaceus (Fogo Selvagem): II. Current and historic epidemiologic studies. J Invest Dermatol. 1989;92:4.
19. Mustafa MB, Porter SR, Smoller BR, Sitaru C. Oral mucosal manifestations of autoimmune skin diseases. Autoimmun Rev. 2015;14:930.
20. Kavala M, Topaloğlu Demir F, Zindanci I, et al. Genital involvement in pemphigus vulgaris (PV): correlation with clinical and cervicovaginal pap smear findings. J Am Acad Dermatol. 2015;73:655.
21. Kavala M, Altıntaş S, Kocatürk E, et al. Ear, nose and throat involvement in patients with pemphigus vulgaris: correlation with severity, phenotype and disease activity. J Eur Acad Dermatol Venereol. 2011;25:1324.
22. Torchia D, Romanelli P, Kerdel FA. Erythema multiforme and Stevens-Johnson syndrome/toxic epidermal necrolysis associated with lupus erythematosus. J Am Acad Dermatol. 2012;67:417.
23. Amagai M. Pemphigus. In: Bolognia JL, Jorizzo JL, Schaffer JV, et al., editors. Dermatology, 3rd ed. vol 1. Elsevier, Saunders; 2012. p. 2776. ISBN: 9780702051821.
24. Shinkuma S, Nishie W, Shibaki A, et al. Cutaneous pemphigus vulgaris with skin features similar to the classic mucocutaneous type: a case report and review of the literature. Clin Exp Dermatol. 2008;33:724.
25. Payne AS, Stanley JR. Pemphigus. In: Goldsmith LA, Katz SI, Gilchrest BA, Paller AS, Leffell DJ, Wolff K, editors. Fitzpatrick's dermatology in general medicine, vol. 1. 8th ed. New York: McGraw Hill; 2012. https://accessmedicine.mhmedical.com/content.aspx?bookid=392&sectionid=41138687. Accessed January 14, 2018.
26. Lebeau S, Müller R, Masouyé I, et al. Pemphigus herpetiformis: analysis of the autoantibody profile during the disease course with changes in the clinical phenotype. Clin Exp Dermatol. 2010;35:366.
27. Martin LK, Werth V, Villanueva E, et al. Interventions for pemphigus vulgaris and pemphigus foliaceus. Cochrane Database Syst Rev. 2009;(1):CD006263.
28. Beissert S, Werfel T, Frieling U, et al. A comparison of oral methylprednisolone plus azathioprine or mycophenolate mofetil for the treatment of pemphigus. Arch Dermatol. 2006;142:1447.
29. Bystryn JC, Steinman NM. The adjuvant therapy of pemphigus. An update. Arch Dermatol. 1996;132:203.
30. Kasperkiewicz M, Schmidt E, Zillikens D. Current therapy of the pemphigus group. Clin Dermatol. 2012;30:84.
31. Atzmony L, Hodak E, Leshem YA, et al. The role of adjuvant therapy in pemphigus: a systematic review and meta-analysis. J Am Acad Dermatol. 2015;73:264.
32. Ratnam KV, Phay KL, Tan CK. Pemphigus therapy with oral prednisolone regimens. A 5-year study. Int J Dermatol. 1990;29:363.
33. Harman KE, Albert S, Black MM, British Association of Dermatologists. Guidelines for the management of pemphigus vulgaris. Br J Dermatol. 2003;149:926.
34. Murrell DF, Dick S, Ahmed AR, et al. Consensus statement on definitions of disease, end points, and therapeutic response for pemphigus. J Am Acad Dermatol. 2008;58:1043.
35. Kneisel A, Hertl M. Autoimmune bullous skin diseases. Part 2: diagnosis and therapy. J Dtsch Dermatol Ges. 2011;9:927.
36. Hertl M. Pemphigus vulgaris. CME Dermatol. 2009;4:94.
37. Caldarola G, Kneisel A, Hertl M, Feliciani C. Herpes simplex virus infection in pemphigus vulgaris: clinical and immunological considerations. Eur J Dermatol. 2008;18:440.

Stevens-Johnson Syndrome and Toxic Epidermal Necrolysis

4

Farhan Huq, Talib Omer, and Solomon Behar

Background

Stevens-Johnson syndrome/toxic epidermal necrolysis (SJS/TEN) is a rare but devastating febrile mucocutaneous type-IV hypersensitivity reaction following drug administration. Overall mortality for TEN remains high at 25–34% [1, 2]. Drug-reactive T-lymphocytes drive the release of cytotoxic mediators, ultimately resulting in widespread keratinocyte apoptosis and separation at the dermal-epidermal junction [3]. Treatment is supportive and is ideally done in the setting of a burn intensive care unit, with the aim of supporting the vital organs, while reepithelialization can take place [1].

Presentation, Diagnosis, and Associated Clinical Symptoms

SJS is defined by <10% body involvement. TEN (also referred to as Lyell syndrome) is the more extensive variant and involves >30% of the body surface area. The intermediary range between 10% and 30% is known as SJS/TEN overlap.

Initiation of a causative drug, most commonly allopurinol, aromatic anticonvulsants, sulfonamides, aminopenicillins, cephalosporins, tetracyclines, quinolones, imidazole antifungals, lamotrigine (Fig. 4.1), nevirapine, abacavir, or oxicam NSAIDs, occurs 4–21 days prior to the drug eruption [1, 2, 4, 5]. But re-exposure of

F. Huq
Department of Dermatology, University of Michigan, Ann Arbor, MI, USA

T. Omer (✉)
Department of Emergency Medicine, Keck School of Medicine, University of Southern California, Los Angeles, CA, USA

S. Behar
Pediatric Emergency Medicine, Long Beach Memorial/Miller Children's Hospital & Children's Hospital Los Angeles, Los Angeles, CA, USA

© Springer International Publishing AG, part of Springer Nature 2018
E. Rose (ed.), *Life-Threatening Rashes*, https://doi.org/10.1007/978-3-319-75623-3_4

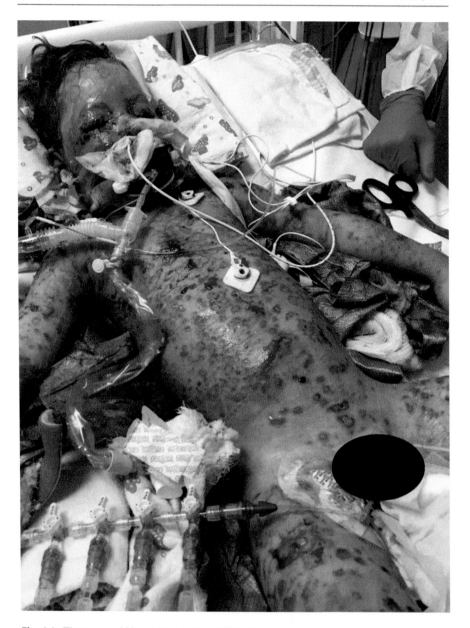

Fig. 4.1 Three-year-old boy who developed TEN after being started on lamotrigine for seizures. (Photo credit: Justin Greenberg, DO, University of Southern California, Keck School of Medicine, Los Angeles, CA)

an offending medication can precede SJS/TEN by hours [1, 4]. Though medications are by far the most frequent cause of SJS/TEN, other causative factors include measles-mumps rubella vaccination, *Mycoplasma pneumonia* infection, *dengue* virus, *cytomegalovirus* reactivation, or IV contrast administration [4].

Epidemiology: Incidence and Prevalence

SJS is more common than SJS/TEN overlap, which is more common than TEN. SJS has an incidence of 1.2–6 cases per million persons per year [4]. TEN has an incidence of 0.4–1.2 cases per million per year; SJS is roughly three times more prevalent than TEN [4]. Overall, SJS/TEN incidence ranges between 1.2 and 12.7 cases per million person per year [6, 7]. HIV-infected individuals have a much higher chance of developing SJS/TEN, where it affects 1 out of every 1000 individuals, possibly due to the use of drugs such as rifampin, sulfonamide antibiotics, and various antiretrovirals (most commonly nevirapine) [8].

Mortality generally correlates with increased cutaneous involvement. In the USA, mean adjusted mortality is 4.8% (range = 3.7–7.6) for SJS, 19.4% (range = 15.7–22.3) for SJS/TEN, and 14.8% (range = 7.7–19.0) for TEN [8].

SJS/TEN is associated with nonwhite race, particularly Asians (odds ratio = 3.27) and blacks (odds ratio = 2.01) [6]. Predictors of mortality include increased age, increased number of chronic conditions, infection (septicemia, pneumonia, tuberculosis), hematological malignancy (non-Hodgkin's lymphoma, leukemia), and renal failure [6].

Clinical Presentation

Please refer to Table 4.1 for a systems-based summary of clinical findings. Ninety percent of patients have concomitant mucosal involvement (ocular, genitourinary, or oral). Oral mucosa is more commonly involved than ocular, anal, or genital mucosa [9] (Fig. 4.2a). Mucosal involvement develops shortly before or concomitantly with skin changes in almost all cases [10]. Dermal changes appear as dusky red skin macules or patches that progress to bullae (Fig. 4.3), skin sloughing (Figs. 4.4 and 4.5), and mucosal erosions (2b, 3 and 6). Epidermal sheets bunch into

Table 4.1 Cutaneous and extracutaneous manifestations of SJS/TEN

Organ system	Manifestations
Ocular	Conjunctival hyperemia, sicca syndrome, sandy sensation, symblepharon, corneal scarring, corneal xerosis, trichiasis, blindness, subconjunctival fibrosis, photophobia, vision loss
Otolaryngologic	Hypopharyngeal stenosis, nasal septal synechiae, auditory canal stenosis, pinna synechiae
Oral dermatologic	Dental growth abnormalities, gingival and labial synechiae Macular rash, bullous eruption/epidermal separation, permanent dyspigmentation, eruptive melanocytic nevi, onycholysis, onychodystrophy, loss of fingernails, and hair thinning
Respiratory	Bronchiolitis obliterans, bronchiectasis, and chronic obliterative bronchitis
Gastrointestinal/hepatic	Esophageal strictures and webs; rarely, small bowel obstruction, persistent intestinal ulcers, chronic cholestasis, ischemic hepatitis
Gynecologic	Vulvar and vaginal adenosis, vaginal stenosis, fusion of the labia minora and majora, hematocolpos, hydrocolpos
Renal	Glomerulonephritis

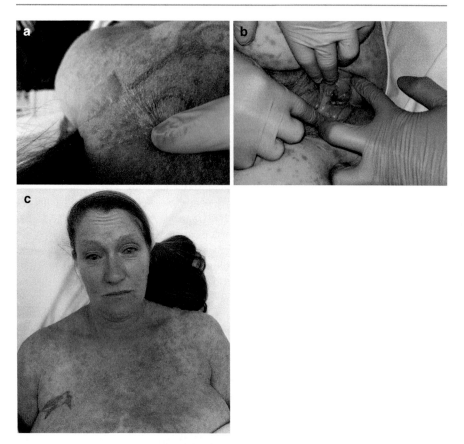

Fig. 4.2 (**a**) shows the Nikolsky sign on the back of a middle-aged female with SJS-TEN without known trigger. (Photo credit: Talib Omer, MD PhD; University of Southern California, Keck School of Medicine, Los Angeles, CA). (**b**) She also had vaginal mucus membrane involvement. (Photo credit: Talib Omer, MD PhD; University of Southern California, Keck School of Medicine, Los Angeles, CA). (**c**) Large parts of the torso and her eyes were affected as well. (Photo credit: Talib Omer, MD PhD; University of Southern California, Keck School of Medicine, Los Angeles, CA)

thinly rolled sheets that rim the edges of ruptured bullae, reminiscent of wet cigar paper [4]. Prodromal symptoms include flu-like symptoms of fever, cough, rhinorrhea, anorexia, malaise, conjunctivitis, dysuria, and/or uveitis which may precede the rash by several days [11].

A symmetrical, painful macular exanthem appears on the face and trunk (Figs. 4.1, 4.2c, 4.6 and 4.7). Nikolsky sign (Fig. 4.2b) develops, whereby gentle stroking of the skin produces separation of the epidermis and the basal layer and blisters form. Asboe-Hansen sign, where pressure on a bulla causes extension to the unaffected adjacent skin, may also be seen [1].

Loss of the dermal barrier integrity leads to extensive fluid loss, electrolyte shifts, and increased susceptibility to infections, often caused by *Pseudomonas* and

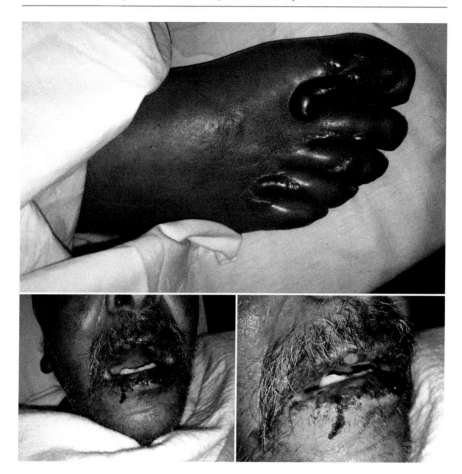

Fig. 4.3 Figure shows involvement of lips, mucus membranes, and feet in a patient with SJS. (Photo credit: Talib Omer, MD PhD and Neil Rifenbark, MD; University of Southern California, Keck School of Medicine, Los Angeles, CA)

S. Aureus [11]. The most serious complications include sepsis (most common cause of death), severe hypovolemia and hypovolemic shock, severe electrolyte derangement, acute respiratory distress syndrome, multiple organ dysfunction syndrome, abdominal compartment syndrome caused by aggressive fluid resuscitation, and bowel necrosis.

Other complications that may be seen are dyspigmentation, eruptive melanocytic nevi, onycholysis (separation of the nail plate from the nail bed), onychodystrophy (change in nail morphology), loss of fingernails, and hair thinning [1].

Ocular, oral, oropharyngeal, dermatologic, respiratory, gastrointestinal/hepatic, gynecologic, and renal involvement has been described in the literature, including corneal and colonic perforation [12, 13]. Apposing inflamed and denuded mucosa can lead to synechiae/scar formation, adhesions, stenosis, stricturing, or even perforation [12, 13].

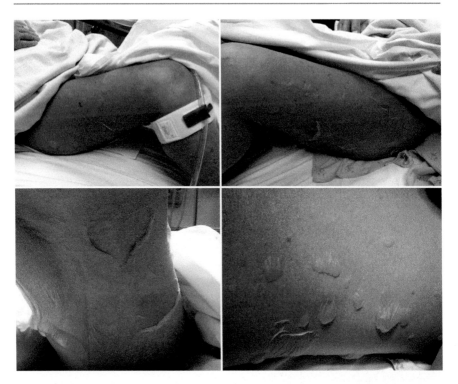

Fig. 4.4 Dermal changes appear as dusky red skin macules or patches that progress to bullae and skin sloughing. Epidermal sheets bunch into thinly rolled sheets that rim the edges of ruptured bullae, reminiscent of wet cigar paper (Photo credit: Tracie Pearson, MD; University of Michigan Department of Dermatology)

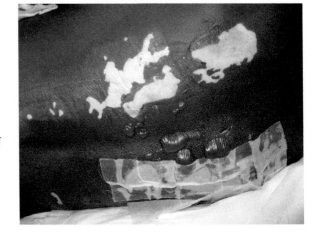

Fig. 4.5 Figure shows bullae and skin sloughing of the posterior trunk in a patient with SJS-TEN. (Photo credit: Heather Murphy-Lavoie, MD; Louisiana State University School of Medicine)

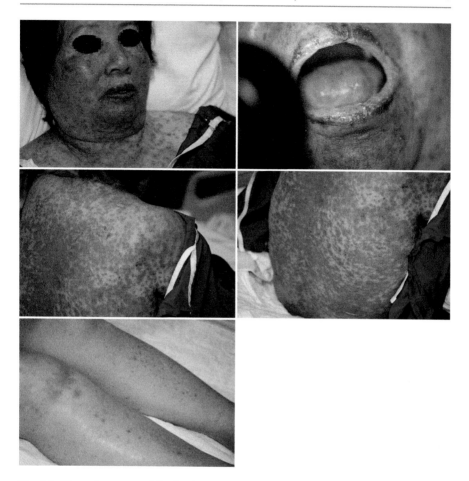

Fig. 4.6 Figure shows truncal distribution while sparing distal extremities, in contrast to erythema multiforme. (Photo credit: Arjun Dupati, MD; University of Michigan Department of Dermatology)

Atypical Presentation

The appearance of SJS may vary significantly. In some rare cases, only mucus membrane involvement may be observed. At times, SJS/TEN may be indistinguishable from other illnesses. In a case report, a patient developed high fever, pancytopenia, diarrhea with mucosal erosions, and an erythematous exanthema with flaccid blisters following orthotopic liver transplantation [14]. Although skin biopsies suggested diagnosis of SJS/TEN overlap, postmortem chimerism analysis revealed a distribution of >40%, indicating TEN [14].

Another case series illustrates the difficulty of diagnosis in pediatric patients with underlying systemic lupus erythematosus (LE) who developed bullous eruptions [15]. A series of three patients with pediatric systemic LE presented with

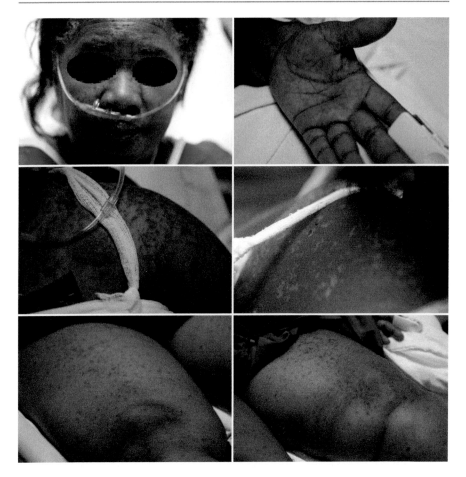

Fig. 4.7 Healing SJS/TEN with pigmented skin. (Photo credit: Elizabeth Thompson, MD; University of Michigan Department of Dermatology)

severe worsening of skin disease resembling TEN. However, the initial photo-distribution of the eruption, subacute progression, limited mucosal involvement, mild systemic symptoms, supportive biopsy and laboratory results, and lack of culprit drugs were more suggestive of a TEN-like cutaneous LE [15].

Common Mimics and Differential Diagnosis

Erythema Multiforme

In contrast to SJS/TEN, erythema multiforme (EM) demonstrates multiple target or iris lesions and typically involves less than 10% of the body surface area [16]. EM is usually self-limiting, and complete recovery takes between 1 and 4 weeks. EM is tied to infectious causes 90% of the time, particularly HSV and *Mycoplasma pneumoniae*, though it may be drug-induced in <10% of cases [3, 16, 17]. Patients with EM develop raised lesions symmetrically on distal extremities, whereas SJS/TEN lesions are more often flat or purpuric with trunk and/or widespread distribution [17]. Prodromal symptoms are rare, and few, if any, systemic symptoms are present, but these may include fever, malaise, cough, headache, rhinitis, sore throat, myalgia, arthralgia, nausea, and vomiting [1, 16]. Oral mucosal involvement occurs in approximately 70% of cases; the lips, alveolar mucosa, and palate can be involved [16]. See Chap. 5 for more information.

Staphylococcal Scalded Skin Syndrome

Please refer to Table 4.2 for common differential diagnoses to consider in addition to SJS/TEN. Although staphylococcal scalded skin syndrome (SSSS) is predominantly a pediatric disease affecting those <5 years of age, it can also be seen in immunosuppressed adults or those with renal failure [1]. Early on in the classification scheme, SJS/TEN was mistakenly thought to be a related clinical entity [3]. Epidermolytic toxins released by *S. Aureus* cause superficial intraepidermal blistering at the level of the epidermal granular layer, a more superficial level than that of SJS/TEN, and as a result, it lacks the associated necrosis, inflammation, or prolonged healing [18]. Antecedent *staph* infection is not always detected [18]. The superficial blisters usually occur in areas of friction or body orifices [18]. Also, a key differentiating feature is a distinct lack of mucosal surface involvement [18]. See Chap. 10 for more information.

Acute Graft Vs. Host Disease

Differentiating graft vs. host disease and SJS/TEN may be extremely challenging. Histologically, (GVHD) is indistinguishable from TEN, as both entities demonstrate full thickness epidermal necrosis, pauci-inflammatory dermal infiltrate, and subepidermal blistering [1, 19]. Bone marrow transplant recipients frequently also receive medications known to incite TEN, and high-dose chemotherapy-induced neutropenia can lead to oral mucositis [18]. GVHD typically occurs 2–6 weeks after a hematopoietic stem cell transplant. It presents as a symmetric acral morbilliform and sometimes a lichenoid eruption; it is predominantly distributed on the upper back, palms, soles, pinnae, and cheeks; however, the bullae spread in an acral to proximal direction, and the early eruption is folliculocentric (distributed around hair follicles) [1, 18, 20]. Acral involvement of the palms and soles and an erythematous to violaceous discoloration of the ears are very suggestive of GVHD [20, 21]. In contrast, TEN usually begins on the trunk and spreads distally [18]. A dermal CD8+/CD4+ T-lymphocyte ratio of ≥ 4 in the appropriate clinical setting may be a useful guide for one to consider a diagnosis of TEN over stage 4 skin GVHD [19].

Table 4.2 Differential diagnosis of SJS/TEN; IF denotes direct immunofluorescence

Disease	Fever	Mucositis	Morphology	IF	Onset	Miscellaneous features
Drug-induced pemphigoid	No	Rare	Tense bullae (sometimes hemorrhagic)	+	Acute	Diuretic a common cause, especially spironolactone; often pruritic
Staphylococcal scalded skin syndrome	Yes	Absent	Erythema, skin tenderness, periorificial crusting	−	Acute	Affects children under 5, adults on dialysis, and those on immunosuppressive therapy
Drug-induced pemphigus	No	Usually absent	Erosions, crusts, patchy erythema (resembles pemphigus foliaceus)	±	Gradual	Commonly caused by penicillamine and other "thiol" drugs; resolves after inciting agent is discontinued
Drug-triggered pemphigus	No	Present	Mucosal erosions, flaccid bullae	+	Gradual	Caused by "non-thiol" drugs; persists after discontinuation of drug; may require long-term immunosuppressive therapy
Paraneoplastic pemphigus	No	Present (usually severe)	Polymorphous skin lesions, flaccid bullae	+	Gradual	Associated with malignancy, especially lymphoma; resistant to treatment
Acute graft versus host disease	Yes	Present	Morbilliform rash, bullae, and erosions	−	Acute	Closely resembles TEN
Acute generalized exanthematous pustulosis	Yes	Rare	Superficial pustules (resembles pustular psoriasis)	−	Acute	Self-limiting on discontinuation of drug
Drug-induced linear IgA bullous dermatosis	No	Rare	Tense, subepidermal bullae (resembles pemphigoid)	+	Acute	Vancomycin most commonly implicated drug; pruritus often present

Drug-Induced Linear IgA Bullous Dermatitis

Drug-induced linear IgA bullous dermatitis can produce an extensive bullous eruption similar to SJS/TEN [1]. EM-like lesions, pruritic urticarial plaques, and tense
bullae of the trunk and limbs may occur suddenly, but mucosal involvement is rare
[1]. Histologically, lack of keratinocyte necrosis and a predominantly neutrophilic
infiltrate help distinguish drug-induced linear bullous dermatitis from bullous fixed
drug eruption, bullous EM, and SJS/TEN, which also have a subepidermal split [22].

Table 4.3 SCORTEN
criteria [23]

Variable	Value
Age > 40 years	1 point
Heart rate ≥ 120/min	1 point
Comorbid malignancy	1 point
Epidermal detachment ≥10% of BSA on day 1	1 point
Blood urea nitrogen >28 ng/dL	1 point
Glucose >252 mg/dL	1 point
Bicarbonate <20 mEq/L	1 point

Table 4.4 SCORTEN
mortality [23]

SCORTEN	Mortality rate (%)
0–1	3.2
2	12.1
3	35.3
4	58.3
≥ 5	90

Disease Prognosis

The SCORTEN (SCORe of Toxic Epidermal Necrosis) is a prognostic score and was developed to assess disease severity and predict mortality risk (Table 4.4) in patients with TEN. Scoring can be done on any of the first 5 days of admission but is most valid on days 1 and 3 post-admission [23, 24]. However, mortality risk may be underestimated in patients with respiratory involvement [23].

Management

The cornerstone of management of SJS/TEN is the discontinuation of the suspected causative medication; early identification and discontinuation are linked with improved survival [1, 3, 4]. Additional supportive treatment recommendations are detailed in Table 4.5. From there, however, the lack of systematic data and dearth of controlled trials makes systemic medication administration controversial [3].

Septicemia is the most frequent cause of death in TEN patients [26, 27]. However, *prophylactic antibiotics are not recommended*; their use has been implicated in emergence of resistant organisms as well as increased mortality [27, 28]. However, when there is clinical suspicion for an early infection based on hematologic parameters (such as rising white cell count and inflammatory markers) or clinical signs (such as fever, tachycardia, tachypnea, hypotension, altered mentation, etc.), blood cultures should be obtained and parenteral antibiotic therapy should be initiated. The mainstay of management for TEN in many ways mirrors that of burn care. For more severe cases (with SCORTEN ≥2), transfer to a tertiary burn center should be considered. Early referral to a burn unit is beneficial to TEN patients, reducing

Table 4.5 Supportive care recommendations [13, 25]

Supportive therapy	Recommendations
Fluid resuscitation	Lactated Ringer's to maintain urinary output of 0.5–1.0 cc/kg/h
Nutritional support	Intense monitoring of calorie and protein intake. Inpatient nutritional consultation. Enteral therapy titrated according to prealbumin and C-reactive peptides every 3 days. Consider nasogastric tube placement and feedings if more than 20% TBSA epidermal loss or mucosal involvement
Wound care	Debridement to remove sloughed epidermis, fibrinous exudate, and debris. Use anti-shear wound care. Consider a silver-impregnated antimicrobial dressing (Acticoat/Excalt). Facial dressing with 2% mupirocin or plain petroleum gauze
Ophthalmic care	Aggressive corneal lubrication. Frequent ocular exams utilizing fluorescein dye to assess for denudation and ulceration of the conjunctiva and cornea, along with early ophthalmology service consultation if indicated. An amniotic membrane graft may be necessary with severe ocular involvement
Pain control	Multimodal therapy with opioid and nonopioid analgesics; consider adjunctive anxiolytics prior to wound care

overall mortality, as well as the incidence of bacteremia, septicemia, and length of hospitalization [29].

Systemic Corticosteroids

Historically, high-dose corticosteroids have been used to treat SJS/TEN, despite lack of demonstrated efficacy. Dexamethasone 100 mg IV for 3 days and methylprednisolone 1000 mg IV for 3 days have decreased mortality in small case series, but the dearth of data supporting their use lead the most recent UK guidelines to not recommend corticosteroid therapy [3, 30, 31]. Furthermore, some data suggests that lower doses of corticosteroids given 48 hours or more prior to admission can cause an increase in infections, length of stay, and mortality [18].

Intravenous Immune Globulin

Intravenous immune globulin (IVIG) is created from a plasma pool of several thousand donors and consists mainly of IgG [18]. Initially, evidence suggested that IVIG could inhibit in vitro Fas-FasL-mediated keratinocyte apoptosis; however, subsequent studies have been conflicting regarding its clinical efficacy [32]. One meta-analysis examining 13 studies did not find a statistical reduction in mortality but suggested that there was a strong inverse correlation between IVIG dosage and standardized mortality rates [33]. Another recent meta-analysis including nine studies showed no difference in mortality between IVIG and supportive care [34]. The European consensus guidelines suggest that if IVIG is considered, a total dose of at least 3 g/kg, fractionated over 3–5 days, should be administered [35].

Cyclosporine

Cyclosporine is a calcineurin inhibitor that can block cytotoxic T-cell lymphocytes and their resultant apoptotic cascade [1, 36]. A prospective study of 29 patients, of which 10 patients had SJS, 12 had SJS/TEN overlap, and 7 had TEN, indicates that cyclosporine may be effective [36]. Though the prognostic score predicted 2.75 deaths, none occurred; however the study was too small to be statistically significant ($P = 0.1$) [36]. Patients were treated with cyclosporine solution, administered orally through a nasogastric catheter at an initial dose of 1.5 mg/kg twice daily for 10 days, 1 mg/kg twice daily for the 10 following days, and finally 0.5 mg/kg twice daily for 10 days for a total treatment period of a 30 days [36]. In the same study, cyclosporine was stopped after more than 10 days in three cases for side effects including posterior leukoencephalopathy ($n = 1$), neutropenia ($n = 1$), and nosocomial pneumonia ($n = 1$), and dosage was tapered earlier than scheduled in two patients for alteration in renal function [36].

TNF–α Antagonists

TNF–α is a potent pro-inflammatory cytokine involved in protection against a variety of infectious agents. TNF–α inhibitors are thought to block direct cytotoxicity and apoptosis in TEN [3, 37]. In several case reports, a single 5 mg/kg or 300 mg dose of infliximab led to the resolution of cutaneous lesions in individuals with TEN [37–40]. Etanercept, another TNF-α inhibitor delivered in a single 50 mg subcutaneous injection, led to rapid reepithelialization and no mortalities for a series of ten patients [41]. Though etanercept and infliximab have been promising, thalidomide is contraindicated. Notably, an earlier randomized controlled study utilizing thalidomide vs. placebo was terminated prematurely due to excess mortality in the thalidomide group—ten of 12 patients died compared with three of ten in the placebo group [42].

Granulocyte Colony Stimulating Factor (G–CSF)

In two cases of extensive TEN affecting >80% body surface area with neutropenia, G-CSF was administered and full recovery was seen [43]. Topical G-CSF has been shown to promote wound healing in chronic leg ulcers and nonhealing ulcers of necrobiosis lipoidica; for the aforementioned two cases of TEN, accelerated reepithelialization was seen within 3 days of introducing G-CSF [43].

Pediatric Considerations

For children, data on management and prognosis of SJS/TEN is scarce. The incidences of SJS, SJS-TEN, and TEN were a mean 5.3, 0.8, and 0.4 cases per million children per year in the USA, respectively [44]. Mortality in the pediatric population was 0% for SJS, 4% for SJS/TEN, and 16% for TEN [44]. In one case report, after failure of glucocorticoids (hydrocortisone at 18 mg/kg/day) and immunoglobulins (initially 0.5 g/kg/day, subsequently increased to 1 g/kg/day), two cycles of plasmapheresis were able to inhibit progression of cutaneous lesions [45]. A case series of ten children with a mean age of 8.1, seven having SJS and three with TEN, showed that three to five sessions of hemoperfusion along with full-dose prednisone (1.5–2.0 mg/kg/day) halted disease progression for cases refractory to methylprednisolone (10–30 mg/kg/day for 3 days) and IVIG (1 g/kg/day) [46].

Complications

As previously mentioned in this chapter, SJS/TEN is a multi-organ disease process with myriad potential complications and long-term sequelae described in the literature (see Table 4.1). These may result from multiple pathophysiological mechanisms, including directly apposed denuded mucosal epithelium, massive fluid shifts, or direct end-organ drug toxicity [47, 48].

Cutaneous and ocular sequelae are the most common, occurring approximately 44% of the time [47]. Cutaneous complications include chronic eczema, persistent skin pigmentary changes (including hyperpigmentation and hypopigmentation), and chronic nail changes, such as anonychia (absence of nails), dystrophic nails, and longitudinal nail ridges [47]. Ophthalmic sequelae such as pterygium (pink conjunctival hyperplasia onto the cornea), dry eye syndrome with epiphora (excessive tearing), foreign body sensation, hyperemia, chronic conjunctivitis, trichiasis (ingrowth or inversion of the eyelashes), corneal erosions, and symblepharon/synechia (partial or complete adhesion of the palpebral conjunctiva to the bulbar conjunctiva) [47, 49].

Extracutaneous and extraocular manifestations can also occur. Respiratory complications, such as chronic obliterative bronchitis and bronchiectasis, presumably due to respiratory mucosal epithelial involvement, may present months following resolution of the initial rash [47, 48]. Patients may also complain of cough, dyspnea, and/or wheezing [48].

Gastrointestinal complications, ranging from esophageal dysmotility/dysphagia to esophageal strictures, can be occurring as early as 1 month following the onset of SJS/TEN [48]. It is thought that nasogastric tube usage and oral medications during the acute phase may contribute [48]. Chronic hepatic involvement may manifest as cholestasis [48]. Hepatocellular necrosis and ischemic hepatitis are other GI complications that are surmised to stem from fluid losses from SJS/TEN [48].

Subsequent renal complications are also possible. Though progressive membranous glomerulonephritis can also occur in the acute phase of illness, other patients have been shown to have deterioration of chronic kidney disease after SJS/TEN [47]. Chronic nephritis is thought to be due to direct drug nephrotoxicity rather than a direct effect of SJS/TEN [48]. Finally, otolaryngologic and genitourinary complications, though rare, may also follow SJS/TEN (Table 4.1). Physicians should be vigilant for post-SJS/TEN sequelae; a low threshold for seeking multidisciplinary/specialist care should always be maintained.

Key Points

- SJS is defined by <10% body involvement. TEN (also referred to as Lyell syndrome) is the more extensive variant and involves >30% of the body surface area. The intermediary range between 10% and 30% is known as SJS/TEN overlap.
- Dermal changes appear as dusky red skin macules or patches that progress to bullae, skin sloughing, and mucosal erosions. A symmetrical, painful macular exanthem appears on the face and trunk. Nikolsky sign develops, whereby gentle stroking of the skin produces separation of the epidermis and the basal layer and blisters form. Asboe-Hansen sign, where pressure on a bulla causes extension to the unaffected adjacent skin, may also be seen.
- Mucosal involvement occurs in 90% of cases, most commonly the oral mucosa.
- Early discontinuation of the precipitating drug is paramount and ideally treatment in a specialized burn unit. Aside from this, management is controversial. Modalities for treatment include high-dose corticosteroids, IVIG, etanercept, infliximab, G-CSF, and hemoperfusion.

Bibliography

1. Schwartz RA, McDonough PH, Lee BW. Toxic epidermal necrolysis: part II. Prognosis, sequelae, diagnosis, differential diagnosis, prevention, and treatment. J Am Acad Dermatol. 2013;69(2):187.e1–16–quiz203–4. https://doi.org/10.1016/j.jaad.2013.05.002.
2. Mockenhaupt M, Viboud C, Dunant A, et al. Stevens-Johnson syndrome and toxic epidermal necrolysis: assessment of medication risks with emphasis on recently marketed drugs. The EuroSCAR-study. J Invest Dermatol. 2008;128(1):35–44. https://doi.org/10.1038/sj.jid.5701033.
3. Harris V, Jackson C, Cooper A. Review of toxic epidermal necrolysis. Int J Mol Sci. 2016;17(12):2135. https://doi.org/10.3390/ijms17122135.
4. Schwartz RA, McDonough PH, Lee BW. Toxic epidermal necrolysis: Part I. Introduction, history, classification, clinical features, systemic manifestations, etiology, and immunopathogenesis. J Am Acad Dermatol. 2013;69(2):173.e1–13–quiz185–6. https://doi.org/10.1016/j.jaad.2013.05.003.
5. Husain Z, Reddy BY, Schwartz RA. DRESS syndrome: part I. Clinical perspectives. J Am Acad Dermatol. 2013;68(5):693.e1–14–quiz706–8. https://doi.org/10.1016/j.jaad.2013.01.033.
6. Hsu DY, Brieva J, Silverberg NB, Silverberg JI. Morbidity and mortality of Stevens-Johnson syndrome and toxic epidermal necrolysis in United States adults. J Invest Dermatol. 2016;136(7):1387–97. https://doi.org/10.1016/j.jid.2016.03.023.
7. Frey N, Jossi J, Bodmer M, et al. The epidemiology of Stevens-Johnson syndrome and toxic epidermal necrolysis in the UK. J Invest Dermatol. 2017;137(6):1240–7. https://doi.org/10.1016/j.jid.2017.01.031.

8. Mittmann N, Knowles SR, Koo M, Shear NH, Rachlis A, Rourke SB. Incidence of toxic epidermal necrolysis and Stevens-Johnson syndrome in an HIV cohort: an observational, retrospective case series study. Am J Clin Dermatol. 2012;13(1):49–54. https://doi.org/10.2165/11593240-000000000-00000.

9. Schneider JA, Cohen PR. Stevens-Johnson syndrome and toxic epidermal necrolysis: a concise review with a comprehensive summary of therapeutic interventions emphasizing supportive measures. Adv Ther. 2017;34(6):1235–44. https://doi.org/10.1007/s12325-017-0530-y.

10. Harr T, French LE. Toxic epidermal necrolysis and Stevens-Johnson syndrome. Orphanet J Rare Dis. 2010;5(1):39. https://doi.org/10.1186/1750-1172-5-39.

11. Downey A, Jackson C, Harun N, Cooper A. Toxic epidermal necrolysis: review of pathogenesis and management. J Am Acad Dermatol. 2012;66(6):995–1003. https://doi.org/10.1016/j.jaad.2011.09.029.

12. Baccaro LM, Sakharpe A, Miller A, Amani H. The first reported case of ureteral perforation in a patient with severe toxic epidermal necrolysis syndrome. J Burn Care & Res: Off Publ Am Burn Assoc. 2014;35(4):e265–8. https://doi.org/10.1097/BCR.0b013e31829a4374.

13. Saeed HN, Chodosh J. Ocular manifestations of Stevens-Johnson syndrome and their management. Curr Opin Ophthalmol. 2016;27(6):522–9. https://doi.org/10.1097/ICU.0000000000000312.

14. Jeanmonod P, Hubbuch M, Grünhage F, et al. Graft-versus-host disease or toxic epidermal necrolysis: diagnostic dilemma after liver transplantation. Transpl Infect Dis. 2012;14(4):422–6. https://doi.org/10.1111/j.1399-3062.2012.00746.x.

15. Yu J, Brandling-Bennett H, Co DO, Nocton JJ, Stevens AM, Chiu YE. Toxic epidermal necrolysis-like cutaneous lupus in pediatric patients: a case series and review. Pediatrics. 2016;137(6):e20154497-e20154497. https://doi.org/10.1542/peds.2015-4497.

16. Williams PM, Conklin RJ. Erythema multiforme: a review and contrast from Stevens-Johnson syndrome/toxic epidermal necrolysis. Dent Clin N Am. 2005;49(1):67–76–viii. https://doi.org/10.1016/j.cden.2004.08.003.

17. Lim VM, Do A, Berger TG, et al. A decade of burn unit experience with Stevens-Johnson syndrome/toxic epidermal necrolysis: clinical pathological diagnosis and risk factor awareness. Burns: J Int Soc Burn Injuries. 2016;42(4):836–43. https://doi.org/10.1016/j.burns.2016.01.014.

18. Pereira FA, Mudgil AV, Rosmarin DM. Toxic epidermal necrolysis. J Am Acad Dermatol. 2007;56(2):181–200. https://doi.org/10.1016/j.jaad.2006.04.048.

19. Naik H, Lockwood S, Saavedra A. A pilot study comparing histological and immunophenotypic patterns in stage 4 skin graft vs host disease from toxic epidermal necrolysis. J Cutan Pathol. 2017;1(7797):268–4. https://doi.org/10.1111/cup.12986.

20. Cices AD, Carneiro C, Majewski S, et al. Differentiating skin rash after stem cell transplantation: graft versus host disease, cutaneous reactions to drugs and viral exanthema. Curr Derm Rep. 2016;5(1):12–7. https://doi.org/10.1007/s13671-016-0126-9.

21. Correia O, Delgado L, Barbosa IL, et al. CD8+ lymphocytes in the blister fluid of severe acute cutaneous graft-versus-host disease: further similarities with toxic epidermal necrolysis. Dermatology (Basel). 2001;203(3):212–6.

22. Wiadrowski TP, Reid CM. Drug-induced linear IgA bullous disease following antibiotics. Australas J Dermatol. 2001;42(3):196–9.

23. Bastuji-Garin S, Fouchard N, Bertocchi M, Roujeau JC, Revuz J, Wolkenstein P. SCORTEN: a severity-of-illness score for toxic epidermal necrolysis. J Invest Dermatol. 2000;115(2):149–53. https://doi.org/10.1046/j.1523-1747.2000.00061.x.

24. Guégan S, Bastuji-Garin S, Poszepczynska-Guigné E, Roujeau J-C, Revuz J. Performance of the SCORTEN during the first five days of hospitalization to predict the prognosis of epidermal necrolysis. J Invest Dermatol. 2006;126(2):272–6. https://doi.org/10.1038/sj.jid.5700068.

25. McCullough M, Burg M, Lin E, Peng D, Garner W. Steven Johnson syndrome and toxic epidermal necrolysis in a burn unit: a 15-year experience. Burns: J Int Soc Burn Injuries. 2017;43(1):200–5. https://doi.org/10.1016/j.burns.2016.07.026.

26. Atiyeh BS, Dham R, Yassin MF, El-Musa KA. Treatment of toxic epidermal necrolysis with moisture-retentive ointment: a case report and review of the literature. Dermatol Surg: Off Publ Am Soc Dermatol Surg [et al]. 2003;29(2):185–8.
27. Mahar PD, Wasiak J, Cleland H, et al. Secondary bacterial infection and empirical antibiotic use in toxic epidermal necrolysis patients. J Burn Care & Res: Off Publ Am Burn Assoc. 2014;35(6):518–24. https://doi.org/10.1097/BCR.0000000000000062.
28. Schulz JT, Sheridan RL, Ryan CM, MacKool B, Tompkins RG. A 10-year experience with toxic epidermal necrolysis. J Burn Care Rehabil. 2000;21(3):199–204.
29. Gerull R, Nelle M, Schaible T. Toxic epidermal necrolysis and Stevens-Johnson syndrome: a review. Crit Care Med. 2011;39(6):1521–32. https://doi.org/10.1097/CCM.0b013e31821201ed.
30. Kardaun SH, Jonkman MF. Dexamethasone pulse therapy for Stevens-Johnson syndrome/toxic epidermal necrolysis. Acta Derm Venereol. 2007;87(2):144–8. https://doi.org/10.2340/00015555-0214.
31. Hirahara K, Kano Y, Sato Y, et al. Methylprednisolone pulse therapy for Stevens-Johnson syndrome/toxic epidermal necrolysis: clinical evaluation and analysis of biomarkers. J Am Acad Dermatol. 2013;69(3):496–8. https://doi.org/10.1016/j.jaad.2013.04.007.
32. Viard I, Wehrli P, Bullani R, et al. Inhibition of toxic epidermal necrolysis by blockade of CD95 with human intravenous immunoglobulin. Science. 1998;282(5388):490–3.
33. Barron SJ, Del Vecchio MT, Aronoff SC. Intravenous immunoglobulin in the treatment of Stevens-Johnson syndrome and toxic epidermal necrolysis: a meta-analysis with meta-regression of observational studies. Int J Dermatol. 2015;54(1):108–15. https://doi.org/10.1111/ijd.12423.
34. Zimmermann S, Sekula P, Venhoff M, et al. Systemic Immunomodulating therapies for Stevens-Johnson syndrome and toxic epidermal necrolysis. JAMA Dermatol. 2017;153(6):514–9. https://doi.org/10.1001/jamadermatol.2016.5668.
35. Enk AH, Hadaschik EN, Eming R, et al. European guidelines (S1) on the use of high-dose intravenous immunoglobulin in dermatology. J Eur Acad Dermatol Venereol. 2016;30(10):1657–69. https://doi.org/10.1111/jdv.13725.
36. Valeyrie-Allanore L, Wolkenstein P, Brochard L, et al. Open trial of ciclosporin treatment for Stevens-Johnson syndrome and toxic epidermal necrolysis. 2010;163(4):847–53. https://doi.org/10.1111/j.1365-2133.2010.09863.x.
37. Hunger RE, Hunziker T, Buettiker U, Braathen LR, Yawalkar N. Rapid resolution of toxic epidermal necrolysis with anti-TNF-α treatment. J Allergy Clin Immunol. 2005;116(4):923–4. https://doi.org/10.1016/j.jaci.2005.06.029.
38. Scott-Lang V, Tidman M, McKay D. Toxic epidermal necrolysis in a child successfully treated with infliximab. Pediatr Dermatol. 2012;31(4):532–4. https://doi.org/10.1111/pde.12029.
39. Zárate-Correa LC, Carrillo-Gómez DC, Ramírez-Escobar AF, Serrano-Reyes C. Toxic epidermal necrolysis successfully treated with infliximab. J Investig Allergol Clin Immunol. 2013;23(1):61–3.
40. Fischer M, Fiedler E, Marsch WC, Wohlrab J. Antitumour necrosis factor-alpha antibodies (infliximab) in the treatment of a patient with toxic epidermal necrolysis. Br J Dermatol. 2002;146(4):707–9. https://doi.org/10.1046/j.1365-2133.2002.46833.x.
41. Paradisi A, Abeni D, Bergamo F, Ricci F, Didona D, Didona B. Etanercept therapy for toxic epidermal necrolysis. J Am Acad Dermatol. 2014;71(2):278–83. https://doi.org/10.1016/j.jaad.2014.04.044.
42. Wolkenstein P, Latarjet J, Roujeau J-C, et al. Randomised comparison of thalidomide versus placebo in toxic epidermal necrolysis. Lancet. 1998;352(9140):1586–9. https://doi.org/10.1016/S0140-6736(98)02197-7.
43. de Sica-Chapman A, Williams G, Soni N, Bunker CB. Granulocyte colony-stimulating factor in toxic epidermal necrolysis (TEN) and Chelsea & Westminster TEN management protocol [corrected]. Br J Dermatol. 2010;162(4):860–5. https://doi.org/10.1111/j.1365-2133.2009.09585.x.
44. Hsu DY, Brieva J, Silverberg NB, Paller AS, Silverberg JI. Pediatric Stevens-Johnson syndrome and toxic epidermal necrolysis in the United States. J Am Acad Dermatol. 2017;76(5):811–817.e814. https://doi.org/10.1016/j.jaad.2016.12.024.

45. Hinc-Kasprzyk J, Polak-Krzemińska A, Głowacka M. Ożóg-Zabolska I. The use of plasmapheresis in a 4-year-old boy with toxic epidermal necrosis. Anaesthesiol Intensive Ther. 2015;47(3):210–3. https://doi.org/10.5603/AIT.2015.0034.
46. Wang Y-M, Tao Y-H, Feng T, Li H. Beneficial therapeutic effects of hemoperfusion in the treatment of severe Stevens-Johnson syndrome/toxic epidermal necrolysis: preliminary results. Eur Rev Med Pharmacol Sci. 2014;18(23):3696–701.
47. Yang C, Cho Y, Chen K, Chen Y, Song H, Chu C. Long-term sequelae of Stevens-Johnson syndrome/toxic epidermal necrolysis. Acta Derm Venereol. 2016;96(4):525–9. https://doi.org/10.2340/00015555-2295.
48. Saeed H, Mantagos IS, Chodosh J. Complications of Stevens-Johnson syndrome beyond the eye and skin. Burns : J Int Soc Burn Injuries. 2016;42(1):20–7. https://doi.org/10.1016/j.burns.2015.03.012.
49. Kohanim S, Palioura S, Saeed HN, et al. Acute and chronic ophthalmic involvement in Stevens-Johnson syndrome/toxic epidermal necrolysis - a comprehensive review and guide to therapy. II. Ophthalmic disease. Ocul Surf. 2016;14(2):168–88. https://doi.org/10.1016/j.jtos.2016.02.001.

Erythema Multiforme

5

David Burbulys and Kelly D. Young

Background

Erythema multiforme (EM) is an uncommon, acute, widespread, immune-mediated hypersensitivity reaction that results in a self-limited mucocutaneous syndrome. This syndrome is classically characterized by a polymorphous cutaneous rash that presents with acrally distributed, concentrically colored, distinct target or iris-like lesions (Fig. 5.1). This may be accompanied by oral, genital, or ocular mucosal erosions or bullae (Fig. 5.2). Erythema multiforme major (EM-M) is the designation used to describe the syndrome with mucosal involvement, while erythema multiforme minor (EM-m) is the more common form and reserved for the condition without mucosal involvement [1–3]. Despite clinical and histopathologic similarities, EM is now regarded as a distinct clinical entity from Stevens-Johnson syndrome (SJS) and toxic epidermal necrolysis (TEN) [4–7].

There are several precipitating factors associated with developing EM, including infections (nearly 90%), medications (10%), and less common triggers such as genetic predisposition, autoimmune disease, neoplastic conditions, immunizations, pregnancy, menstruation, radiation, food additives, and chemical exposures [8–55] (Table 5.1). In contradistinction, SJS and TEN are most commonly associated with medication use [56–59]. In some series, an idiopathic etiology is cited up to 60% of the time, demonstrating that triggers may be difficult to identify. Of the identified causes, acute or recurrent HSV infection is implicated in 70–80% of cases and is the most common precipitant in all forms of EM [8–10, 60]. *Mycoplasma pneumoniae* is linked to 10%

D. Burbulys (✉) · K. D. Young
Health Sciences Clinical Professor of Emergency Medicine, David Geffen School of Medicine at UCLA, Los Angeles, CA, USA

Harbor-UCLA Medical Center, Department of Emergency Medicine, Torrance, CA, USA
e-mail: burbulys@emedharbor.edu; kyoung@emedharbor.edu

© Springer International Publishing AG, part of Springer Nature 2018
E. Rose (ed.), *Life-Threatening Rashes*, https://doi.org/10.1007/978-3-319-75623-3_5

Fig. 5.1 Classical target lesion of erythema multiforme from minocycline exposure. (By Dr. Gary M. White. (Own work) [Public domain], via Regionalderm.com, modified from http://www.regionalderm.com/Regional_Derm/RD_Large/Erythema_mult_g2.jpg)

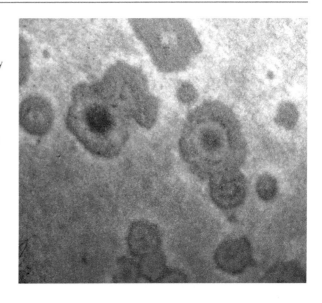

Fig. 5.2 Mucosal changes seen in erythema multiforme major following ciprofloxacin exposure. (By Dr. H.S. Shilpashree, (Own work) [Public domain], from https://openi.nlm.nih.gov/detailedresult.php?img=PMC3543559_JPP-3-339-g001&query=erythema+multiforme&it=xg&req=4&npos=120)

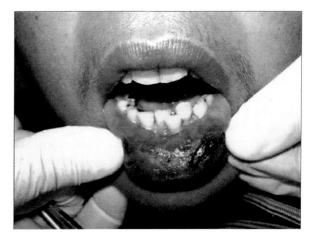

of infection-mediated cases, especially in children [11, 12, 61] (Fig. 5.3). The most common drugs triggering EM are antibiotics (sulfonamides, penicillins), NSAIDS, and antiepileptics (barbiturates, carbamazepine) [1–3, 62]. There are no proposed etiologic differences for EM-m and EM-M, but there are for recurrent and persistent EM.

The incidence of EM is unknown but generally thought to be much less than 1% [1, 63]. HSV-associated EM commonly occurs in young adults (20–40 years) and *Mycoplasma pneumoniae*-associated EM in children. Other less common etiologic forms may be seen in older adults. In older studies there appears to be a slight female predominance while in more recent studies a slight male predominance, perhaps due to a higher incidence of HIV coinfection and a slight racial predilection

Table 5.1 Causes of acute, intermittent erythema multiforme

Infections (90%)	Herpes simplex virus 1 and 2[a] *Mycoplasma pneumoniae*[a] Fungal infections[a]	Adenovirus Coxsackie virus *Cytomegalovirus* Epstein-Barr virus Echovirus Hepatitis viruses (B and C) Human immunodeficiency virus Influenza virus *Legionella pneumophila* *Mycobacterium* *Parapoxvirus* Parvovirus Pneumococcus *Salmonella* Streptococci Varicella zoster virus
Medications (10%)	Sulfonamides[a] Nonsteroidal anti-inflammatory drugs[a] Penicillins[a] Anticonvulsants (barbiturates, carbamazepine, phenytoin)[a]	Allopurinol Corticosteroids (systemic) Cephalosporins Imidazole Phenothiazines Quinolones Terbinafine Tetracycline Valproic acid
Vaccines	Bacille Calmette-Guerin Hepatitis B Smallpox	
Immune conditions	Complex aphthosis Graft versus host disease Inflammatory bowel disease Polyarteritis nodosa Sarcoidosis	
Malignancies	Gastric carcinoma Leukemia Lymphoma Renal carcinoma	
Other	Food additives (benzoates, nitrobenzene) Chemicals (perfumes, terpenes) Menstruation (progestins) Radiation and ultraviolet light	

[a]Common

in some Asian groups [1, 62–66]. Genetic susceptibility is likely, with several specific human leukocyte antigen types overrepresented [1–3]. This is better described in HSV-associated, recurrent, and persistent EM.

EM is thought to be mediated through a type 4c hypersensitivity reaction due to a cell-mediated immune response that targets the skin and mucosa epithelial cells and small blood vessels displaying the specific antigens [62]. In HSV-associated

Fig. 5.3 Atypical erythema multiforme associated with mycoplasma pneumoniae infection. (Courtesy Dr. Taylor McCormick (Own work), Denver Health Medical Center, Denver, CO)

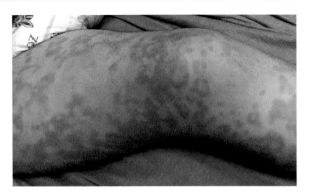

EM, the syndrome begins after viral DNA fragments are transported through the blood to distant skin sites by mononuclear cells. These DNA fragment products are expressed on keratinocytes and recruit CD4+ helper T cells which then respond with the production of gamma interferon. This initiates a cascade of inflammatory mediators and further attracts autoreactive T cells, which lead to the pathologic lesions [67–72]. Drug-associated EM lesions are noted to be positive for tumor necrosis factor alpha and not gamma interferon, suggesting varying pathophysiologic mechanism depending on etiology [73].

There may be associated prodromal symptoms in the more severe form of EM. EM may occur with varying degrees of severity and is commonly recurrent and rarely persistent. The diagnosis is clinical, though histopathologic testing may be useful to distinguish EM from other clinically important imitators. The syndrome is generally self-limited and resolves in 3–6 weeks without sequelae. Symptomatic therapy is frequently all that is required except in the rare severe forms where hospitalization may be needed. In recurrent and persistent subtypes of EM, long-term HSV suppressive antiviral therapy is recommended [1–3].

Classic Clinical Presentation

Prodrome

Prodromal symptoms may be seen in the more significant EM cases that have widespread cutaneous or mucosal lesions. The prodrome generally develops 1 week prior to the onset of rash and may consist of mild malaise, myalgias, fever, headache, nausea, cough, rhinorrhea, sore throat, or arthralgias [1–3].

Cutaneous Lesions

As the name "multiforme" suggests, there may be a host of cutaneous and mucosal manifestations. The initial cutaneous lesions begin as sharply demarcated red or pink macules that then progress to round erythematous papules. The classic papules develop into target or iris-like lesions after 3–4 days. Target lesions characteristically have three distinct zones and range in size from 2–10 mm. The zones consist of a dark-red, brown, dusky, or violaceous central area, often with a small blister, crust, or superficial area of necrosis, surrounded by a near-normal colored ring of edema, and then a lighter-red halo of erythema (Fig. 5.4). In some areas, lesions may enlarge gradually into several centimeter large plaques (Fig. 5.5). The extent of the rash is variable, but lesions are traditionally distributed over the extremities in

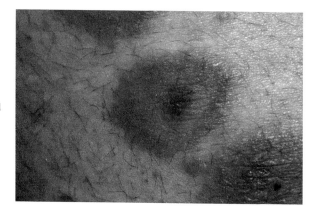

Fig. 5.4 The three zones seen in the classic target lesion of erythema multiforme from minocycline exposure. (By Dr. Gary M. White. (Own work) [Public domain], via Regionalderm.com, modified from http://www.regional-derm.com/Regional_Derm/ RD_Large/Erythema_mult_ g2.jpg)

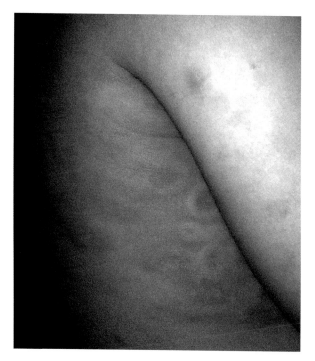

Fig. 5.5   Large plaque-like lesion of erythema multiforme. (Courtesy of Dr. Yaron Ivan (Own work), Florida Hospital for Children Emergency Center, Orlando, FL)

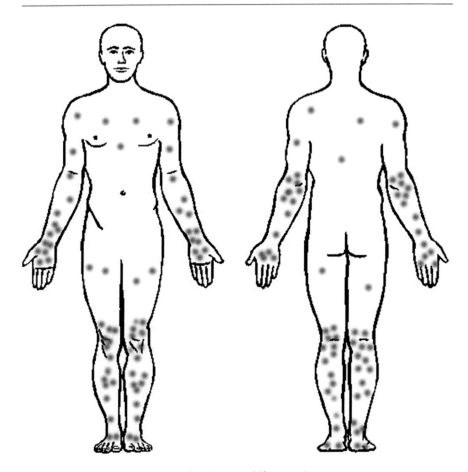

Fig. 5.6 Classical acral distribution of erythema multiforme rash

an acral pattern and are commonly clustered over the elbows and knees and on the extensor surfaces of the forearms and shins (Fig. 5.6). The dorsum of the hands and feet are frequently affected, as are the palms and soles (Fig. 5.7). As the syndrome progresses, less densely scattered lesions are noted to develop centripetally on the trunk and face at times. EM lesions frequently develop in areas of previous trauma or sunburn (Fig. 5.8). Edema of the nail folds may be seen (Fig. 5.9). The lesions are generally asymptomatic but rarely may be pruritic or mildly painful. Complete recovery typically occurs in 1–4 weeks without scarring. Transient hyper- or hypopigmentation may be seen for weeks to months following resolution [1–3] (Fig. 5.10).

Fig. 5.7 Typical target
lesion of erythema multi-
forme. (Courtesy of Dr.
Solomon Behar (Own work),
LAC+USC Medical Center
and Children's Hospital, Los
Angeles, CA)

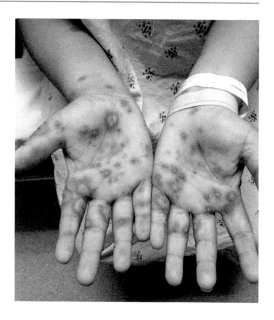

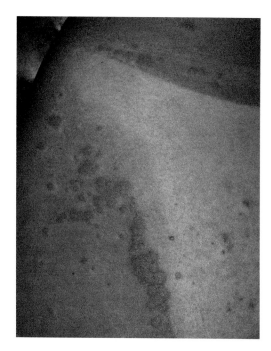

Fig. 5.8 Atypical photodistributed
lesions of erythema multiforme
associated with herpes simplex virus
reactivation. (By Dr. Gary
M. White. (Own work) [Public
domain], via Regionalderm.com,
modified from http://www.
regionalderm.com/Regional_Derm/
RD_Large/Erythema_mult_g2.jpg)

Fig. 5.9 Atypical acral rash
of erythema multiforme with
hand and nail fold edema.
(By James Heilman, MD
(Own work) [Public domain]
[CC BY-SA 3.0 (http://
creativecommons.org/
licenses/by-sa/3.0) or GFDL
(http://www.gnu.org/
copyleft/fdl.html)], via
Wikimedia Commons from
https://commons.wikimedia.
org/wiki/File%3AErythema_
multiforme_minor_of_the_
hand.jpg)

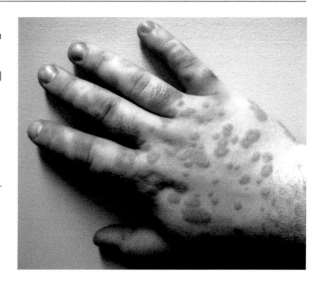

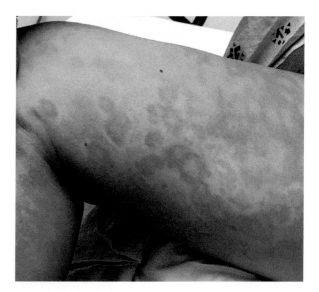

Fig. 5.10 Resolving EM
lesions. (Courtesy Dr. Emily
Rose (Own work),
LAC+USC Medical Center
and Children's Hospital, Los
Angeles, CA)

Mucosal Lesions

Mucosal involvement occurs in 25–70% of EM cases and is subtyped as EM
major (EM-M). Mucosal lesions generally occur concurrently with the cutaneous
rash but may precede or follow it by a few days. The presence of mucosal manifestation alone is infrequently seen. Involvement of the vermillion lip, oral labial
mucosa, gingiva, buccal mucosa, palate, and tongue is most common. Ocular,

Fig. 5.11 Mucosal involvement in erythema multiforme major following diclofenac sodium exposure. (By Dr. Isaac Joseph (Own work) [Public domain], modified from https://openi.nlm.nih.gov/detailedresult.php?img=PMC3303512_JOMFP-16-145-g002&query=erythema+multiforme&req=4&npos=191)

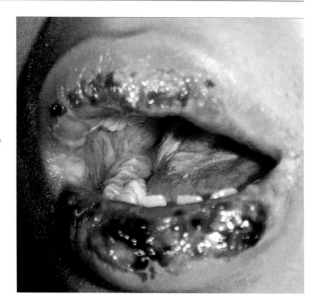

genital, pharyngeal, and upper respiratory mucosal involvement is rare in EM and should lead one to consider the diagnosis of SJS/TEN. Erythematous mucosa progresses to multiple superficial erosions and areas of ulceration and pseudomembrane formation. Vesicles or bullae are common, as is hemorrhagic crusting of the lips [74–78] (Fig. 5.11). Nikolsky's sign is not present, differentiating EM-M from SJS/TEN [79]. The lesions are mildly to significantly painful and at times may compromise fluid and food intake or speech. These lesions frequently take up to 6 weeks to heal, generally without scarring. Ocular, pulmonary, and GI involvement has rarely been known to cause long-term sequelae such as blindness or stricture [80, 81].

Recurrent EM

Most patients with EM have a single isolated incidence. Some patients may experience multiple recurrences, which are often frequent and long lasting. In one study, the average recurrence rate was six times per year (2–24) with a mean duration of 6–10 years [82]. A variety of inciting factors have been identified. As with isolated EM, HSV infection has been implicated in 61–100% of the cases. Other causes may include recurrent infections with *Mycoplasma pneumoniae* or *Candida* vulvovaginitis. Chronic infections with hepatitis C or chronic exposure to agents such as the food preservative benzoic acid or ultraviolet light have also been reported [54, 82–86]. Recurrent EM is frequently difficult to treat, and atypical presentation is more common (Fig. 5.12).

Fig. 5.12 Atypical lesions associated with persistent erythema multiforme associated with Epstein-Barr virus infection. (From by Dr. Gary M. White. (Own work) [Public domain], via Regionalderm.com, from http://www.regionalderm.com/Regional_Derm/RD_Large/Erythema_mult_g2.jpg)

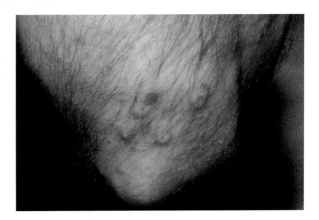

Persistent EM

Persistent EM is rare and is characterized by the continual occurrence of typical and atypical EM lesions for months to years. Lesions are often widespread and may be more papulonecrotic or bullous. Persistent EM is frequently associated with chronic infections, chronic inflammatory disorders, or malignancies. These include HSV, Epstein-Barr virus, hepatitis C, inflammatory bowel disease, leukemia, lymphoma, gastric adenocarcinoma, or renal cell carcinoma [17, 40, 87]. Addressing the underlying etiology is the most effective management of persistent EM.

Atypical Presentation

Lesion variability between patients is common; diverse types of macules, papules, vesicles, bullae and urticarial lesions, or plaques are frequently encountered [88–92]. Classic target lesions usually occur at some point during the syndrome, although atypical target lesions with only the central darker zone and surrounding erythematous border but no intervening pale edematous zone are common (Fig. 5.13). The distribution of the rash is generally fixed but may also be variable and progress slowly over several days. As the rash approaches resolution, polycyclic, annular, and geographic distributions rather than acral distributions may be seen [41, 93–96]. Classic lesions are asymptomatic but at times may burn or be mildly pruritic.

Mucosal involvement may be nonexistent or significant but is predominantly limited to the oral surfaces. Extensive involvement of the ocular, genital, pulmonary, or GI mucosa should raise the concern for SJS/TEN rather than EM. There is considerable morphological overlap between EM-m/EM-M and SJS/TEN syndromes, and, until recently, they were considered to represent a spectrum of severity for the same disease processes. An international consensus clinical classification system now differentiates EM-m/EM-M and SJS/TEN into two distinct entities based on different precipitants, clinical characteristics, pathophysiology, and treatment [4–7] (Table 5.2).

Fig. 5.13 Atypical target lesion of erythema multiforme. (By Dr. Grook Da Oger (Own work) [Public domain], CC BY-SA 3.0, modified from https://commons.wikimedia.org/w/index.php?curid=15900875. https://commons.wikimedia.org/wiki/File%3AErythema_Multiforme_EM_01_ajustement_niveaux_auto.jpg)

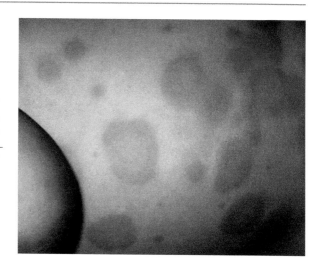

Table 5.2 Erythema multiforme and Stevens-Johnson syndrome, two distinct clinical entities

	Erythema multiforme	Stevens-Johnson syndrome
Triggers	Predominantly infections (HSV)	Predominantly medications
Prodrome	Rare, mild	Common, flu-like
Cutaneous lesions	Typical and atypical target-like papules or plaques	Atypical target-like macules with widespread blister and bullous lesions
Distribution	Acral	Truncal
Tender	No	Frequently
Skin detachment	No	Common
Mucosal involvement	None or mild; generally limited to one or two oral surfaces	May be severe and widespread
Systemic symptoms	Absent	Prominent
Mechanisms	CD4+ T cells, gamma-interferon	CD8+ T cells, tumor necrosis factor alpha
Biopsy	More dermal inflammation and keratinocyte necrosis	Minimal inflammation with sheets of epidermal necrosis
Prognosis	Benign and self-limited	Significant morbidity and mortality possible
Associations	Uncommon except when recurrent	HIV, cancer, and connective tissue disease
Recurrence	Common	No

Associated Systemic Symptoms

Systemic symptoms are rarely encountered with EM. The syndrome is generally limited to the cutaneous or mucosal surfaces. Prodromal symptoms may be seen in severe cases of EM-M, with symptoms such as mild malaise, myalgias, fever, headache, nausea, cough, rhinorrhea, sore throat, and arthralgias presenting 1 week before the onset of cutaneous lesions. It is unclear if they are a component of the syndrome or the result of a precipitant HSV infection. As EM is frequently associated with a host of other acute or chronic infectious diseases, inflammatory or autoimmune syndromes, or malignancies, specific signs and symptoms attributed to those underlying causes may also be noted. These are more common with recurrent or persistent EM [1–3].

Time Course of Disease

There may be a recognized antecedent infection or exposure, or prodromal syndrome, which prefaces rash development by approximately 1 week. A papular eruption appears and spreads in a symmetric acral fashion, generally developing into pathognomonic target lesions within 3 days. Lesions remain fixed in position for several days to 1 week and then may spread centripetally. The lesions begin to heal with complete resolution in 2–3 weeks. There may be hyper- or hypopigmentation lasting for 1–2 months following healing. Mucosal involvement generally starts at the same time as cutaneous lesions but may precede or trail by a few days. Mucosal lesions generally take longer to heal and resolve 1–2 weeks after resolution of the cutaneous rash [1–3].

Common Mimics and Differential Diagnosis

Many diseases and syndromes have characteristics that may be difficult to differentiate from EM [76, 97–109] (Table 5.3). The most common targetoid mimics are SJS/TEN, urticaria, polymorphic light eruptions, fixed drug eruptions, and small

Table 5.3 Differential diagnosis of erythema multiforme

Target-like	Figurate erythema
	Fixed drug eruption
	Lupus erythematosus
	Pityriasis rosea
	Polymorphic light eruption
	Stevens-Johnson syndrome
	Toxic epidermal necrolysis
	Urticaria
	Urticarial vasculitis
	Viral exanthems
Bullous-like	Autoimmune bullous disease (bullous pemphigoid, paraneoplastic pemphigus, and pemphigus vulgaris)
	Dermatitis herpetiformis
	Drug eruption
	Linear IgA bullous dermatosis
	Pemphigoid gestationis
	Stevens-Johnson syndrome
	Toxic epidermal necrolysis
Mucosal-like	Stevens-Johnson syndrome
	Toxic epidermal necrolysis

vessel vasculitis. Important bullous mimics are the autoimmune vesiculobullous disorders. The diagnosis of EM is largely based on historical features and physical findings; there are no pathognomonic laboratory investigations. Histopathologic features and direct and indirect immunofluorescence findings are not definitive in EM but may be helpful to identify other potential disorders.

SJS/TEN

In SJS constitutional symptoms are common. The rash is characterized by atypical macular rather than papular targetoid lesions and is frequently quite tender. These lesions classically begin on the trunk and spread distally rather than beginning acrally. Mucosal involvement is often severe and frequently involves multiple sites in addition to the mouth. Nikolsky's sign may be present. The rash is generally in response to medication exposure or rarely following infection. Pathology reveals extensive epidermal necrosis with a paucity of inflammatory cells.

Urticaria

With urticaria there may be systemic histaminic signs and symptoms and a history of exposure depending on the underlying etiology. The rash is widespread and notably transient and migratory with elevated papules, plaques, or wheals with central zones of normal skin or erythema. There may be angioedema. Pruritus is common. Resolution of each lesion is rapid and new ones develop frequently. Pathology demonstrates prominent papillary edema with a perivascular and interstitial infiltrate of eosinophils, mast cells, and lymphocytes.

Polymorphous Light Eruption

Polymorphous light eruptions present mainly in young women with a variety of lesions, including erythematous papules, plaques, and targetoid lesions following ultraviolet sunlight exposure. It is generally pruritic. This condition may be associated with cutaneous lupus erythematosus. Pathology shows dermal edema and a perivascular lymphocytic infiltrate.

Fixed Drug Eruption

Fixed drug eruptions characteristically recur at the same site each time a particular medication is taken. The lesion is usually a dusky plaque without central clearing and may be associated with a central bullous area and is frequently solitary. Repeat exposures often lead to more lesions, predominantly on the extremities. Mucosal and genital involvement may be seen. Histopathology resembles that seen in EM, but the cellular infiltrate extends deeper, and melanin incontinence is more prominent.

Cutaneous Small Vessel Vasculitis

This entity encompasses several syndromes including Henoch-Schonlein purpura (HSP) and urticarial vasculitis. The rash is often urticarial or with targetoid lesions but more commonly presents with palpable purpura. It is precipitated by medications, infection, chronic inflammatory conditions, or malignancy. The lower extremities are most affected. Pathology reveals leukocytoclastic vasculitis. Perivascular IgA deposits are seen specifically in HSP.

Autoimmune Vesiculobullous Disease

Bullous pemphigoid is frequently chronic, predominantly seen in elderly patients, and often associated with preexisting skin diseases or malignancy. The rash features urticarial, erythematous plaques and large, tense bullae that are pruritic. Upon rupture, bullae are replaced with crusted erosions. There may be mucosal lesions. Pathology shows a prominent eosinophilic infiltrate and a variable dermal neutrophilic infiltrate with a split under the epidermis. Direct immunofluorescence demonstrates anti-basement membrane autoantibodies, and indirect immunofluorescence shows circulating pemphigoid autoantibodies.

Paraneoplastic pemphigus is rare and universally associated with malignancy. Painful mucosal lesions predominate and are severe and intractable and affect all mucosal surfaces. Cutaneous lesions are chronic, highly variable, and polymorphous in appearance. The prominent bullae slough easily and may be intensely pruritic or painful. Pathology reveals suprabasilar acanthosis, dead keratinocytes, and an inflammatory reaction. Direct immunofluorescence reveals desmosome autoantibody deposition, and indirect immunofluorescence may show anti-plakin antibodies.

Other

Other targetoid EM mimics include erythema annulare centrifugum, Rowell's syndrome (lupus erythematosus), Sweet's syndrome (acute febrile neutrophilic dermatosis), pityriasis rosea, and viral exanthems. Other bullous EM mimics include pemphigus vulgaris and mucus membrane pemphigoid. Other mucosal EM mimics include primary herpetic gingivostomatitis, oral lichen planus, and complex aphthosis.

Key Physical Exam Findings and Diagnostic Features

There are no specific objective exam or diagnostic criteria required for the diagnosis of EM other than the classic presentation and diagnostic features described above (Fig. 5.14). Clinicians should look for evidence of precipitating HSV or *Mycoplasma pneumoniae* infections or medication use. Key exam findings include a

Fig. 5.14 Classic violaceous target lesions of
erythema multiforme by
Puppy123456 (Own work)
[Public domain], via
Wikimedia Commons.
(Modified from https://
commons.wikimedia.org/
wiki/File%3AEM_on_legs.
jpg)

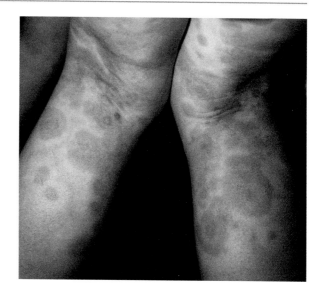

polymorphous rash with typical cutaneous target lesions and sometimes mucosal
involvement, usually confined to the mouth. In patients with recurrent or persistent
EM, a thorough history and exam should also be undertaken to identify less common significant underlying causative etiologies.

Diagnosis

The diagnosis of EM is clinical. No diagnostic or laboratory tests have been identified that are specific in confirming the diagnosis. If the diagnosis is unclear, then a
careful history and physical exam may reveal findings that point to one of the mimic
diagnoses. In this case, appropriate laboratory studies, skin biopsies, and pathologic
investigation may be helpful. In cases of severe EM, nonspecific increased erythrocyte sedimentation rate, C-reactive protein, white blood cell count, and liver enzyme
levels have been reported.

Tzanck smear or HSV PCR may be useful in oral, skin, or genital lesions that are
thought to represent acute HSV. When respiratory symptoms are present, chest
radiograph and serologic testing and throat swab for PCR for *Mycoplasma pneumoniae* may be helpful. In idiopathic cases of recurrent or persistent EM, serologic
testing for HSV should strongly be considered. In these cases, selected laboratory
testing and imaging to rule out underlying infections and inflammatory, autoimmune, or malignant disorders should also be considered [1, 2, 110–112].

Pathologic testing of cutaneous or mucosal EM lesional biopsies has similar features but may be influenced by the evolutionary stage of the lesion. Earlier stage
lesions are preferred. Hematoxylin and eosin staining may show epidermal keratinocyte destruction with hydropic degeneration of the basal keratinocytes and

spongiosis and bullae formation in the epidermal layers. Mild focal necrosis is also seen, but not with large sheets as in SJS/TEN. In the upper dermis and along the dermo-epidermal junction, there is moderate to dense perivascular lymphocytic infiltration, edema, and generalized eosinophilic infiltrates. Direct immunofluorescence is not specific but may show deposition of immune proteins C3 and fibrin along the dermo-epidermal junction and IgM, C3, and fibrin around blood vessels. When autoimmune bullous disease is considered, perilesional normal skin should also be included for direct immunofluorescence staining [113–116].

Management

Acute EM treatment varies by the severity of the disease and whether it is isolated or recurrent (Table 5.4). In patients with mild acute EM-m, therapy is symptomatic. Treatment of HSV has been shown to decrease recurrent EM rates but has not been

Table 5.4 Erythema multiforme treatment

Erythema multiforme minor	Treat underlying infection Symptomatic treatment with antihistamines, analgesics, and topical moderate potency corticosteroids for cutaneous lesions
Erythema multiforme major, outpatient	Treat underlying infection Symptomatic treatment with antihistamines, analgesics, and topical moderate potency corticosteroids for cutaneous lesions Symptomatic treatment with topical analgesics, antiseptics, and high potency corticosteroids for mucosal lesions
Erythema multiforme major, inpatient	Treat underlying infection Treat fluid and electrolyte disturbances, maintain nutrition, control pain, and consider a brief, rapidly tapered course of oral corticosteroids
Recurrent or persistent erythema multiforme	Continual treatment for HSV with acyclovir, valacyclovir, or famciclovir Search for and treat underlying cause
Proposed systemic agents for recurrent or persistent erythema multiforme	Antimalarial drugs (hydroxychloroquine)[a] Azathioprine[a] Cyclosporine[a] Dapsone[a] Mycophenolate mofetil[a] Adalimumab Apremilast Cimetidine Corticosteroids Immunoglobulin Interferon alpha PUVA (photochemotherapy) Rituximab Thalidomide Tofacitinib

[a]Common

shown to affect the course of acute isolated cases of EM [117]. The syndrome is otherwise self-limited and resolves in a few weeks without consequence. Topical corticosteroids and oral antihistamines for any associated itching or burning are all that are required. In patients with EM-M and moderately painful oral erosions, high potency topical corticosteroid gel and topical analgesics such as phenol or lidocaine may be helpful in select populations. Topical antiseptics should also be employed [2, 111, 118].

Those with extensive oral involvement may be severely symptomatic and unable to maintain hydration, and systemic corticosteroids might be considered to decrease the severity and shorten the course of the disease. There are no well-controlled studies to guide this recommendation, and systemic corticosteroids may only partially suppress the disease, prolonging the duration and increasing the risk of chronicity [119]. A prudent course may be to start a moderate daily dose of oral prednisone until there is improvement and then rapidly taper the course over 2–3 weeks. Patients who are unable to maintain oral intake may require hospitalization for fluid or electrolyte disturbances, nutritional support, and pain control. Ocular involvement is rare, but patients that manifest this should be referred to an ophthalmologist promptly as complications such as scarring and visual impairment may occur. Topical corticosteroids and frequent use of lubricants are often employed [1, 2].

Recurrent EM treatment should begin with a thorough investigation for underlying causes. If an offending drug is identified, it should be eliminated for life. If another cause is identified, it should be specifically treated. Systemic antiviral medication is a first-line therapy for HSV-associated recurrent EM and should also be strongly considered for idiopathic recurrent EM. Continuous therapy has been shown to be highly effective in several small studies employing a 6-month trial of acyclovir twice daily, showing improvement in up to 90% of patients [117]. When therapy was discontinued, several patients experienced recurrence and required long-term treatment. There is suggestion in the literature that larger doses or alternative antivirals, such as valacyclovir or famciclovir, may be effective in resistant patients [120–123]. For patients who experience recurrent EM despite continuous antiviral therapy, alternative systemic agents should be considered. The most common recommendations include azathioprine, mycophenolate mofetil, or dapsone. Several other immunosuppressive agents or immunomodulators have been suggested, many of which have significant side effects [124–136]. Given the rarity of the syndrome, there will likely never be large, randomized, controlled trials to guide therapy, and informed decision-making with patients and subspecialty consultation will be required.

Complications

Complications are rare. Denuded epithelial or mucosal surfaces may become superinfected. Ocular mucosal lesions may lead to corneal clouding or scarring and visual impairment. Significant pulmonary or GI mucosal involvement may lead to chronic respiratory insufficiency or esophageal strictures, but these are exceedingly rare. Immunosuppressive medication may lead to opportunistic infection or malignancy [137–141].

Bottom Line: Erythema Multiforme Clinical Pearls
EM is a widespread hypersensitivity reaction of varying severity. HSV is the most common precipitant, and the possibility of HSV infection should be considered. There may be a preceding prodromal period. The rash is acral, polymorphous, and the defining lesions have a characteristic target appearance. There may (EM major) or may not (EM minor) be oral mucosal involvement. The disorder is self-limited and resolves without sequelae in 3–6 weeks in most cases. Symptomatic therapy is generally all that is required. Severe disease may require hospitalization for hydration, analgesia, antiviral therapy, and systemic corticosteroids. A minority of cases recur frequently over several years or may be continuous. HSV is still the most common precipitant and chronic suppressive antiviral therapy should be instituted. At times, long-term corticosteroids, immunosuppressive agents, or immunomodulators may be needed. In these instances, a search for associated chronic infections, inflammatory conditions, or malignancy should be considered. Severe or widespread mucosal involvement suggests SJS, which is a distinct disease entity, rather than EM-M.

Bibliography

1. Samim F, et al. Erythema multiforme: a review of epidemiology, pathogenesis, clinical features, and treatment. Dent Clin N Am. 2013;57(4):583–96.
2. Sokumbi O, Wetter DA. Clinical features, diagnosis, and treatment of erythema multiforme: a review for the practicing dermatologist. Int J Dermatol. 2012;51(8):889–902.
3. Lamoreux MR, Sternbach MR, Hsu WT. Erythema multiforme. Am Fam Physician. 2006;74(11):1883–8.
4. Tomasini C, et al. From erythema multiforme to toxic epidermal necrolysis. Same spectrum or different diseases? G Ital Dermatol Venereol. 2014;149(2):243–61.
5. Schneider G, et al. A systematic review of validated methods for identifying erythema multiforme major/minor/not otherwise specified, Stevens-Johnson syndrome, or toxic epidermal necrolysis using administrative and claims data. Pharmacoepidemiol Drug Saf. 2012;21(Suppl 1):236–9.
6. Watanabe R, et al. Critical factors differentiating erythema multiforme majus from Stevens-Johnson syndrome (SJS)/toxic epidermal necrolysis (TEN). Eur J Dermatol. 2011;21(6):889–94.
7. Williams PM, Conklin RJ. Erythema multiforme: a review and contrast from Stevens-Johnson syndrome/toxic epidermal necrolysis. Dent Clin N Am. 2005;49(1):67–76. viii
8. Kamala KA, Ashok L, Annigeri RG. Herpes associated erythema multiforme. Contemp Clin Dent. 2011;2(4):372–5.
9. Aurelian L, Ono F, Burnett J. Herpes simplex virus (HSV)-associated erythema multiforme (HAEM): a viral disease with an autoimmune component. Dermatol Online J. 2003;9(1):1.
10. Singla R, Brodell RT. Erythema multiforme due to herpes simplex virus. Recurring target lesions are the clue to diagnosis. Postgrad Med. 1999;106(5):151–4.
11. Langley A, et al. Erythema multiforme in children and mycoplasma pneumoniae aetiology. J Cutan Med Surg. 2016;20(5):453–7.

12. Vargas-Hitos JA, Manzano-Gamero MV, Jimenez-Alonso J. Erythema multiforme associated with mycoplasma pneumoniae. Infection. 2014;42(4):797–8.
13. Schalock PC, Brennick JB, Dinulos JG. Mycoplasma pneumoniae infection associated with bullous erythema multiforme. J Am Acad Dermatol. 2005;52(4):705–6.
14. Petrosino MI, et al. Erythema multiforme syndrome associated with acute acquired cyto-megalovirus infection. Arch Med Sci. 2016;12(3):684–6.
15. Gallina L, et al. Erythema multiforme after orf virus infection. Epidemiol Infect. 2016;144(1):88–9.
16. Woolley IJ, Korman TM. Acute HIV infection presenting as erythema multiforme in a 45-year-old heterosexual man. Med J Aust. 2015;203(3):137.
17. Turnbull N, et al. Persistent erythema multiforme associated with Epstein-Barr virus infection. Clin Exp Dermatol. 2014;39(2):154–7.
18. Park IH, et al. A case of erythema multiforme followed by herpes zoster. Infection. 2014;42(4):799–800.
19. Lee YB, et al. Two cases of erythema multiforme associated with molluscum contagiosum. Int J Dermatol. 2009;48(6):659–60.
20. Olut AI, et al. Erythema multiforme associated with acute hepatitis B virus infection. Clin Exp Dermatol. 2006;31(1):137–8.
21. Gutierrez-Galhardo MC, et al. Erythema multiforme associated with sporotrichosis. J Eur Acad Dermatol Venereol. 2005;19(4):507–9.
22. Fuhrman L. Dermatological manifestations of hepatitis C. Dermatol Nurs. 2000;12(3):175–80. 184-6
23. Vilas-Sueiro A, et al. Erythema multiforme associated with phenytoin and cranial radiation therapy (EMPACT syndrome) in a patient with lung Cancer. Actas Dermosifiliogr. 2016;107(2):169–70.
24. Sahraei Z, Mirabzadeh M, Eshraghi A. Erythema multiforme associated with misoprostol: a case report. Am J Ther. 2016;23(5):e1230–3.
25. Sawamura S, et al. Crizotinib-associated erythema multiforme in a lung cancer patient. Drug Discov Ther. 2015;9(2):142–3.
26. Massot A, Gimenez-Arnau A. Cutaneous adverse drug reaction type erythema multiforme major induced by eslicarbazepine. J Pharmacol Pharmacother. 2014;5(4):271–4.
27. Edwards D, et al. Erythema multiforme major following treatment with infliximab. Oral Surg Oral Med Oral Pathol Oral Radiol. 2013;115(2):e36–40.
28. Isik SR, et al. Multidrug-induced erythema multiforme. J Investig Allergol Clin Immunol. 2007;17(3):196–8.
29. Layton D, et al. Serious skin reactions and selective COX-2 inhibitors: a case series from prescription-event monitoring in England. Drug Saf. 2006;29(8):687–96.
30. Moisidis C, Mobus V. Erythema multiforme major following docetaxel. Arch Gynecol Obstet. 2005;271(3):267–9.
31. Carrillo-Jimenez R, Zogby M, Treadwell TL. Erythema multiforme associated with bupro-pion use. Arch Intern Med. 2001;161(12):1556.
32. Roujeau JC, Stern RS. Severe adverse cutaneous reactions to drugs. N Engl J Med. 1994;331(19):1272–85.
33. Schofield JK, et al. Recurrent erythema multiforme: tissue typing in a large series of patients. Br J Dermatol. 1994;131(4):532–5.
34. Khalil I, et al. HLA DQB1*0301 allele is involved in the susceptibility to erythema multi-forme. J Invest Dermatol. 1991;97(4):697–700.
35. Grunnet KM, et al. Autoimmune progesterone dermatitis manifesting as mucosal erythema multiforme in the setting of HIV infection. JAAD Case Rep. 2017;3(1):22–4.
36. Torchia D, Romanelli P, Kerdel FA. Erythema multiforme and Stevens-Johnson syndrome/toxic epidermal necrolysis associated with lupus erythematosus. J Am Acad Dermatol. 2012;67(3):417–21.
37. Doherty C, Ulitsky O, Petronic-Rosic V. Erythema multiforme-like presentation of chronic graft versus host disease. J Am Acad Dermatol. 2008;59(5 Suppl):S127–8.

38. Ghosh I, et al. Erythema multiforme associated with metastatic breast cancer. Indian J Dermatol. 2013;58(6):485–6.
39. Ohtani T, Deguchi M, Aiba S. Erythema multiforme-like lesions associated with lesional infiltration of tumor cells occurring with adult T-cell lymphoma/leukemia. Int J Dermatol. 2008;47(4):390–2.
40. Tzovaras V, et al. Persistent erythema multiforme in a patient with extrahepatic cholangiocarcinoma. Oncology. 2007;73(1–2):127–9.
41. Davidson DM, Jegasothy BV. Atypical erythema multiforme--a marker of malignancy? Report of a case occurring with renal cell carcinoma. Cutis. 1980;26(3):276–8.
42. Monastirli A, et al. Erythema multiforme following pneumococcal vaccination. Acta Dermatovenerol Alp Pannonica Adriat. 2017;26(1):25–6.
43. Storie EB, Perry A. Erythema multiforme following smallpox vaccination. Mil Med. 2014;179(1):e113–5.
44. Wiwanitkit S, Wiwanitkit V. Erythema multiforme after rabies vaccination. Pediatr Dermatol. 2013;30(6):e299.
45. Samad I, Chong VH, Lim SS. Erythema multiforme secondary to H1N1 vaccine. South Med J. 2011;104(1):73–4.
46. Katoulis AC, et al. Erythema multiforme following vaccination for human papillomavirus. Dermatology. 2010;220(1):60–2.
47. Karincaoglu Y, et al. Erythema multiforme due to diphtheria-pertussis-tetanus vaccine. Pediatr Dermatol. 2007;24(3):334–5.
48. Studdiford J, et al. Erythema multiforme after meningitis vaccine: patient safety concerns with repeat immunization. Pharmacotherapy. 2006;26(11):1658–61.
49. Bernardini ML, et al. Erythema multiforme following live attenuated trivalent measles-mumps-rubella vaccine. Acta Derm Venereol. 2006;86(4):359–60.
50. Loche F, et al. Erythema multiforme associated with hepatitis B immunization. Clin Exp Dermatol. 2000;25(2):167–8.
51. Raghunath RS, Venables ZC, Millington GW. The menstrual cycle and the skin. Clin Exp Dermatol. 2015;40(2):111–5.
52. Koley S, et al. Erythema multiforme following application of hair dye. Indian J Dermatol. 2012;57(3):230–2.
53. Kim H, et al. Erythema multiforme major due to occupational exposure to the herbicides alachlor and butachlor. Emerg Med Australas. 2011;23(1):103–5.
54. Nasabzadeh TJ, et al. Recurrent erythema multiforme triggered by progesterone sensitivity. J Cutan Pathol. 2010;37(11):1164–7.
55. Yoshitake T, et al. Erythema multiforme and Stevens-Johnson syndrome following radiotherapy. Radiat Med. 2007;25(1):27–30.
56. Techasatian L, et al. Drug-induced Stevens-Johnson syndrome and toxic epidermal necrolysis in children: 20 years study in a tertiary care hospital. World J Pediatr. 2017;13(3):255–60.
57. Abdulah R, et al. Incidence, causative drugs, and economic consequences of drug-induced SJS, TEN, and SJS-TEN overlap and potential drug-drug interactions during treatment: a retrospective analysis at an Indonesian referral hospital. Ther Clin Risk Manag. 2017;13:919–25.
58. Miliszewski MA, et al. Stevens-Johnson syndrome and toxic epidermal necrolysis: an analysis of triggers and implications for improving prevention. Am J Med. 2016;129(11):1221–5.
59. Hidajat C, LoicD. Drug-mediated rash: erythema multiforme versus Stevens-Johnson syndrome. BMJ Case Rep. 2014; 2014.
60. Weston WL. Herpes-associated erythema multiforme. J Invest Dermatol. 2005;124(6):xv–xvi.
61. Terraneo L, et al. Unusual eruptions associated with mycoplasma pneumoniae respiratory infections: review of the literature. Dermatology. 2015;231(2):152–7.
62. Ilkit M, Durdu M, Karakas M. Cutaneous id reactions: a comprehensive review of clinical manifestations, epidemiology, etiology, and management. Crit Rev Microbiol. 2012;38(3):191–202.

63. Chan HL, et al. The incidence of erythema multiforme, Stevens-Johnson syndrome, and toxic epidermal necrolysis. A population-based study with particular reference to reactions caused by drugs among outpatients. Arch Dermatol. 1990;126(1):43–7.
64. Siedner-Weintraub Y, et al. Paediatric erythema multiforme: epidemiological, clinical and laboratory characteristics. Acta Derm Venereol. 2017;97(4):489–92.
65. Moreau JF, et al. Epidemiology of ophthalmologic disease associated with erythema multiforme, Stevens-Johnson syndrome, and toxic epidermal necrolysis in hospitalized children in the United States. Pediatr Dermatol. 2014;31(2):163–8.
66. Kamaliah MD, et al. Erythema multiforme, Stevens-Johnson syndrome and toxic epidermal necrolysis in northeastern Malaysia. Int J Dermatol. 1998;37(7):520–3.
67. Pollack BP, Sapkota B, Haun PL. Activating transcription factor 3 (ATF3) expression is increased in erythema multiforme and is regulated by IFN-gamma in human keratinocytes. Exp Dermatol. 2010;19(8):e310–3.
68. Gober MD, et al. The herpes simplex virus gene Pol expressed in herpes-associated erythema multiforme lesions upregulates/activates SP1 and inflammatory cytokines. Dermatology. 2007;215(2):97–106.
69. Ono F, et al. CD34+ cells in the peripheral blood transport herpes simplex virus DNA fragments to the skin of patients with erythema multiforme (HAEM). J Invest Dermatol. 2005;124(6):1215–24.
70. Kokuba H, et al. Erythema multiforme lesions are associated with expression of a herpes simplex virus (HSV) gene and qualitative alterations in the HSV-specific T-cell response. Br J Dermatol. 1998;138(6):952–64.
71. Aurelian L, Kokuba H, Burnett JW. Understanding the pathogenesis of HSV-associated erythema multiforme. Dermatology. 1998;197(3):219–22.
72. Imafuku S, et al. Expression of herpes simplex virus DNA fragments located in epidermal keratinocytes and germinative cells is associated with the development of erythema multiforme lesions. J Invest Dermatol. 1997;109(4):550–6.
73. Kokuba H, Aurelian L, Burnett J. Herpes simplex virus associated erythema multiforme (HAEM) is mechanistically distinct from drug-induced erythema multiforme: interferon-gamma is expressed in HAEM lesions and tumor necrosis factor-alpha in drug-induced erythema multiforme lesions. J Invest Dermatol. 1999;113(5):808–15.
74. Said S, Golitz L. Vesiculobullous eruptions of the oral cavity. Otolaryngol Clin N Am. 2011;44(1):133–60. vi
75. Scully C, Bagan J. Oral mucosal diseases: erythema multiforme. Br J Oral Maxillofac Surg. 2008;46(2):90–5.
76. Farthing P, Bagan JV, Scully C. Mucosal disease series. Number IV. Erythema multiforme. Oral Dis. 2005;11(5):261–7.
77. Ayangco L, Rogers RS 3rd. Oral manifestations of erythema multiforme. Dermatol Clin. 2003;21(1):195–205.
78. Dryankova MM, Popova CL. Erythema multiforme--oral manifestations. Folia Med (Plovdiv). 2001;43(1–2):57–63.
79. Mignogna MD, et al. Nikolsky's sign on the gingival mucosa: a clinical tool for oral health practitioners. J Periodontol. 2008;79(12):2241–6.
80. Celentano A, et al. Oral erythema multiforme: trends and clinical findings of a large retrospective European case series. Oral Surg Oral Med Oral Pathol Oral Radiol. 2015;120(6):707–16.
81. Chang YS, et al. Erythema multiforme, Stevens-Johnson syndrome, and toxic epidermal necrolysis: acute ocular manifestations, causes, and management. Cornea. 2007;26(2):123–9.
82. Schofield JK, Tatnall FM, Leigh IM. Recurrent erythema multiforme: clinical features and treatment in a large series of patients. Br J Dermatol. 1993;128(5):542–5.
83. Wetter DA, Davis MD. Recurrent erythema multiforme: clinical characteristics, etiologic associations, and treatment in a series of 48 patients at Mayo Clinic, 2000 to 2007. J Am Acad Dermatol. 2010;62(1):45–53.
84. Dumas V, et al. Recurrent erythema multiforme and chronic hepatitis C: efficacy of interferon alpha. Br J Dermatol. 2000;142(6):1248–9.

85. Cohen PR. Herpes simplex virus-induced recurrent erythema multiforme. J Gt Houst Dent Soc. 1995;66(9):17–8.
86. Brice SL, et al. The herpes-specific immune response of individuals with herpes-associated erythema multiforme compared with that of individuals with recurrent herpes labialis. Arch Dermatol Res. 1993;285(4):193–6.
87. Wanner M, et al. Persistent erythema multiforme and CMV infection. J Drugs Dermatol. 2007;6(3):333–6.
88. Ladizinski B, Lee KC. Oral ulcers and targetoid lesions on the palms. JAMA. 2014;311(11):1152–3.
89. Stollery N. Annular lesions. Practitioner. 2012;256(1752):30–1.
90. Wolf R, Lipozencic J. Shape and configuration of skin lesions: targetoid lesions. Clin Dermatol. 2011;29(5):504–8.
91. Hughey LC. Approach to the hospitalized patient with targetoid lesions. Dermatol Ther. 2011;24(2):196–206.
92. Loh KY. A 'target' skin lesion. Aust Fam Physician. 2008;37(11):946.
93. Keller N, et al. Nonbullous erythema multiforme in hospitalized children: a 10-year survey. Pediatr Dermatol. 2015;32(5):701–3.
94. Elfatoiki FZ, Chiheb S. Atypical erythema multiforme. Pan Afr Med J. 2015;20:436.
95. Katta R. Taking aim at erythema multiforme. How to spot target lesions and less typical presentations. Postgrad Med. 2000;107(1):87–90.
96. Gessesse B, Mulugeta E. Multiforme skin lesions in Yekatit 12 Hospital, 1976-1994. Ethiop Med J. 2000;38(1):43–7.
97. Feller L, et al. Immunopathogenic oral diseases: an overview focusing on pemphigus vulgaris and mucous membrane pemphigoid. Oral Health Prev Dent. 2017;15(2):177–82.
98. Caccavale S, Ruocco E. Acral manifestations of systemic diseases: drug-induced and infectious diseases. Clin Dermatol. 2017;35(1):55–63.
99. Yong AA, Tey HL. Paraneoplastic pemphigus. Australas J Dermatol. 2013;54(4):241–50.
100. Yachoui R, Cronin PM. Systemic lupus erythematosus associated with erythema multiforme-like lesions. Case Rep Rheumatol. 2013;2013:212145.
101. Rosenkrantz W. Immune-mediated dermatoses. Vet Clin North Am Equine Pract. 2013;29(3):607–13.
102. Mathur AN, Mathes EF. Urticaria mimickers in children. Dermatol Ther. 2013;26(6):467–75.
103. Lo Schiavo A, et al. Bullous pemphigoid: etiology, pathogenesis, and inducing factors: facts and controversies. Clin Dermatol. 2013;31(4):391–9.
104. Emer JJ, et al. Urticaria multiforme. J Clin Aesthet Dermatol. 2013;6(3):34–9.
105. Beer K, Beer MS, Appelbaum D. Granuloma annulare masquerading as erythema multiforme. J Drugs Dermatol. 2013;12(6):694–7.
106. Kempton J, et al. Misdiagnosis of erythema multiforme: a literature review and case report. Pediatr Dent. 2012;34(4):337–42.
107. Rochael MC, et al. Sweet's syndrome: study of 73 cases, emphasizing histopathological findings. An Bras Dermatol. 2011;86(4):702–7.
108. Guerrier G, Daronat JM, Deltour R. Unusual presentation of acute annular urticaria: a case report. Case Rep Dermatol Med. 2011;2011:604390.
109. Ogilvie P, et al. Pemphigoid gestationis without blistersHautarzt. 2000;51(1):25–30.
110. Cretu A, et al. Erythema multiforme--etiopathogenic, clinical and therapeutic aspects. Rev Med Chir Soc Med Nat Iasi. 2015;119(1):55–61.
111. Shabahang L. Characteristics of adult outpatients with erythema multiforme. Pak J Biol Sci. 2010;13(22):1106–9.
112. Leaute-Labreze C, et al. Diagnosis, classification, and management of erythema multiforme and Stevens-Johnson syndrome. Arch Dis Child. 2000;83(4):347–52.
113. Fukiwake N, et al. Detection of autoantibodies to desmoplakin in a patient with oral erythema multiforme. Eur J Dermatol. 2007;17(3):238–41.
114. Carrozzo M, Togliatto M, Gandolfo S. Erythema multiforme. A heterogeneous pathologic phenotype. Minerva Stomatol. 1999;48(5):217–26.

115. Cote B, et al. Clinicopathologic correlation in erythema multiforme and Stevens-Johnson syndrome. Arch Dermatol. 1995;131(11):1268–72.
116. Howland WW, et al. Erythema multiforme: clinical, histopathologic, and immunologic study. J Am Acad Dermatol. 1984;10(3):438–46.
117. Tatnall FM, Schofield JK, Leigh IM. A double-blind, placebo-controlled trial of continuous acyclovir therapy in recurrent erythema multiforme. Br J Dermatol. 1995;132(2):267–70.
118. Sanchis JM, et al. Erythema multiforme: diagnosis, clinical manifestations and treatment in a retrospective study of 22 patients. J Oral Pathol Med. 2010;39(10):747–52.
119. AlFar MY, et al. The use of corticosteroids in management of herpes associated erythema multiforme. J Pak Med Assoc. 2015;65(12):1351–3.
120. Staikuniene J, Staneviciute J. Long-term valacyclovir treatment and immune modulation for herpes-associated erythema multiforme. Cent Eur J Immunol. 2015;40(3):387–90.
121. Routt E, Levitt J. Famciclovir for recurrent herpes-associated erythema multiforme: a series of three cases. J Am Acad Dermatol. 2014;71(4):e146–7.
122. Inoue K, et al. Herpes virus-associated erythema multiforme following valacyclovir and systemic corticosteroid treatment. Eur J Dermatol. 2009;19(4):386–7.
123. Kerob D, et al. Recurrent erythema multiforme unresponsive to acyclovir prophylaxis and responsive to valacyclovir continuous therapy. Arch Dermatol. 1998;134(7):876–7.
124. Davis MD, Rogers RS 3rd, Pittelkow MR. Recurrent erythema multiforme/Stevens-Johnson syndrome: response to mycophenolate mofetil. Arch Dermatol. 2002;138(12):1547–50.
125. Viard I, et al. Inhibition of toxic epidermal necrolysis by blockade of CD95 with human intravenous immunoglobulin. Science. 1998;282(5388):490–3.
126. Muller CS, Hinterberger LR, Vogt T. Successful treatment of Rowell syndrome using oral cyclosporine A. Int J Dermatol. 2011;50(8):1020–2.
127. Oak AS, Seminario-Vidal L, Sami N. Treatment of antiviral-resistant recurrent erythema multiforme with dapsone. Dermatol Ther. 2017;30(2).
128. Kieny A, Lipsker D. Efficacy of interferon in recurrent valaciclovir-refractory erythema multiforme in a patient not infected with hepatitis C virus. Clin Exp Dermatol. 2016;41(6):648–50.
129. Chen CW, et al. Persistent erythema multiforme treated with thalidomide. Am J Clin Dermatol. 2008;9(2):123–7.
130. Hoffman LD, Hoffman MD. Dapsone in the treatment of persistent erythema multiforme. J Drugs Dermatol. 2006;5(4):375–6.
131. Geraminejad P, et al. Severe erythema multiforme responding to interferon alfa. J Am Acad Dermatol. 2006;54(2 Suppl):S18–21.
132. Bakis S, Zagarella S. Intermittent oral cyclosporin for recurrent herpes simplex-associated erythema multiforme. Australas J Dermatol. 2005;46(1):18–20.
133. Conejo-Mir JS, et al. Thalidomide as elective treatment in persistent erythema multiforme: report of two cases. J Drugs Dermatol. 2003;2(1):40–4.
134. Mahendran R, Grant JW, Norris PG. Dapsone-responsive persistent erythema multiforme. Dermatology. 2000;200(3):281–2.
135. Kurkcuoglu N, Alli N. Cimetidine prevents recurrent erythema multiforme major resulting from herpes simplex virus infection. J Am Acad Dermatol. 1989;21(4 Pt 1):814–5.
136. Jones RR. Azathioprine therapy in the management of persistent erythema multiforme. Br J Dermatol. 1981;105(4):465–7.
137. Viarnaud A, et al. Severe sequelae of erythema multiforme: three cases. J Eur Acad Dermatol Venereol. 2017.
138. Sokumbi O, el-Azhary RA, Langman LJ. Therapeutic dose monitoring of mycophenolate mofetil in dermatologic diseases. J Am Acad Dermatol. 2013;68(1):36–40.
139. Dore J, Salisbury RE. Morbidity and mortality of mucocutaneous diseases in the pediatric population at a tertiary care center. J Burn Care Res. 2007;28(6):865–70.
140. Sen P, Chua SH. A case of recurrent erythema multiforme and its therapeutic complications. Ann Acad Med Singap. 2004;33(6):793–6.
141. Carucci LR, Levine MS, Rubesin SE. Diffuse esophageal stricture caused by erythema multiforme major. AJR Am J Roentgenol. 2003;180(3):749–50.

Measles

6

Loren Yamamoto

Background

Measles (also known as rubeola) is a highly contagious and serious viral disease. Transmission is via direct contact with infectious droplets or by airborne spread [1]. The measles virus is an RNA virus, genus *Morbillivirus*, family *Paramyxoviridae*.

Since the MMR (measles-mumps-rubella) vaccine is highly efficacious at preventing measles, substantial immunity is present in most modern communities. Even for those children whose parents have declined/refused immunization, substantial herd immunity exists to protect them; however, as the number of nonimmunized children increases, outbreaks and epidemics of measles become more likely. Given the high level of immunization in most areas, a case of measles is an uncommon event. Pediatricians/practitioners practicing in the era prior to measles vaccine (prior to the 1970s) encountered children with measles frequently and hence were skilled at identifying cases of measles. Most pediatricians/practitioners in the current era are likely to have encountered a small number of measles cases resulting in sparse clinical experience with this entity.

The purpose of this chapter is to help pediatricians/practitioners who are part of the current generation, in which measles is uncommon, to recognize a case of measles.

Classic Clinical Presentation

The significant clinical findings in measles are fever, cough, coryza (nasal congestion), rash (exanthem), mouth findings (enanthem), and conjunctival injection.

L. Yamamoto
University of Hawai'i John A. Burns School of Medicine, Honolulu, HI, USA

Kapi'olani Medical Center For Women & Children, Honolulu, HI, USA
e-mail: Loreny@hawaii.edu; Loreny@kapiolani.org

© Springer International Publishing AG, part of Springer Nature 2018
E. Rose (ed.), *Life-Threatening Rashes*, https://doi.org/10.1007/978-3-319-75623-3_6

Atypical Presentation

Since measles is very uncommon due to immunization, variations on the classic presentation might be more common than the classic presentations in unimmunized children. Immunocompromised patients will have a more severe course.

Time Course of the Disease

Patients are contagious for about 9 days from the period 4 days before the rash onset to 4–6 days after appearance of the rash [1–3]. The incubation period is 8–12 days; however, from onset of rash in the index case to the onset of rash in susceptible contacts is 7–21 days, mean of 14 days [1, 2]. See Table 6.1.

Key Physical Exam Findings and Diagnostic Features

The characteristic features of measles are its rash (exanthem) and mouth findings (enanthem). See Figs. 6.1, 6.2, 6.3, 6.4, and 6.5 for characteristic clinical features. Clinicians must be familiar with these visual diagnostic features as the diagnosis is made clinically. Pediatricians/practitioners in the current era have seen many cases of roseola and Kawasaki disease. Since these two entities have many aspects in common with measles, this experience can be very helpful in recognizing measles. See Table 6.2 for comparison and contrasting features of these disease entities.

The rash pattern of measles is described as "morbilliform," which is defined as "measles-like"; hence, it is not very helpful from a descriptive standpoint. The rash on the torso of an infant with roseola is very morbilliform. The back is more typically morbilliform than the anterior torso and face. Freeze the image of the roseola rash in your mind since this is the typical morbilliform rash pattern in measles as well, except that in measles, it will be on the face as well. See the series of measles rash images. In Kawasaki disease, the rash is described as "polymorphous" which means that it could have many different patterns, but a few of the dominant patterns that are seen are erythema multiforme-like and morbilliform patterns.

Table 6.1 Timing of exposure, incubation, contagiousness, and clinical findings [1–3]

Day 0	Exposure
Day 0–10	Incubation
Day 7–10	Onset of contagious potential
Day 10	Prodromal phase, mild fever, early Koplik spots
Day 11	High fever, conjunctivitis, cough, coryza, Koplik spots, mouth/lip/tongue redness
Day 13	Morbilliform rash beginning on the forehead
Day 14–15	Morbilliform rash spreads downward and outward. Cough/coryza improving
Day 18–20	Rash fading, desquamating. No longer contagious

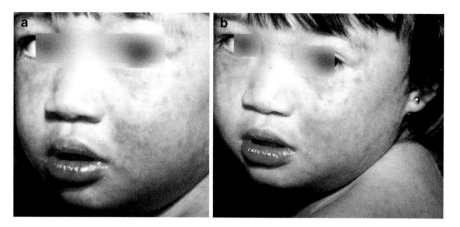

Fig. 6.1 (a, b) These two pictures are of the same child. They show the facial morbilliform rash, conjunctival injection, and red, cracked lips

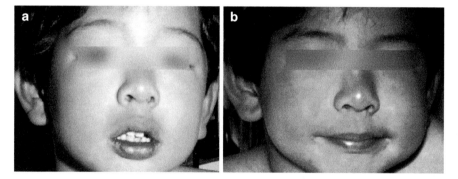

Fig. 6.2 (a, b) These two pictures are of the same child. They show a more confluent rash. Note the forehead involvement. The lips are red and cracked

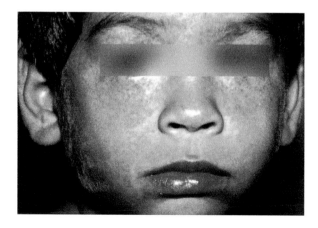

Fig. 6.3 This picture shows the morbilliform rash on his face. His lips are red, but not cracked

Fig. 6.4 This picture shows the facial morbilliform rash on an infant's face. Note the forehead involvement. His lips are red and cracked. Nasal crusting is noted

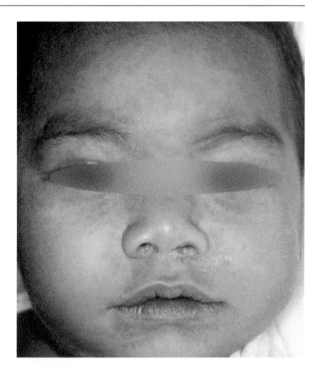

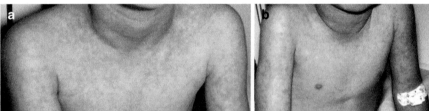

Fig. 6.5 (**a**, **b**) These two pictures are of the same child. Morbilliform rash on the upper torso. The neck rash appears to be more confluent

The direction of spread of the rash can be helpful. The rash of measles begins on the forehead and spreads downward and outward over 3 days (see Fig. 6.6) [1, 2]. Remembering an egg dripping down the head is a visual aid for how the rash of measles progresses. The rash of roseola follows the resolution of a febrile period and starts on the neck and torso, rapidly spreading to the face and extremities, such that the entirety of the rash is often the presenting chief of complaint. The rash of measles is classically non-pruritic.

The conjunctival injection of measles and Kawasaki disease can be difficult to distinguish. While there is sometimes perilimbic sparing (less injection around the corneal limbus) with Kawasaki disease, this is often not present. Consider the

Table 6.2 Measles clinical findings compared to roseola and Kawasaki disease

	Measles	Roseola	Kawasaki disease
Fever:	*High*	Resolved	*High*
Skin:			
Rash pattern	*Morbilliform*	*Morbilliform*	Polymorphous
Rash starting point	Starts on the face	Face/torso	Variable
Rash spread	Downward, outward	Rapid spread	Variable
Rash pruritic	Non-pruritic	Variable	Variable
Conjunctivitis	*Yes*	No	*Yes*
Mouth:			
Red lips	*Yes*	No	*Yes*
Red tongue/mucosa	*Yes*	No	*Yes*
Koplik spots	<u>**Pathognomonic**</u>	No	No
Respiratory symptoms	<u>**Severe**</u>	Minor	Minor

Bold/italic items indicate clinical findings similar or identical in measles plus one of the other entities. Bold/underlined items indicate clinical findings that are present in measles, but not the other two entities

conjunctival injection to be similar. Patients with measles almost always have significant conjunctival injection.

The mouth findings (enanthem) of measles and Kawasaki disease both have redness of the lips, tongue, and oral mucosa. The strawberry phenomena which sometimes refers to its redness (ripe strawberry) or the speckled pattern on the tongue (seeds on a strawberry) is variable in both. In the early stages of measles, Koplik spots are present. These are pathognomonic for measles, but they are not likely to be present late in the disease course. They can be useful in identifying early cases such as those children who might be brought in for clinical attention during an epidemic outbreak. Koplik spots are described as "grains of sand in a red sea." The small spots are bluish white, white, or pale yellow and roughly the size of grains of sand, which are visible over the inflamed, red buccal mucosa. Koplik spots can also be seen on the palate, lips, gums, conjunctiva, and vaginal mucosa. See the Koplik spots series of images (Figs. 6.7, 6.8, 6.9, 6.10, and 6.11).

While using the similarities of roseola and Kawasaki disease can be helpful with the rash, eye, and mouth findings, measles results in cough and coryza (nasal congestion) that separate it from these other two entities. Saying say this another way, children with measles are coughing significantly with significant nasal congestion/mucus. If the respiratory symptoms are minimal, consider Kawasaki disease. Conversely, if a suspected Kawasaki disease patient has severe respiratory symptoms, think about the possibility that this could be measles. To simplify this further, think about measles in a morbilliform Kawasaki-like patient with significant cough/coryza. Look for Koplik spots.

Immunization and travel histories can be useful and very helpful. A patient with a reliable complete immunization history is very likely to be immune to

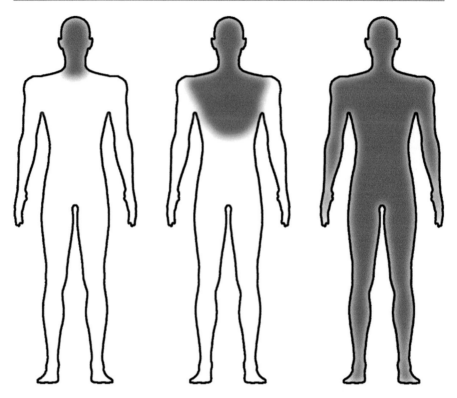

Fig. 6.6 Direction of spread in the rash of measles. The rash typically begins on the head and spreads "down and out"

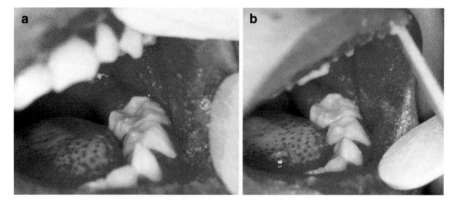

Fig. 6.7 (**a–e**) These five pictures are of the same child. The Koplik spots are on his buccal mucosa. The oral mucosa, gums, lips, and tongue are red

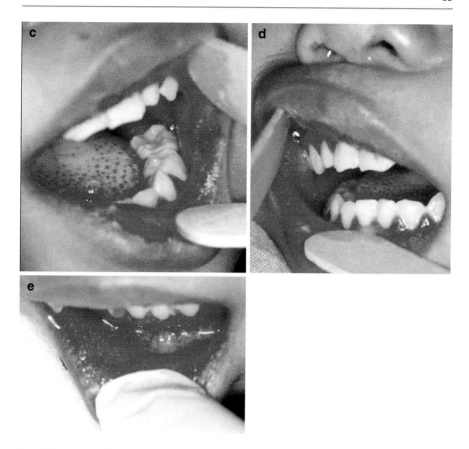

Fig. 6.7 (continued)

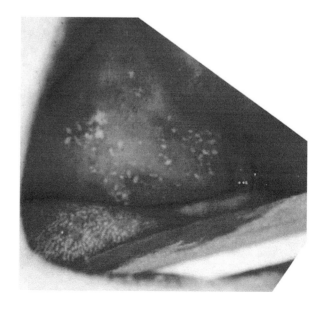

Fig. 6.8 The Koplik spots are bigger in this picture which is showing the left buccal mucosa and a tongue blade depressing his tongue

Fig. 6.9 A reflective steel retractor (appears black on the right of the image) is holding his lip open to show the Koplik spots in the left buccal mucosa. The mucosa does not appear to be very red in this image. The Koplik spots appear to be fading at this point

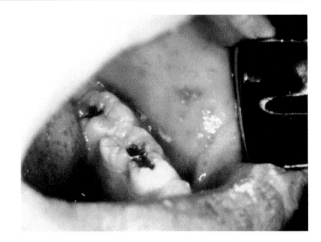

Fig. 6.10 Koplik spots on the left buccal mucosa. The papillae on the tongue appear prominent resembling strawberry seeds

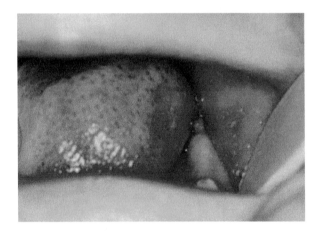

measles. The immunization reliability in other countries might not be as good as that in the United States. All of the measles cases that I have seen in my career in Hawaii came from Japan, Korea, and Micronesia. Measles is still common in many parts of the world including some countries in Europe, Asia, the Pacific, and Africa [4].

Nonimmunized children residing in areas in which measles is nonexistent are similarly not likely to acquire measles; however, travel into these areas from measles endemic areas can easily occur. It is unrealistic to expect that the likelihood of exposure is nil, and measles is a potentially serious disease that is preventable. Measles outbreaks can occur even in populations in which less than 10% of the population is susceptible (i.e., nonimmunized) [3]. The United States has experienced many outbreaks of measles. A well-publicized outbreak occurred at a California amusement park that attracts international visitors, where a large number of people are concentrated into a confined area [5].

Fig. 6.11 Koplik spots in a 6-month-old infant. Note the crusting nasal secretions

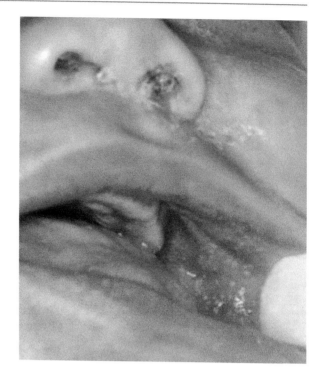

Diagnosis

The initial diagnosis is made by visual recognition of clinical features and confirmed with serum testing that typically results several days after the clinical encounter. Serum IgM antibody to measles is diagnostic, but it might not be detectable initially. Reverse transcriptase polymerase chain reaction (RT-PCR) is diagnostic as well. In most instances, a lab will not be capable of delivering a stat result disabling immediate laboratory confirmation in the outpatient (clinic, office, ED) setting. In practice, a clinical diagnosis must be made.

Common Mimics and Differential Diagnosis

Kawasaki disease bears the greatest similarity to measles. These can usually be distinguished by the morbilliform rash and cough/coryza of measles. While Kawasaki disease can exhibit a morbilliform rash, its rash pattern is more often non-morbilliform, and its respiratory symptoms are less severe. Rubella differs from measles since its rash is milder, its fever is low grade, and the enanthem is classically "Forchheimer spots" on the soft palate. Koplik spots are pathognomonic for measles. A known measles outbreak and suspected or confirmed exposure increase the likelihood of measles in a nonimmunized patient. Lymphadenopathy or lymphadenitis can appear in measles, Kawasaki disease, and rubella.

Management

While many children endured measles in the outpatient setting prior to the era of immunization, measles should be considered to be a serious disease. The case fatality rate was 1% in the mid-twentieth century, but this has declined to 0.1% as overall nutrition and medical care improved. Hospitalization decisions should be based on clinical risk, immunocompetence, and social factors that affect clinical risk. Community contagious considerations can affect hospitalization decisions as well. Immunocompromised patients should be hospitalized since they are at high risk for complications.

Low levels of vitamin A are associated with higher morbidity and mortality. Treatment with vitamin A is indicated for all patients with measles since randomized trials have demonstrated reduced morbidity and mortality with vitamin A therapy [1, 2].

No specific antiviral treatment for measles is approved for routine use. Measles virus is susceptible to ribavirin in vitro which has been used to treat some high-risk patients with measles [1, 2]. Gamma globulin might have some benefit in high-risk patients [2].

Complications

Complications are listed in Table 6.3 [2, 3]. Measles affects the respiratory tract directly, and patients can also develop bacterial pneumonia with *Streptococcus pneumoniae*, *Haemophilus influenzae*, and *Staphylococcus aureus*.

Acute encephalitis is more common in adolescents and adults, compared to children. It occurs at an overall rate of 1–3 per 1000 cases [2]. Subacute sclerosing panencephalitis (SSPE) is a rare complication that has a delayed onset of several years resulting in prolonged neurodegeneration and death [2].

Table 6.3 Complications of measles

Respiratory complications: pneumonia, tracheitis, croup, respiratory failure, otitis media, latent tuberculosis activation
Cardiac complications: myocarditis
GI complications: diarrhea, vomiting, dehydration, appendicitis, abdominal pain
Neurologic complications: febrile seizures, acute encephalitis, deafness, intellectual disabilities, SSPE (subacute sclerosing panencephalitis)
Hematologic complications: hemorrhagic measles, thrombocytopenia
Infection complications: bacteremia, sepsis, cellulitis, toxic shock syndrome, pneumonia, immunosuppression, latent tuberculosis activation
Ophthalmic complications: blindness in vitamin A-deficient children

Measles is a major cause of acquired blindness worldwide, mostly occurring in low-income countries. This risk is higher in vitamin A-deficient children. It is generally accepted that patients with measles should be treated with vitamin A to eliminate any risk of vitamin A deficiency to reduce the risk of blindness. Promoting vitamin A supplementation in children with measles is a high priority by the World Health Organization to reduce the risk of blindness. However, a Cochrane review examining two trials of vitamin A treatment failed to show any reduction in blindness with vitamin A treatment. This could be due to the study being performed in a largely non-vitamin A-deficient cohort with a relatively small sample size [6].

> **Bottom Line: Measles Clinical Pearls**
> Measles is a serious infectious disease that is preventable via immunization, and thus most clinicians have very little experience with measles. The rash is similar to roseola. It starts from the forehead and proceeds downward like an egg dripping down the head. The fever, conjunctival injection, red lips, and red tongue are similar to Kawasaki disease. Cough and coryza are significant. Koplik spots are pathognomonic. The diagnosis is clinical and management is supportive. Measles is highly contagious, and management includes consideration of the public health implications of an outbreak (and protecting immunocompromised from exposure).

Photo/Image Credits The pictures shown in this chapter are courtesy of the collections from Dr. Raul Rudoy and Dr. Mitsuo Tottori. These are all from very old and fading 35 mm slides that required cleaning, restoring, transparency scanning, and image adjusting. The image adjusting can change the actual color. Best efforts were made to make these color adjustments as close to what I thought they should be. All images in this chapter are copyright 2017 Loren Yamamoto, University of Hawaii Department of Pediatrics.

References

1. Committee on Infectious Diseases, American Academy of Pediatrics; Kimberlin DW, Brady MT, Jackson MA, Long SS. Section 3: summaries of infectious diseases: measles. Red Book Online: Red Book 2015 Report of the Committee on Infectious Diseases. 30th ed. 2015. Am Acad Pediatr (Elk Grove Village, IL). https://redbook.solutions.aap.org/chapter.aspx?sectionid=88187186&bookid=1484. Reviewed 4 July 2017.
2. Mason WH. Chapter 246. Measles. In: Kliegman RM, Stanton BF, St. Geme III JW, et al., editors. Nelson textbook of pediatrics. 20th ed. Philadelphia: Elsevier, Inc; 2016. p. 1542–8.
3. Rota PA, Moss WJ, Takeda M, et al. Measles. Nat Rev Dis Primers. 2016;2:1–16. Article number: 16049. doi:https://doi.org/10.1038/nrdp.2016.49.
4. Centers for Disease Control and Prevention. Measles cases and outbreaks. https://www.cdc.gov/measles/cases-outbreaks.html. Reviewed 4 July 2017.

5. Zipprich J, Winter K, Hacker J, et al. Measles outbreak — California, December 2014–February 2015. Morbidity and Mortality Weekly Report (MMWR). 2015;64(06):153–4. https://www.cdc.gov/mmwr/preview/mmwrhtml/mm6406a5.htm?s_cid=mm6406a5_w. Reviewed 4 July 2017.
6. Bello S, Meremikwu MM, Ejemot-Nwadiaro RI, Oduwole O. Routine vitamin A supplementation for the prevention of blindness due to measles infection in children. Cochrane Database Syst Rev. 2016, Issue 8. Art. No.: CD007719. doi: https://doi.org/10.1002/14651858.CD007719.pub4.

Kawasaki Disease

7

Paul Ishimine and John T. Kanegaye

Background

Kawasaki disease (KD), initially called mucocutaneous lymph node syndrome, was first described in the English literature in 1974 [1]. KD is an acute vasculitis, of small- and medium-sized blood vessels. It occurs almost exclusively in young children but has been documented in adults. KD is a systemic inflammatory illness, and medium-sized arteries, particularly the coronary arteries, may sustain long-term injury. KD is usually self-limited but can lead to significant cardiovascular complications, which can be mitigated with early detection and treatment. KD is the leading cause of acquired heart disease in children in developed countries.

KD is found worldwide [2] with the highest incidence in Asia. Japan has the highest incidence rate, with 265 cases per 100,000 children 0–4 years of age [3]. In contrast, the hospitalization rate for KD in children in California is 25 per 100,000, with the highest hospitalization rates among children of Asian/Pacific Islander ancestry [4]. This disease affects boys more commonly than girls, and the majority of affected children are younger than 5 years of age [5].

The etiology of KD is unknown. Postulated causes include infectious etiologies, genetic causes, and environmental triggers.

P. Ishimine (✉)
Departments of Emergency Medicine and Pediatrics, University of California, San Diego School of Medicine, San Diego, CA, USA
e-mail: pishimine@ucsd.edu

J. T. Kanegaye
Department of Pediatrics, University of California, San Diego School of Medicine, San Diego, CA, USA
e-mail: jkanegaye@rchsd.org

© Springer International Publishing AG, part of Springer Nature 2018
E. Rose (ed.), *Life-Threatening Rashes*, https://doi.org/10.1007/978-3-319-75623-3_7

Classic Clinical Presentation

The classic clinical presentation of KD is based on the presence of ≥5 days of fever and ≥ four of five clinical criteria (see Table 7.1) [6]. These patients are said to have "complete," "typical," or "classic" KD.

Atypical Presentation

Patients who do not fulfill the classic diagnostic criteria may still have KD and are said to have incomplete ("atypical") KD (see Table 7.2). This is more common in young infants than in older children, and the diagnosis of KD is missed more frequently in patients with incomplete KD when compared to those patients with classic symptoms [7, 8]. The American Heart Association (AHA) algorithm for evaluation of suspected incomplete KD performs very well in identifying patients who develop coronary artery aneurysms [6, 9, 10]

Patients with incomplete KD can also be identified in patients with prolonged, unexplained fever and some of classic features who have coronary artery abnormalities on echocardiography (aneurysms are rarely seen before day 10 of illness, but other coronary abnormalities can be seen before the development of aneurysms is noted on ultrasound).

Associated Systemic Symptoms

Although the rash associated with KD is typically the most prominent symptom, KD is a systemic vasculitis, and multiple organ systems can be affected. This is evident in the classic KD diagnostic criteria, which include other non-dermatologic criteria. These patients are frequently irritable. KD patients may have tachycardia and electrocardiographic changes including signs of myocarditis. Patients may also

Table 7.1 Classic clinical criteria [6]

1. Fever persisting at least 5 days[a]
2. Presence of at least four principal features:
Extremity changes (Acute: erythema of palms, soles; edema of hands, feet. Subacute: periungual peeling of fingers and toes in weeks 2 and 3)
Polymorphous exanthem (see key physical exam findings and diagnostic features below)
Bilateral bulbar conjunctival injection without exudate
Changes in lips and oral cavity (e.g., erythema, lip cracking, strawberry tongue, diffuse infection of oral and pharyngeal mucosa)
Cervical lymphadenopathy (> 1.5 cm diameter), usually unilateral
3. Exclusion of other diseases with similar clinical findings

[a]In the presence of ≥ four principal features, diagnosis can be made prior to day 5 of illness. Patients with fever ≥5 days and < four principal criteria can be diagnosed with KD when coronary artery abnormalities are detected by echocardiography or angiography

Table 7.2 Evaluation of suspected incomplete Kawasaki disease

Children with fever ≥5 days and two or three clinical criteria or infants with fever ≥7 days without other explanation
Treat if:
1. CRP ≥ 3.0 mg/dL and/or ESR ≥ 40 mm/h
2. ≥3 laboratory findings:
Age-specific anemia
Platelet count ≥450,000/uL after the seventh day of fever
Albumin ≤3.0 g/dL
Elevated alanine aminotransferase level
Peripheral WBC of ≥16,000/mm³
Urine ≥10 WBC/hpf
Or
Abnormal echocardiogram
Serial reevaluation if:
1. CRP < 3.0 mg/dL and ESR < 40 mm/h
2. CRP ≥ 3.0 mg/dL and/or ESR ≥ 40 mm/h but <3 abnormal laboratory findings
3. Obtain echocardiogram if typical periungual peeling develops

Modified from McCrindle et al. [9]
CRP C-reactive protein, *ESR* Erythrocyte sedimentation rate, *WBC* White blood cell, *Hpf* High-power field

have respiratory symptoms from interstitial pneumonitis and arthritis or arthralgias [11]. Other findings may include vomiting and diarrhea, abdominal pain from hepatitis or gallbladder hydrops, or pancreatitis. Patients with KD can have retropharyngeal phlegmons. An uncommon presentation but pathognomonic feature of KD is erythema and induration at site of previous vaccination with Bacille Calmette-Guerin (BCG) [12].

Time Course of Disease

Because the cause(s) of KD is unknown, the incubation period cannot be determined. Patients usually have a brief period of nonspecific respiratory or gastrointestinal symptoms, followed by the typical signs of KD [13]. There is no clinical feature that consistently begins first, and some features may be only transiently present in the disease course.

Common Mimics and Differential Diagnosis

Because KD is diagnosed based on nonspecific clinical features, the differential diagnosis is extensive (see Table 7.3). The presence of respiratory symptoms, including detection of respiratory viral pathogens, does not exclude the diagnosis of concomitant KD and makes making the diagnosis of KD more challenging [14].

Key Physical Exam Findings and Diagnostic Features

The fever accompanying KD is commonly high, with peak temperatures generally >39°C (102 °F). If left untreated, the fever typically continues for 1–3 weeks. Erythema and painful induration of the palms (Figs. 7.1, and 7.2) and soles occur in the acute phase of disease. Periungual desquamation occurs within 2–3 weeks of onset of the fever and may also involve the palms and soles. Transverse grooves (Beau's lines) may be seen in the fingernails 1–2 months after fever onset. Patients can have variable dermatologic manifestations of KD (Table 7.4) An erythematous rash usually appears within 5 days of fever onset. This rash is most commonly a nonspecific, diffuse maculopapular eruption (Figs. 7.3, and 7.4). The rash is

Table 7.3 Differential diagnosis of Kawasaki disease: diseases and disorders with similar clinical findings [9, 15]

Viral infections (e.g., adenovirus, enterovirus, Epstein-Barr virus, parvovirus, measles)
Staphylococcal and streptococcal toxin-mediated diseases (e.g., scarlet fever, toxic shock syndrome [16], scalded skin syndrome)
Drug hypersensitivity reactions (e.g., Stevens-Johnson syndrome)
Serum sickness
Polyarteritis nodosa
Systemic onset juvenile idiopathic arthritis
Rocky Mountain spotted fever or other rickettsial infections
Leptospirosis

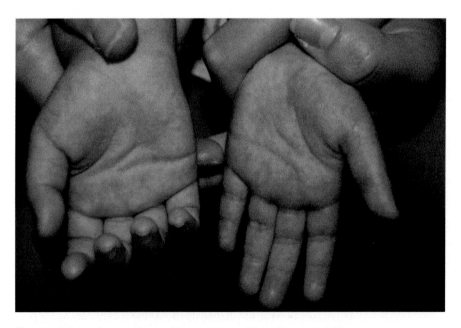

Fig. 7.1 Subtle palmar erythema. (Photo courtesy of John Kanegaye, MD)

Fig. 7.2 Pronounced palmar erythema with edema. (Photo courtesy of Seema Shah, MD)

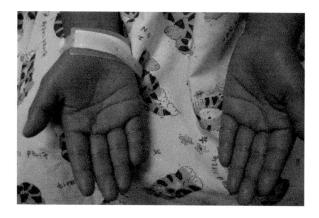

Table 7.4 Dermatologic manifestations of KD [18]

Common:
Acute: Diffuse polymorphous (macular, scarlatiniform, erythema multiforme-like, morbilliform,) rash on trunk and extremities with perineal involvement
Subacute: Periungual desquamation of fingers and toes
Uncommon
Erythroderma
Micropustular eruption
Psoriatic
Urticarial exanthem
Consider alternative diagnoses [9]
Bullae
Petechiae
Vesicles

Fig. 7.3 Truncal eruption consisting of confluent macules and papules. (Photo courtesy of Seema Shah, MD)

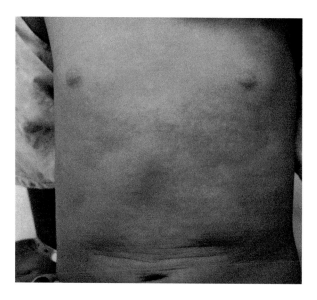

Fig. 7.4 Erythematous, predominantly popular rash with palmar erythema visible on this patient's right hand. (Photo courtesy of John Kanegaye, MD)

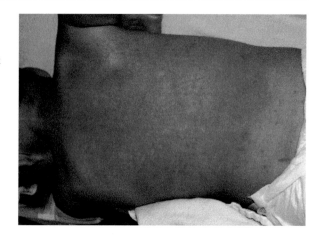

Fig. 7.5 Conjunctival injection with limbic sparing and no discharge. (Photo courtesy of Michael Stoner, MD)

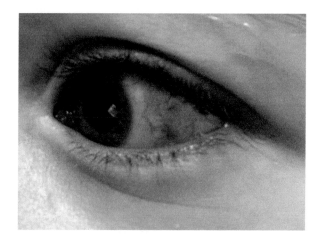

typically extensive, with involvement of the trunk and extremities and accentuation in the groin. However, this rash can be of variable morphology, including rashes similar to urticaria or erythema multiforme. Patients may also have a scarlatiniform rash or erythroderma. However, bullous, vesicular, and petechial rashes are highly unusual with KD [9]. A painless, nonexudative bilateral conjunctival injection with limbic sparing (Fig. 7.5) typically begins shortly after onset of fever. Uveitis may occur with KD with concomitant pain and photophobia. KD also affects the lips and oral cavity, resulting in erythema, fissuring, and peeling of the lips (Fig. 7.6), "strawberry tongue" (Fig. 7.7), and diffuse erythema of the mucosa. Oral ulcerations are not typically seen in KD. Cervical lymphadenopathy is classically unilateral and limited to the anterior cervical triangle with ≥1 lymph node and > 1.5 cm in diameter (Fig. 7.8). Occasionally, cervical lymphadenopathy may be the first and/or only initial clinical finding [17]. However, lymphadenopathy is the least common feature of KD and may be absent.

Fig. 7.6 Cracked, fissured lips with areas of bleeding. (Photo courtesy of John Kanegaye, MD)

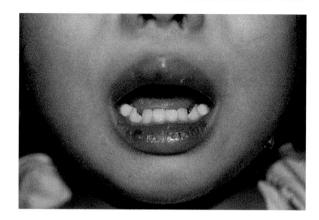

Fig. 7.7 Strawberry tongue. (Photo courtesy of John Kanegaye, MD)

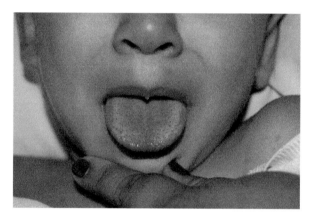

Fig. 7.8 Unilateral cervical node enlargement with overlying erythema. (Photo courtesy of John Kanegaye, MD)

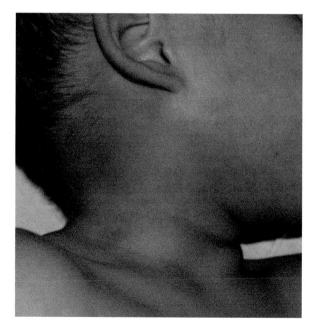

While there are no specific laboratory findings to confirm the diagnosis of KD, laboratory studies can help with the diagnosis. The erythrocyte sedimentation rate and C-reactive protein are almost always elevated in patients with KD, and thus these tests are incorporated into screening algorithms for incomplete KD [6, 9]. Normal values suggest alternative diagnoses. Prior to treatment, leukocytosis and band percentage are highest in the early phases of illness, while the platelet count, absolute and percentage lymphocyte, and absolute eosinophil counts peak between days 11 and 20 of illness. A normocytic, normochromic anemia is common. Liver function tests are frequently abnormal [19]. The gamma-glutamyl transferase and alanine aminotransferase are elevated in 63% and 40% of patients, respectively [20]. Sterile pyuria, defined as ≥8 WBC/mcL for males and ≥ 20 WBC/mcL for females, occurred in 80% of patients with KD (although 54% of concurrent febrile controls also had pyuria by the same criteria) [21]. Pyuria occurs secondary to sloughing of the urethral epithelium and may not be present on a catheterized specimen.

Echocardiography is an important diagnostic modality. The presence of coronary artery aneurysms on echocardiography strongly suggests KD, but a normal echocardiogram does not exclude disease. Echocardiography may also show vessel dilation, systolic and diastolic dysfunction, mitral regurgitation, and aortic root dilation [22].

Management

The main treatment goal in KD is to reduce inflammation to try to prevent development of coronary artery abnormalities. Treatment decreases an incidence of coronary artery aneurysm from 25% to 4–5%. All patients who are diagnosed with KD should receive treatment with intravenous immunoglobulin (IVIG) 2 g/kg in a single infusion as soon as possible [9, 23–25]. Aspirin is given for antiplatelet effect and prevention of thrombus formation. All trials of IVIG efficacy have included concomitant treatment with aspirin. However, aspirin therapy does not appear to lower frequency of coronary abnormalities, and the optimal dose of aspirin is unclear [26, 27]. The 2017 AHA guidelines support treatment with aspirin at either moderate (30–50 mg/kg/day) or high (80–100 mg/kg/day) doses [9].

Although the fever and cutaneous findings resolve quickly in most patients, after initial treatment with IVIG, 10–20% of patients will be resistant to this treatment (defined as persistent or recrudescent fever at least 36 h after completion of IVIG infusion). These patients will require additional anti-inflammatory therapy.

The use of steroids in the treatment of KD is controversial, and the literature contains conflicting results [28, 29]. However, a large meta-analysis concluded that the use of steroids in the acute phase may reduce the rate of coronary artery abnormalities [30]. In particular, the combination of IVIG and glucocorticoids may be more efficacious than IVIG alone in patients at high risk for developing coronary artery aneurysms [31].

KD patients are followed serially with echocardiograms until the dimensions of their coronary arteries stabilize. Depending on the size of the coronary artery aneurysms, long-term therapy may include treatment with antiplatelet medications, anticoagulation, beta-blockers, and statins.

Complications

Patients with KD can present with shock, hemodynamic instability, and multiorgan dysfunction syndrome [32–34]. These patients are at higher risk for refractory KD and coronary artery abnormalities.

The most common complications of KD are coronary artery abnormalities. Coronary aneurysms occur in up to 25% of untreated KD patients (Figs. 7.9, and 7.10). Thrombosis of these aneurysms can lead to myocardial infarctions, dysrhythmias, and sudden death. [35, 36] Coronary artery aneurysms occur more commonly in younger children with KD [37] and in those patient with delays to treatment. The leading cause of death in KD is a thrombotic occlusion in an aneurysmal/stenotic coronary artery.

The risk of cardiac complications is highest in the first year after diagnosis and decreases with time. However, patients with aneurysms, especially those with

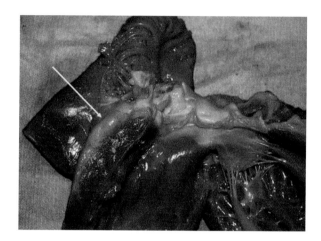

Fig. 7.9 Right coronary artery aneurysm (arrow) in a heart removed during transplant. (Photo courtesy of John Kanegaye, MD)

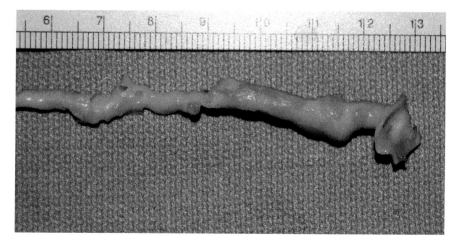

Fig. 7.10 Multiple aneurysms in a right coronary artery. (Photo courtesy of John Kanegaye, MD)

giant aneurysms (>8 mm), are at long-term risk for adverse cardiac events; the 30-year cardiac event rate (death, myocardial infarction, coronary revascularization, or ventricular tachycardia) was 73% [38]. In one study, 5% of patients less than 40 years of age who underwent coronary angiography for suspected myocardial ischemia had aneurysms consistent with preceding KD [39]. Although rates of adverse events among long-term survivors is increased in KD patients with cardiac sequelae compared with non-KD controls, the rates of long-term cardiovascular complications and mortality in KD patients without cardiac complications is not increased [40, 41].

Additional rare complications of KD include macrophage activation syndrome [42], peripheral vasculitis, and sensorineural hearing loss. Recurrence rates of KD range from 1.7% to 3.5% [43].

Bottom Line: Clinical Pearls
- Patients at highest risk for KD are children <5 years of age.
- Patients with classic KD have:
  - Fever for at least 5 days and presence of at least four principal features.
    - Extremity changes.
    - Polymorphous exanthem.
    - Bilateral bulbar nonexudative conjunctivitis.
    - Changes in lips and oral cavity.
    - Cervical lymphadenopathy.
- Patients with fever ≥5 days and two or three classic clinical criteria or infants with fever ≥7 days without other explanation may have incomplete KD.
  - Treat if CRP ≥ 3.0 mg/dL and/or ESR ≥ 40 mm/h.
    - ≥Three laboratory findings:
      - Age-specific anemia.
      - Platelet count ≥450,000/uL after the seventh day of fever.
      - Albumin ≤3.0 g/dL.
      - Elevated alanine aminotransferase (ALT) level.
      - Peripheral white blood cell count (WBC) of ≥16,000/mm³.
      - Urine ≥10 WBC/hpf.
    - Abnormal echocardiogram.
  - Serial reevaluation if:
    - CRP < 3.0 mg/dL and ESR < 40 mm/h.
    - CRP ≥ 3.0 mg/dL and/or ESR ≥ 40 mm/h but <3 abnormal laboratory findings.
    - Obtain echocardiogram if typical periungual peeling develops.
- Consider atypical KD in patients with prolonged fever and irritability, aseptic meningitis, or cervical lymphadenitis unresponsive to antibiotic therapy.
- Young infants more commonly have atypical presentations of KD, are more likely to have a delay in diagnosis and treatment, and are at higher risk for cardiac complications.

References

1. Kawasaki T, Kosaki F, Okawa S, Shigematsu I, Yanagawa H. A new infantile acute febrile mucocutaneous lymph node syndrome (MLNS) prevailing in Japan. Pediatrics. 1974;54:271–6.
2. Singh S, Vignesh P, Burgner D. The epidemiology of Kawasaki disease: a global update. Arch Dis Child. 2015;100:1084–8.
3. Makino N, Nakamura Y, Yashiro M, et al. Descriptive epidemiology of Kawasaki disease in Japan, 2011–2012: from the results of the 22nd nationwide survey. J Epidemiol. 2015;25:239–45.
4. Callinan LS, Holman RC, Vugia DJ, Schonberger LB, Belay ED. Kawasaki disease hospitalization rate among children younger than 5 years in California, 2003–2010. Pediatr Infect Dis J. 2014;33:781–3.
5. Holman RC, Belay ED, Christensen KY, Folkema AM, Steiner CA, Schonberger LB. Hospitalizations for Kawasaki syndrome among children in the United States, 1997–2007. Pediatr Infect Dis J. 2010;29:483–8.
6. Newburger JW, Takahashi M, Gerber MA, et al. Diagnosis, treatment, and long-term management of Kawasaki disease: a statement for health professionals from the Committee on Rheumatic Fever, Endocarditis, and Kawasaki Disease, Council on Cardiovascular Disease in the Young, American Heart Association. Pediatrics. 2004;114:1708–33.
7. Minich LL, Sleeper LA, Atz AM, et al. Delayed diagnosis of Kawasaki disease: what are the risk factors? Pediatrics. 2007;120:e1434–40.
8. Chang FY, Hwang B, Chen SJ, Lee PC, Meng CC, Lu JH. Characteristics of Kawasaki disease in infants younger than six months of age. Pediatr Infect Dis J. 2006;25:241–4.
9. McCrindle BW, Rowley AH, Newburger JW, et al. Diagnosis, treatment, and long-term management of Kawasaki disease: a scientific statement for health professionals from the American Heart Association. Circulation. 2017;135:e927–e99.
10. Yellen ES, Gauvreau K, Takahashi M, et al. Performance of 2004 American Heart Association recommendations for treatment of Kawasaki disease. Pediatrics. 2010;125:e234–41.
11. Gong GW, McCrindle BW, Ching JC, Yeung RS. Arthritis presenting during the acute phase of Kawasaki disease. J Pediatr. 2006;148:800–5.
12. Uehara R, Igarashi H, Yashiro M, Nakamura Y, Yanagawa H. Kawasaki disease patients with redness or crust formation at the Bacille Calmette-Guerin inoculation site. Pediatr Infect Dis J. 2010;29:430–3.
13. Baker AL, Lu M, Minich LL, et al. Associated symptoms in the ten days before diagnosis of Kawasaki disease. J Pediatr. 2009;154:592–5 e2.
14. Turnier JL, Anderson MS, Heizer HR, Jone PN, Glode MP, Dominguez SR. Concurrent respiratory viruses and Kawasaki disease. Pediatrics. 2015;136:e609–14.
15. Cohen E, Sundel R. Kawasaki disease at 50 years. JAMA Pediatr. 2016;170:1093–9.
16. Lin YJ, Cheng MC, Lo MH, Chien SJ. Early differentiation of Kawasaki disease shock syndrome and toxic shock syndrome in a pediatric intensive care unit. Pediatr Infect Dis J. 2015;34:1163–7.
17. Kanegaye JT, Van Cott E, Tremoulet AH, et al. Lymph-node-first presentation of Kawasaki disease compared with bacterial cervical adenitis and typical Kawasaki disease. J Pediatr. 2013;162:1259–63, 63.e1-2.
18. Bayers S, Shulman ST, Paller AS. Kawasaki disease: part I. Diagnosis, clinical features, and pathogenesis. J Am Acad Dermatol. 2013;69:501 e1–11; quiz 11-2.
19. Eladawy M, Dominguez SR, Anderson MS, Glode MP. Abnormal liver panel in acute Kawasaki disease. Pediatr Infect Dis J. 2011;30:141–4.
20. Tremoulet AH, Jain S, Chandrasekar D, Sun X, Sato Y, Burns JC. Evolution of laboratory values in patients with Kawasaki disease. Pediatr Infect Dis J. 2011;30:1022–6.
21. Shike H, Kanegaye JT, Best BM, Pancheri J, Burns JC. Pyuria associated with acute Kawasaki disease and fever from other causes. Pediatr Infect Dis J. 2009;28:440–3.
22. Printz BF, Sleeper LA, Newburger JW, et al. Noncoronary cardiac abnormalities are associated with coronary artery dilation and with laboratory inflammatory markers in acute Kawasaki disease. J Am Coll Cardiol. 2011;57:86–92.

23. Furusho K, Kamiya T, Nakano H, et al. High-dose intravenous gammaglobulin for Kawasaki disease. Lancet. 1984;2:1055–8.
24. Newburger JW, Takahashi M, Beiser AS, et al. A single intravenous infusion of gamma globulin as compared with four infusions in the treatment of acute Kawasaki syndrome. N Engl J Med. 1991;324:1633–9.
25. Newburger JW, Takahashi M, Burns JC, et al. The treatment of Kawasaki syndrome with intravenous gamma globulin. N Engl J Med. 1986;315:341–7.
26. Kim GB, Yu JJ, Yoon KL, et al. Medium- or higher-dose acetylsalicylic acid for acute Kawasaki disease and patient outcomes. J Pediatr. 2017;184:125–9.e1.
27. Dallaire F, Fortier-Morissette Z, Blais S, et al. Aspirin dose and prevention of coronary abnormalities in Kawasaki disease. Pediatrics. 2017;139:e20170098.
28. Newburger JW, Sleeper LA, McCrindle BW, et al. Randomized trial of pulsed corticosteroid therapy for primary treatment of Kawasaki disease. N Engl J Med. 2007;356:663–75.
29. Kobayashi T, Saji T, Otani T, et al. Efficacy of immunoglobulin plus prednisolone for prevention of coronary artery abnormalities in severe Kawasaki disease (RAISE study): a randomised, open-label, blinded-endpoints trial. Lancet. 2012;379:1613–20.
30. Wardle AJ, Connolly GM, Seager MJ, Tulloh RM. Corticosteroids for the treatment of Kawasaki disease in children. The Cochrane Database Syst Rev. 2017;1:Cd011188.
31. Chen S, Dong Y, Kiuchi MG, et al. Coronary artery complication in Kawasaki disease and the importance of early intervention : a systematic review and meta-analysis. JAMA Pediatr. 2016;170:1156–63.
32. Kanegaye JT, Wilder MS, Molkara D, et al. Recognition of a Kawasaki disease shock syndrome. Pediatrics. 2009;123:e783–9.
33. Dominguez SR, Friedman K, Seewald R, Anderson MS, Willis L, Glode MP. Kawasaki disease in a pediatric intensive care unit: a case-control study. Pediatrics. 2008;122:e786–90.
34. Chen PS, Chi H, Huang FY, Peng CC, Chen MR, Chiu NC. Clinical manifestations of Kawasaki disease shock syndrome: a case-control study. J Microbiol Immunol Infect = Wei mian yu gan ran za zhi. 2015;48:43–50.
35. Kato H, Sugimura T, Akagi T, et al. Long-term consequences of Kawasaki disease. A 10- to 21-year follow-up study of 594 patients. Circulation. 1996;94:1379–85.
36. Burns JC, Shike H, Gordon JB, Malhotra A, Schoenwetter M, Kawasaki T. Sequelae of Kawasaki disease in adolescents and young adults. J Am Coll Cardiol. 1996;28:253–7.
37. Salgado AP, Ashouri N, Berry EK, et al. High risk of coronary artery aneurysms in infants younger than 6 months of age with Kawasaki disease. J Pediatr. 2017;185:112–6.e1.
38. Tsuda E, Hamaoka K, Suzuki H, et al. A survey of the 3-decade outcome for patients with giant aneurysms caused by Kawasaki disease. Am Heart J. 2014;167:249–58.
39. Daniels LB, Tjajadi MS, Walford HH, et al. Prevalence of Kawasaki disease in young adults with suspected myocardial ischemia. Circulation. 2012;125:2447–53.
40. Nakamura Y, Aso E, Yashiro M, et al. Mortality among Japanese with a history of Kawasaki disease: results at the end of 2009. J Epidemiol. 2013;23:429–34.
41. Holve TJ, Patel A, Chau Q, Marks AR, Meadows A, Zaroff JG. Long-term cardiovascular outcomes in survivors of Kawasaki disease. Pediatrics. 2014;133:e305–11.
42. Garcia-Pavon S, Yamazaki-Nakashimada MA, Baez M, Borjas-Aguilar KL, Murata C. Kawasaki disease complicated with macrophage activation syndrome: a systematic review. J Pediatr Hematol Oncol. 2017;39:445–51.
43. Maddox RA, Holman RC, Uehara R, et al. Recurrent Kawasaki disease: USA and Japan. Pediatr Int Off J Jpn Pediatr Soc. 2015;57:1116–20.

Toxic Shock Syndrome

8

Elicia Skelton and Anand Swaminathan

Background

Toxic shock syndrome (TSS) is a toxin-mediated systemic inflammatory response syndrome that is classically triggered by either *Staphylococcus aureus* or Group A *Streptococcus* (GAS).

TSS was initially described by Todd et al. in 1978 in a case series of children [1] and became more widely acknowledged in association with highly absorbable tampon use in the early 1980s. Shortly after this widespread recognition, many highly absorbent tampons were withdrawn from the market leading to a decline in staphylococcal TSS cases [2, 3]. Although the incidence of menstrual TSS has decreased dramatically, tampon use – particularly prolonged, continuous use and use of high absorbency materials – still remains a risk factor for developing staphylococcal TSS [4, 5].

Non-menstrual staphylococcal TSS presents very similarly to menstrual TSS and is seen in association with skin lesions, wound infections, indwelling cutaneous catheters, and post-influenza respiratory infections[6, 7]. In both of these forms of staphylococcal TSS, diagnosis is largely clinical, and the organism is infrequently isolated.

Not long after staphylococcal TSS was described, a similar constellation of symptoms associated with Group A *Streptococcus* was reported [8]. Streptococcal and staphylococcal TSS present similarly. However, in streptococcal TSS the source is nearly always identifiable. Streptococcal TSS is often associated with severe skin and deep tissue infections including osteomyelitis, necrotizing fasciitis, myositis, and peritonitis and has also been seen in association with lung infections such as pneumonia. In contrast to staphylococcal TSS, case fatality rates are often much higher in streptococcal TSS (up to 50%).

E. Skelton
Emergency Medicine, Bellevue/NYU Emergency Department, New York, NY, USA

A. Swaminathan (✉)
Emergency Medicine, St. Joseph's Regional Medical Center, Patterson, NJ, USA

© Springer International Publishing AG, part of Springer Nature 2018
E. Rose (ed.), *Life-Threatening Rashes*, https://doi.org/10.1007/978-3-319-75623-3_8

The clinical manifestation of shock and multiorgan failure seen in TSS is attributed to exotoxins produced by both *S. aureus* and GAS. In staphylococcal TSS, the most commonly associated toxins are TSS toxin type 1 (TSST-1), which is implicated in over 90% of menstrual causes, and enterotoxin B. For streptococcal TSS, GAS strains with M protein and pyrogenic exotoxins A and B are most commonly implicated [9–11].

These toxins function as superantigens in the body, which result in the activation of a massive number of T cells and subsequent release of a surplus of cytokines. This cascade ultimately leads to the manifestation of shock and tissue destruction seen in TSS [12].

Classic Clinical Presentation

A list of clinical criteria for TSS was created by the CDC to help classify staphylococcal and streptococcal TSS (see Tables 8.1 and 8.2). However, it should be noted

Table 8.1 Staphylococcal TSS

Clinical criteria	
Must have *all* of the following:	
1. *Fever*: temperature ≥ 102.0 °F (≥38.9 °C)	
2. *Rash*: diffuse macular erythroderma (Figs. 8.1, 8.2, 8.3, 8.4, 8.5, and 8.6)	
3. *Desquamation*: occurring 1–2 weeks after onset of rash. Often involves palmar/plantar surfaces (Fig. 8.7)	
4. *Hypotension*: systolic blood pressure ≤ 90 mmHg (or less than fifth percentile in kids under 16 years)	
5. *Multisystem involvement*	Three or more of the following organ systems:
	(a) Gastrointestinal: vomiting or diarrhea at illness onset
	(b) Muscular: myalgias, creatine phosphokinase at least twice upper limit of normal
	(c) Mucous membranes: hyperemia of vaginal, oropharyngeal, conjunctival membranes (Figs. 8.8, and 8.9)
	(d) Renal: creatinine or blood urea nitrogen at least twice upper limit of normal. Urine with pyuria (≥5 leukocytes per high-power field) in the absence of urinary tract infection
	(e) Hepatic: total bilirubin, alanine aminotransferase enzyme, or aspartate aminotransferase enzyme levels at least twice upper limit of normal
	(f) Hematologic: platelets less than 100,000/mm³
	(g) Central nervous system: disorientation or altered consciousness without focal neurologic deficits when fever/hypotension are absent
Laboratory criteria	
1. Must have negative results on the following tests (if obtained):	
(a) Blood or cerebrospinal fluid cultures (blood culture *may* be positive for *Staphylococcus aureus*)	
(b) Negative serologies for Rocky Mountain spotted fever, leptospirosis, or measles	
Probable case: a case which meets the laboratory criteria and four of the five clinical criteria are present	
Confirmed case: a case which meets the laboratory criteria and in which all five of the clinical criteria described above are present, including desquamation, unless the patient dies before desquamation occurs	

Table 8.2 Streptococcal TSS

Clinical criteria	
Must have *all* of the following:	
1. *Hypotension*: systolic blood pressure ≤ 90 mmHg (or less than fifth percentile in kids under 16 years)	
2. *Multisystem involvement*	Two or more of the following organ systems:
	(a) Renal: creatinine greater than or equal to 2 mg/dL (greater than or equal to 177 μmol/L) for adults or at least twice the upper age limit of normal. In patients with baseline renal dysfunction, a greater than twofold elevation of baseline level creatinine
	(b) Hematologic: platelets less than 100,000/mm³ or disseminated intravascular coagulation
	(c) Hepatic: total bilirubin, alanine aminotransferase enzyme, or aspartate aminotransferase enzyme levels at least twice upper limit of normal. In patients with preexisting liver disease, a greater than twofold increase over the baseline level
	(d) Pulmonary: acute respiratory distress syndrome (defined by acute onset of diffuse pulmonary infiltrates and hypoxemia in the absence of cardiac failure)
	(e) Skin: generalized erythematous macular rash, desquamation, soft tissue necrosis (including necrotizing fasciitis or myositis, or gangrene) (Figs. 8.1, 8.2, 8.3, 8.4, 8.5, 8.6, 8.7, 8.8, and 8.9)
Laboratory criteria	
1. Isolation of Group A *Streptococcus*	
Probable case: a case that meets the clinical case definition in the absence of another identified etiology for the illness and with isolation of Group A *Streptococcus* from a non-sterile site	
Confirmed case: a case that meets the clinical case definition and with isolation of Group A *Streptococcus* from a normally sterile site	

that using these definitions exclusively may underestimate the presence of TSS. The diagnosis is challenging as symptoms tend to be nonspecific and multisystemic. Typical skin erythroderma may not be present initially or at all, and findings such as desquamation often occur later and are absent on initial presentation. Thus providers should maintain a suspicion for TSS even if the exact definition is not met, particularly in the setting of high fever and refractory hypotension and in patients where the source of infection/sepsis cannot be identified [15].

In general, staphylococcal and streptococcal TSS present similarly with a few key differences.

Staphylococcal TSS (Table 8.1)

According to the CDC guidelines, the clinical presentation of staphylococcal TSS must include fever (greater than 102.0F), hypotension (defined by systolic blood pressure less than or equal to 90 mm Hg or less than fifth percentile for children less than 16 years), and skin findings including diffuse macular erythroderma and/or skin desquamation 1–2 weeks after onset of rash. Additionally, multiorgan involvement of three or more of the following organ systems must be present:

gastrointestinal, muscular, mucous membrane, renal, hepatic, hematologic, and central nervous system. Bear in mind that the complete definition of TSS may not be met initially as skin findings may not be present during early presentation to the emergency department. A presumptive diagnosis may be made even in the absence of one or more "hallmark features" [13].

Symptoms often begin with acute onset of headache, fever, myalgias, abdominal pain, and vomiting prior to hospital presentation. By the time patients present to the hospital, headache and vomiting have frequently resolved, and patients will often present with nonspecific symptoms suggestive of multisystem involvement including malaise, weakness, fever, myalgias, sore throat, abdominal pain, and diarrhea. As the symptoms progress, patients may begin to demonstrate signs and symptoms of end-organ failure such as diffuse edema, cyanosis, and decreased urine output. Roughly three-quarters of patients will develop some evidence of non-focal neurologic involvement including somnolence, confusion, and hallucinations. Many patients with menstrual-related TSS may have genitourinary findings including cervical discharge, cervicitis, and bilateral adnexal tenderness.

The classic skin finding associated with early staphylococcal TSS is blanching erythroderma that classically begins on the trunk and spreads to the extremities (Figs. 8.1, 8.2, 8.3, 8.4, and 8.5). It may appear similar in nature to a sunburn and often involves the plantar and palmar surfaces (Fig. 8.6). This rash is typically short-lived and resolves after several days. Diffuse erythoderma and desquamation are less common in streptococcal TSS but still occur frequently (Fig. 8.7). The cutaneous findings associated with streptococcal TSS may be more localized than in staphylococcal TSS. Overlying vesicles, blistering, and bullae may be present, though this is less common and often suggests a more serious skin infection like necrotizing fasciitis. In cases of postoperative TSS, erythema is often most notable surrounding the surgical site.

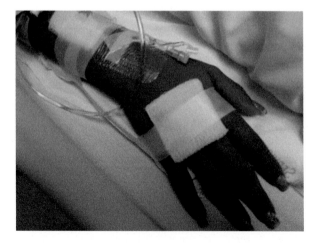

Fig. 8.1 Erythroderma of extremities seen in patient with toxic shock syndrome. (Photograph courtesy of Dr. Carl Kaplan). (Permission to use was given by the physician photographers, and those images were not previously published)

Fig. 8.2 Erythroderma with early desquamation in patient with toxic shock syndrome. (Photograph courtesy of Dr. Nicholas W. Greco). (Permission to use was given by the physician photographers, and those images were not previously published)

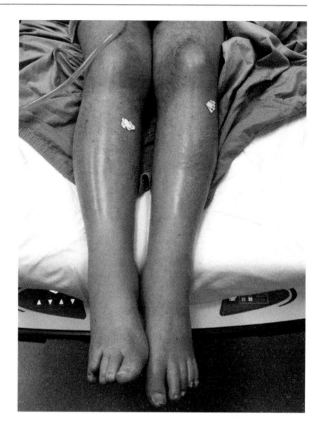

Fig. 8.3 Erythroderma in patient with toxic shock syndrome. (Photograph courtesy of Dr. Nicholas W. Greco). (Permission to use was given by the physician photographers, and those images were not previously published)

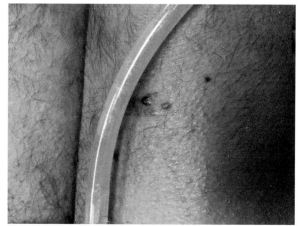

Mucosal involvement usually follows cutaneous involvement and often does not appear until several days into onset of illness. Patients may develop hyperemia and ulcerations of the mucosal membranes including the vagina, oropharynx, and conjunctiva (Figs. 8.8, and 8.9). Roughly 1 week into illness, most patients develop desquamation of the palmar and plantar aspects (Fig. 8.7). In severe cases, loss of hair and nails can occur 2–3 months post illness onset [17].

Fig. 8.4 Erythroderma of the trunk in patient with toxic shock syndrome. (Photograph courtesy of Dr. Nicholas W. Greco). (Permission to use was given by the physician photographers, and those images were not previously published)

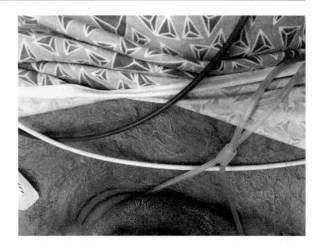

Fig. 8.5 Erythroderma in pediatric patient with toxic shock syndrome. (Source reproduced with permission: Sabella [29])

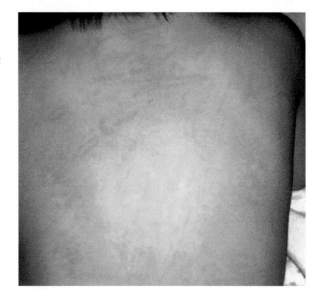

Streptococcal TSS (Table 8.2)

CDC guidelines for clinical diagnosis of streptococcal TSS include hypotension defined by systolic blood pressure less than or equal to 90 mm Hg (or less than fifth percentile for children less than 16 years) and multiorgan involvement characterized by involvement of two or more of the following systems: renal, hepatic, hematologic, pulmonary, or skin (generalized erythematous rash or soft tissue necrosis). Laboratory confirmation of Group A *Streptococcus* is also required [14].

Streptococcal TSS most commonly presents with fever, hypotension, and severe soft tissue pain that is often out of proportion to exam findings, particularly in cases involving necrotizing fasciitis. Though necrotizing fasciitis and streptococcal TSS may occur exclusive of one another, roughly 50% of cases of necrotizing fasciitis

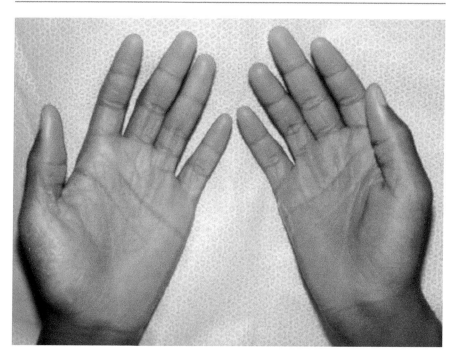

Fig. 8.6 Palmar erythema seen in early toxic shock syndrome. (Photograph courtesy of Dr. Sabella. Source reproduced with permission: Sabella [29])

Fig. 8.7 Desquamation of plantar surface, often seen 7–10 days after onset of illness. (Photograph courtesy of Dr. Sabella. Source reproduced with permission: Sabella [29])

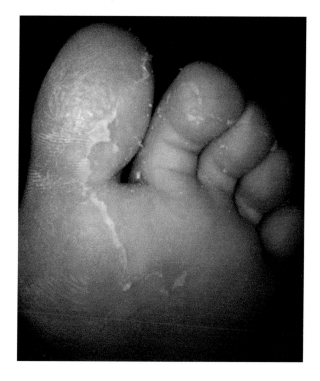

Fig. 8.8 Hyperemia of conjunctival membranes seen in pediatric patient with toxic shock syndrome. (Photograph courtesy of Dr. Sabella. Source reproduced with permission: Sabella [29])

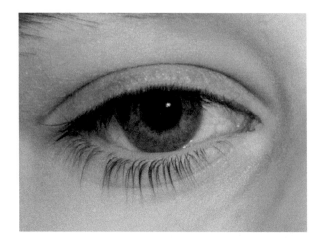

Fig. 8.9 Oral mucosal involvement frequently seen in toxic shock syndrome. (Photograph courtesy of Dr. Sabella. Source reproduced with permission: Sabella [29])

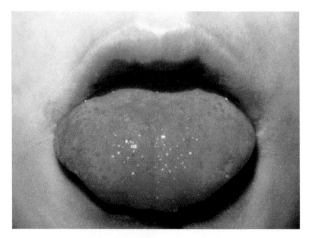

will have concomitant streptococcal TSS [16]. Nonspecific, viral-like syndromes are also commonly seen at the onset of illness.

Atypical Presentation

TSS results in multiorgan dysfunction or failure, and any organ system can be affected. Skin, gastrointestinal, renal, and neurologic findings are common. Cardiovascular findings including pericarditis and cardiomyopathy are less common but may be seen in severe TSS.

Many providers rely on skin findings such as erythroderma and mucosal involvement to key them into the diagnosis. However, rash is not always present, may be subtle, or may occur later in the clinical course lending to difficult diagnosis and atypical presentation on initial ED presentation [18]. Providers should consider the diagnosis of toxic shock syndrome in any patient with hypotension and multiorgan involvement.

Associated Systemic Symptoms

In addition to the classically seen skin manifestations, TSS involves both hypotension and a constellation of associated systemic symptoms indicative of multiorgan failure.

As discussed above, staphylococcal TSS must include fever, hypotension, and skin findings 1–2 weeks after onset of rash. Additionally, multiorgan involvement must be present (see Table 8.1 for more details).

Streptococcal TSS must include the presence of hypotension, multiorgan involvement, and laboratory confirmation of Group A (see Table 8.2 for more details).

Time Course of Disease

Symptoms often begin with acute onset of headache, fever, myalgias, weakness, abdominal pain, and vomiting 1–2 days prior to hospital presentation. Upon hospital presentation (typically day two of illness), headache and vomiting have frequently resolved, but myalgias, abdominal pain, and fever persist. Diarrhea, erythroderma, and hypotension are also very common and begin to develop by the second or third day of illness. By 3–4 hospital days, headache, fever, erythroderma, and GI symptoms have often improved or resolved, but patients may begin to demonstrate confusion, disorientation, or other non-focal neurological findings. Mucocutaneous findings also typically manifest later in the illness and are often not present until on or after the second day of illness. While systemic symptoms generally clear by day 9 of illness, mucocutaneous findings can be severe and long lasting. Nearly all patients will develop desquamatization of the skin between 1 and 2 weeks after illness onset, and some patients may experience loss of hair and nails 2–3 months post illness [17].

Common Mimics and Differential Diagnosis

TSS can be difficult to diagnose, and the presentation mimics a number of other illnesses. A list of common mimics and differential diagnosis can be found in Table 8.3.

Key Physical Exam Findings

Key physical exam findings for staphylococcal TSS include fever, hypotension, and skin findings, most commonly erythroderma (Figs. 8.1, 8.2, 8.3, 8.4, and 8.5), in addition to multiorgan system involvement. Physical exam findings in streptococcal TSS may be less pronounced and include hypotension and multiorgan system involvement (which may include presence or absence of skin findings) in addition to laboratory isolation of Group A *Streptococcus*.

Please see Tables 8.1 and 8.2 for more details.

Table 8.3 Differential diagnosis for toxic shock syndrome

Toxic epidermal necrolysis
Erythema multiforme
Reye syndrome
Kawasaki disease
Tick-borne illness (including Rocky Mountain spotted fever, tick typhus)
Septic shock
Scarlet fever (staphylococcal, streptococcal)
Staphylococcus scalded skin syndrome
Legionnaires disease
Pelvic inflammatory disease
Hemolytic uremic syndrome
Typhoid fever
Meningococcal infections
Infective endocarditis
Infectious mononucleosis
Measles
Listeria

Management

Thorough clinical examination and evaluation are imperative. In addition to looking for any evidence of soft tissue infection, providers should look for and remove all foreign bodies including nasal packing, tampons, and surgical packing that may serve as a source of potential infection. If streptococcal TSS is suspected, early surgical consultation is paramount as these patients often require emergent surgical debridement.

Aggressive supportive care is the bedrock of management in TSS. Vitals including urinary output should be carefully monitored. Aggressive fluid resuscitation is often necessary given the increased vascular permeability seen in this disorder. Vasopressors should be administered as needed to maintain a MAP ≥65 mm Hg. Patients may require supplemental O_2 and intubation if ARDS develops or is present initially.

Despite most sources recommending immediate treatment with broad-spectrum antibiotics, their benefit is unclear. TSS is largely a toxin-mediated systemic inflammatory response, and antibiotics have not been shown to effect the illness acutely. The proposed role of antibiotics is to eradicate the source of circulating toxin in order to prevent further toxin-mediated shock. Clindamycin is a commonly accepted first-line antibiotic in streptococcal TSS as it has been shown to suppress protein synthesis by acting on the 50s ribosomal subunit, thus suppressing production of bacterial toxins [19]. Clindamycin may also have activity against certain staphylococcal TSS strains and should also be considered in cases of staphylococcal TSS or when the source is unknown. In general, the recommended dose is 900 mg IV q8 h [20]. Most resources also recommend patients be empirically covered with vancomycin (15–20 mg/kg/dose q8–12 h) in the setting of suspected methicillin-resistant *S. aureus* (MRSA) or if the strain of *S. aureus* is unknown. Penicillin G or penicillinase-resistant penicillins such as nafcillin and oxacillin (2 g IV q4 h) may be used in combination with clindamycin in patients with methicillin-susceptible *S. aureus* (MSSA) or streptococcal TSS. Treatment is typically continued for at least 1–2 weeks, even in the absence of symptoms (Tintinallis 2011; Rosens 2017/2018 [online]).

IV immune globulin (IVIG) has been proposed as an adjunct treatment due to its ability to help down-regulate the overwhelming inflammatory response in TSS by decreasing cytokine production and neutralizing superantigens. Although there has not been a robust study to date, several case reports and case control studies and one randomized control study suggest that there may be an improvement in mortality and morbidity with the administration of IVIG in streptococcal TSS. Though specific doses have not been well studied, dosing used in the randomized controlled trial by Darenberg et al. involved 1 g/kg on day 1 of initiation followed by 0.5 mg/kg per day on days 2 and 3. Although this study showed improved mortality in those receiving IVIG, it should be noted that the study was terminated early secondary to low incidence of disease and statistical significance was not reached [21–23].

The role of corticosteroids in TSS is unclear. Although they may conceivably mitigate the inflammatory response, clinical and research data is limited on this topic. One study by Todd et al. indicated high-dose steroids may reduce severity and duration of symptoms, but no difference in mortality was shown. It is reasonable to consider high-dose steroids in the setting of refractory vasopressor-dependent shock [24].

Complications

Morbidity can vary depending on the extent of illness. If recognized late or left untreated, multisystemic organ failure can occur including renal, liver, and heart failure. In severe cases of soft tissue infection, debridement and/or amputation may be necessary.

Mortality rates differ drastically between staphylococcal and streptococcal TSS. For staphylococcal TSS, mortality is typically low, with case fatality rates less than 3% in menstrual-related TSS and roughly 5% in non-menstrual TSS [25]. Mortality rate is much higher in streptococcal TSS and has been found to be anywhere from 30% to 80% [26–28].

Bottom Line: Toxic Shock Clinical Pearls

- Toxic shock syndrome (TSS) is a toxin-mediated systemic inflammatory response syndrome that is classically triggered by either *Staphylococcus aureus* or Group A *Streptococcus* (GAS).
- The inflammatory response is attributed to exotoxins produced by both *S. aureus* and GAS that function as superantigens in the body leading to massive cytokine release.

- Staphylococcal TSS involves hypotension, fever, rash, and multiorgan involvement. Streptococcal TSS involves hypotension, multiorgan involvement, and confirmation by laboratory testing.
- The classic skin finding is diffuse macular erythroderma, but this is not always seen in the streptococcal variety of TSS and may vary in appearance depending on the time course of the illness.
- TSS can be difficult to diagnose as symptoms tend to be nonspecific and multisystemic, and typical skin findings may not be present on initial evaluation in the emergency department. Early recognition of TSS is crucial in preventing severe morbidity and mortality. Providers should maintain a high index of suspicion for TSS even if the exact definition is not met, particularly in the setting of high fever and refractory hypotension and in patients where the source of infection/sepsis cannot be identified.
- Thorough physical examination including evaluation for skin/soft tissue infection and removal of all foreign bodies is necessary. Early surgical consultation is crucial particularly in patients with concern for streptococcal TSS with consideration of debridement.
- As with all critically ill patients in shock, supportive care including aggressive fluid resuscitation and maintenance of adequate mean arterial pressures is key.
- Early empiric treatment with clindamycin and either vancomycin (if MRSA suspected) or antistaphylococcal penicillin (if MSSA). The use of IVIG has not been validated, but studies suggest benefits in morbidity and mortality. There is no evidence to suggest corticosteroid use at this time but may be considered in severe cases of TSS or in cases of shock refractory to vasopressors.

References

1. Todd J, Fishaut M, Kapral F. Toxic-shock syndrome associated with phage-group-I Staphylococci. Lancet. 1978;312:1116–8.
2. Centers for Disease Control (CDC). Reduced incidence of menstrual toxic-shock syndrome–United States, 1980–1990. Tech Rep. 1990;25:421–3
3. Broome CV. Epidemiology of toxic shock syndrome in the United States: overview. Rev Infect Dis. 1989;11:S14–21.
4. Shands KN, Schmid GP, Dan BB. Toxic-shock syndrome in menstruating women: association with tampon use and Staphylococcus aureus and clinical features in 52 cases. N Engl J Med. 1980;303:1436–42.
5. Davis JP, Chesney PJ, Wand PJ. Toxic-shock syndrome: epidemiologic features, recurrence, risk factors, and prevention The New England. J Med. 1980:1429–35.
6. DeVries AS, Lesher L, Schlievert PM, Al E. Staphylococcal toxic shock syndrome 2000–2006: epidemiology, clinical features, and molecular characteristics. PLoS One. 2011;6(8):e22997.
7. MacDonald KL, Osterholm MT, Hedberg CW, Al E. Toxic shock syndrome. A newly recognized complication of influenza and influenza-like illness. JAMA. 1987;257:1053–8.

8. Cone LA, Woodard DR, Schlievert PM. Clinical and bacteriologic observations of a toxic shock-like syndrome due to Streptococcus pyogenes. N Engl J Med. 1987;317:146–9.
9. Perry S, Reid R. Toxic shock syndrome and streptococcal toxic shock syndrome. In: Tintinalli J, Stapczynski J, Ma O, Cline D, Cydulka R, Meckler G, editors. Tintinalli's Emergency Medicine: a comprehensive study guide. 7th ed. New York: McGraw-Hill Education LLC; 2011. Ch. 145. p. 999–1003.
10. Fernández-Frackelton M. Toxic shock syndrome. In: Hockberger R, Walls RM, Gausche-Hill M, editors. Rosen's emergency medicine: concepts and clinical practice. 9th ed. Elsevier; 2017. Ch. 121. p. 1593–7.
11. Stevens DL. Invasive group A streptococcus infections clinical infectious disease. Clin Infect Dis. 1992;14:2–11.
12. Low Donald E. Toxic shock syndrome. Crit Care Clin. 2013;29:651–75.
13. Centers for Disease Control. Toxic Shock Syndrome (Other Than Streptococcal) (TSS) 2011 Case definition. MMWR Tech Rep. 2011. https://wwwn.cdc.gov/nndss/conditions/toxic-shock-syndrome-other-than-streptococcal/case-definition/2011/.
14. Centers for Disease Control: Streptococcal Toxic Shock Syndrome (STSS) (Streptococcus pyogenes) 2010 case definition. MMWR Tech Rep. 2010. https://wwwn.cdc.gov/nndss/conditions/streptococcal-toxic-shock-syndrome/case-definition/2010/.
15. Burnham JP, Kollef MH. Understanding toxic shock syndrome. Intensive Care Med. 2015;41:1707–10.
16. Kaul R, McGeer A, Low DE, Green K, Schwartz B. Population-based surveillance for group A streptococcal necrotizing fasciitis: clinical features, prognostic indicators, and microbiologic analysis of seventy-seven cases. Ontario Group A Streptococcal Study. Am J Med. 1997;103:18–24.
17. Chesney PJ, Davism JP, Purdy WK, Wand PJ, Chesney RW. Clinical manifestations of toxic shock syndrome. JAMA. 1981;246:741–8.
18. John C, Niermann M, Sharon B, Peterson M, Kranz D, Schlievert P. Staphylococcal toxic shock syndrome erythroderma is associated with superantigenicity and hypersensitivity. Clin Infect Dis. 2009;49:1893–6.
19. Schlievert PM, Kelly JA. Clindamycin-induced suppression of toxic-shock syndrome--associated exotoxin production. J Infect Dis. 1984;149(3):471.
20. Kalyan S, Chow AW. Staphylococcal toxic shock syndrome toxin-1 induces the translocation and secretion of high mobility group-1 protein from both activated T cells and monocytes. Mediators Inflamm. 2008;2008:1.
21. Kaul R, McGeer A, Norrby-Teglund A, Al E. Intravenous immunoglobulin therapy in streptococcal toxic shock syndrome – a comparative observational study. Clin Infect Dis. 1999;28:800–7.
22. Barry W, Hudgins L, Donta ST, Pesanti EL. Intravenous immunoglobulin therapy for toxic shock syndrome. JAMA. 1992;267:3315–6.
23. Darenberg J, Ihendyane N, Sjölin J, et al. Intravenous immunoglobulin G therapy in streptococcal toxic shock syndrome: a European randomized, double-blind, placebo-controlled trial. Clin Infect Dis. 2003;37:333–40.
24. Todd J, Ressman M, Caston S, Todd B, Wiesenthal A. Corticosteroid therapy for patients with toxic shock syndrome. JAMA. 1984;252:3399–402.
25. Hajjeh RA, Reingold A, Weil A, et al. Toxic shock syndrome in the United States: surveillance update 1979–1996. Emerg Infect Dis. 1999;5:807–10.
26. Davies H, McGeer A, Schwartz B, et al. Invasive group A streptococcal infections in Ontario. Can N Engl J Med. 1996;335:547–54.
27. Stevens DL, Tanner MH, Winship J. Severe group A streptococcal infections associated with a toxic shock- like syndrome and scarlet fever toxin A. N Engl J Med. 1989;321:1–7.
28. Demers B, Simor A, Vellend H. Severe invasive group A streptococcal infections in Ontario, Canada: 1987–1991. Clin Infect Dis. 1993;16:792–800.
29. Sabella C. Toxic shock syndromes. In: Usatine RP, Sabella C, Smith M, Mayeaux EJ, Jr., Chumley HS, Appachi E, editors. The color atlas of pediatrics. New York: McGraw-Hill; http://accesspediatrics.mhmedical.com.ezproxy.med.nyu.edu/content.aspx?bookid=1443&sectionid=79849415. Accessed 24 July 2017.

Scarlet Fever

9

Nathaniel Johnson and James Dill

Background

Scarlet fever, also known as "scarlatina," is a complication of streptococcal pharyngitis, though scarlet fever may also follow skin infections caused by Group A strep (GAS). It typically affects children between 5 and 15 years of age, with most of those cases occurring in children less than 10. Exposure to *S. pyogenes* produces a pyrogenic erythrotoxin (usually type A, B, or C) that causes a delayed-type hypersensitivity reaction, resulting in the classic rash described below [1, 7]. GAS is usually spread by contact with nasal or oral secretions from infected patient or (less commonly) GAS carriers [6]. It may also be transmitted through skin contact, via fomites, and even (rarely) by food vectors. Of note, 15–20% of children are asymptomatic carriers of the organism [8]. Though GAS is responsible for 20–30% of sore throat visits in children [1, 10], scarlet fever affects a minority of patients with GAS infections.

Clinical Presentation

Sore throat and fever typically precede scarlet fever by a few days. The sore throat appears erythematous, most notably involving the tonsils and posterior oropharynx. Also present may be white discoloration of the oropharynx with swelling, and areas of yellow or white purulence [3, 8]. Other symptoms may include chills, cervical lymphadenopathy, abdominal pain, and vomiting. An enanthem of bright red tongue (often referred to as a "strawberry tongue") (Fig. 9.1) and Forchheimer spots may also be transiently present in the oropharynx, which are small, red spots on the soft palate (petechiae) (Fig. 9.2).

N. Johnson · J. Dill (✉)
Emergency Medicine/Pediatrics, University of Arizona, Tucson, AZ, USA
e-mail: njohnson@aemrc.arizona.edu; jdill@aemrc.arizona.edu

© Springer International Publishing AG, part of Springer Nature 2018
E. Rose (ed.), *Life-Threatening Rashes*, https://doi.org/10.1007/978-3-319-75623-3_9

Fig. 9.1 "Strawberry" tongue. (Photo courtesy of Afag Azizova)

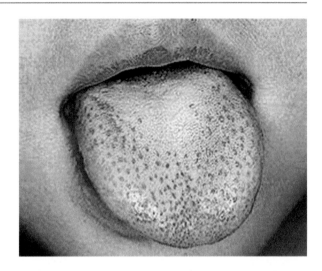

Fig. 9.2 Forchheimer spots. (Photo courtesy of Dr. Jack Springer, MD)

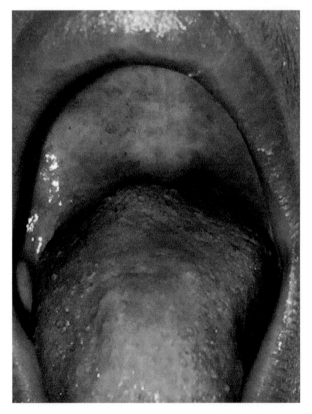

The rash (exanthem) usually begins on the face or chest, sometimes behind the ears and on the neck, but may also appear first in the axilla and/or groin. It then typically spreads to the chest and trunk and the rest of the body (Fig. 9.3). If present on the face, the rash classically has the appearance of red cheeks and a pale area around the mouth (circumoral pallor) (Fig. 9.4). The rash is red, fine, and rough-textured

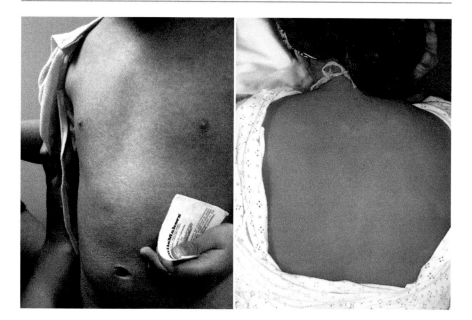

Fig. 9.3   Scarlatiniform rash

Fig. 9.4   Circumoral
pallor. (Photo courtesy of
Dr. Jack Springer, MD)

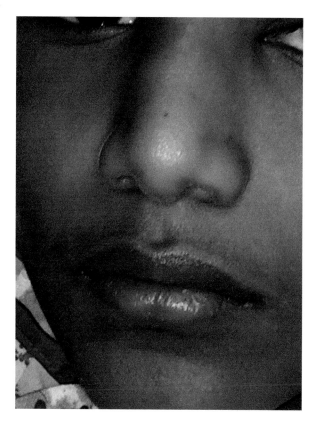

Fig. 9.5 Pastia's lines

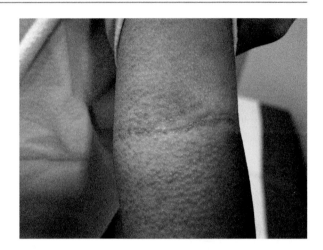

(sandpaper-like) and will blanch when pressure is applied. The rash tends to be more pronounced in the skin folds, where the skin lines come together. This creates distinct bright pink or red linear markings at the skin folds known as Pastia's lines (Fig. 9.5).

Associated Systemic Symptoms

In addition to sore throat and the diagnostic rash of scarlet fever, patients commonly report fever, fatigue, headaches, enlarged and tender lymph nodes, and abdominal pain. Symptoms of conjunctivitis, cough, rhinorrhea, diarrhea, herpangina/stomatitis, and nasal congestion, if present, are likely more indicative of a viral infectious process than GAS infection, even if other symptoms of strep are concurrent.

Severe headache, abdominal pain, and/or sore throat/neck pain, particularly if seen in conjunction with hypotension, tachycardia, tachypnea, altered mentation, abnormal WBC count, and/or high fevers, may indicate less common but more severe complications of GAS infection. These include abscess, necrotizing deep soft tissue infection, meningitis, and bacterial sepsis.

Time Course

The incubation period after exposure until the development of scarlet fever symptoms is usually between 1 and 4 days [9]. The rash typically begins 1–2 days after GAS infection, as the organism needs to be actively producing the toxin for the hypersensitivity reaction to occur. However, it should be noted that the rash may appear up to 7 days after the onset of infection or even prior to the beginning of other symptoms, such as the sore throat itself [7]. After about 3–4 days, the rash begins to fade and skin peeling (desquamation) begins. Typically, this presents as flaking on the face with progression to peeling around the palms and fingers. After desquamation, Pastia's lines can persist as pigmented lines.

Common Mimics and Differential Diagnosis

GAS infections are the most commonly seen bacterial pharyngitis in pediatric patients older than 3 years of age [1]. However, the majority of pharyngitis seen and diagnosed in pediatric patients is viral in etiology. Many viral infections that cause pharyngitis share diagnostic features with GAS pharyngitis but the diagnostic rash of scarlet fever should be a distinguishing feature from most viral exanthems.

The presentation of scarlet fever may be mistaken for the progression of classic Kawasaki disease. Distinguishing between the two is essential, as both have potentially severe sequelae, and the treatment of each differ substantially. Similarities between the two include potentially similar timeline of symptom progression, as well as the symptoms themselves—the reddened ("strawberry") tongue, eventual skin desquamation, sore throat, and a rash. Noninfectious conjunctivitis can be present with Kawasaki disease, which may help with differentiating between the two entities. However, this symptom is not always present [19, 20]. Other distinguishing features are described further below (Table 9.1).

Additionally, Forchheimer spots are not diagnostic of scarlet fever, as they can be present in 20% of patients with rubella and are also sometimes present in measles. The differentiation between these infections would be based on characteristics of the illness in question and the characteristic rashes found in each.

Key Physical Findings and Diagnostic Features

The initial suspicion for the diagnosis of scarlet fever is based on clinical symptoms and signs—most notably the rash. However, The Infectious Diseases Society of America (IDSA) no longer recommends treating strep throat empirically based solely on signs and symptoms, as the ability to diagnose GAS based on signs and symptoms alone is generally poor [1, 11]. The Modified Centor Score (Table 9.2), a validated scoring system for identifying the likelihood of the presence of strep

Table 9.1 Differentiation of scarlet fever vs. Kawasaki disease

Scarlet fever	Kawasaki disease
Fever responds to antipyretics	Fever does *not* respond to antipyretics
Tender adenopathy	Painless adenopathy
Rash blanches, fine texture, Pastia's lines	Nonspecific polymorphous rash
Verify with rapid antigen test/culture	Evaluate with serial ECHOs
Treated with antibiotics	Treated with high-dose ASA, IVIG
Can lead to RF, PSGN, suppurative/nonsuppurative complications	Can cause aneurysm formation, depressed cardiac activity

Table 9.2 Modified Centor
Criteria [22]

Criteria	Point
Temperature > 38 C	+1
Absence of cough	+1
Tender anterior chain lymph nodes	+1
Tonsillar swelling/exudate	+1
3–14 years old	+1
15–44 years old	+0
45 years old and older	−1

[a]Two or more points and testing should be considered

pharyngitis, can be helpful in guiding decision-making for testing with the intent to treat; however, clinical acumen is still essential in deciding if testing is necessary [2].

There are several methods for diagnosis of GAS infection. Throat culture is the diagnostic gold standard and, when obtained properly, has a sensitivity of 90–95% [12]. Cultures should be swabbed from either the tonsils or the posterior pharyngeal wall. However, this can be difficult with an uncooperative child, and false negatives can result, particularly if there has been previous recent treatment with antibiotics [1, 5].

The yield of positive results can be increased by adding an anaerobic culture medium, though this approach is controversial [13]. Throat cultures should be incubated at 35C–37C for a minimum of 18–24 h, though continued overnight incubation at room temperatures for up to 48 h can increase positive yields [9].

Rapid antigen detection tests (RADTs) in the emergency department have significantly increased the number of people appropriately treated beyond culture alone; however, with sensitivities of 70–90%, the sensitivity of this testing approach is inferior to agar cultures [14–16].

ASA titers can be helpful to diagnose the nonsuppurative sequelae of GAS infections; however, they aren't useful in the acute setting as they can take between 3 and 8 weeks to reach peak levels after a GAS infection [17, 18].

Management

There is no additional treatment for scarlet fever other than the management for GAS pharyngitis. Once diagnosed, the treatment goal is primarily aimed at reducing risk of subsequent acute rheumatic fever (ARF). If untreated, the risk of ARF following GAS infection is estimated to be around 0.5–3%; but host factors (including genetic predisposition), environment, and prevalence of certain GAS bacteria subtypes in the involved community all contribute to this risk [25].

The reduction of symptoms and the prevention of subsequent nonsuppurative and suppurative complications of GAS infection are also considerations.

Reduction of symptoms focuses primarily on treating the associated pharyngitis and constitutional symptoms of strep infections. The mainstay of this care is over-the-counter analgesics, particularly NSAIDs, and can also include steroids (for pharyngitis). Initiation of antibiotics has only a modest effect on symptom relief, reducing symptom burden by an estimated 16–24 h [23].

Table 9.3 GAS infection antibiotic regimens [1]

Medication	Route	Dose	Duration
Penicillin V	Oral	Children: 250 mg BID/TID Adolescents/adults: 250 mg QID OR 500 mg BID	10 days
Amoxicillin	Oral	50 mg/kg up to max 1000 mg Qday 25 mg/kg up to max 500 mg BID	10 days
Benzathine penicillin G	IM	<27 kg: 600 k U 27 kg and higher: 1200 k U	Once

Table 9.4 GAS infection antibiotic regimens, penicillin allergy [1]

Medication	Route	Dose	Duration
Cefadroxil	Oral	30 mg/kg up to max 1000 mg Qday	10 days
Cephalexin	Oral	20 mg/kg/dose up to max 500 mg/dose BID	10 days
Clindamycin	Oral	7 mg/kg/dose up to max 300 mg/dose TID	10 days
Azithromycin	Oral	12 mg/kg up to max 500 mg Qday	5 days
Clarithromycin	Oral	7.5 mg/kg/dose up to max 250 mg/dose BID	10 days

Antibiotics of choice include penicillin VK, amoxicillin, or cephalosporins, clindamycin, and macrolides for penicillin-allergic patients (Tables 9.3 and 9.4). Oral medication duration remains 10 days, with the exception of shorter treatment duration for azithromycin. The use of macrolide antibiotics is NOT recommended unless patients have a history of severe hypersensitivity reaction (i.e., anaphylaxis) to penicillin antibiotics. While there is no documented GAS resistance to penicillin antibiotics, there is variable (as high as 97% in some studies) GAS resistance to azithromycin. These resistance patterns appear to be temporally and geographically variable [21].

Complications

Scarlet fever itself, today, is typically benign. This is dramatic change from the beginning of the prior century when mortality was as high as 30%. Similarly, morbidity and mortality from acute rheumatic fever/disease (ARF) has also seen a significant decrease in the past 100 years. Concurrently, however, invasive strep infections have been on the rise. These trends are dynamic and hinge on multiple factors that include host population, environment, and pathogen types—particularly M protein type [24, 25].

Treatment of the causative organism (GAS) aims primarily to reduce the subsequent risk of rheumatic fever (RF). In RF, carditis is a serious complication, and, worldwide, it is the most common cause of acquired heart disease. Rheumatic heart disease presents as a new murmur, pericardial friction rub, and/or CHF.

Treating GAS infections does NOT appear to decrease risk of post-strep glomerulonephritis (PSGN). PSGN is caused by glomerular immune complex deposition following GAS infections of the skin or pharynx. It presents with edema, gross hematuria or discolored urine, and/or hypertension.

GAS infections, including and in addition to scarlet fever, can lead to other complications not related to acute rheumatic fever. These include the suppurative complications—peritonsillar abscess, retropharyngeal abscess, sinusitis, otitis media, other soft tissue abscesses and necrotizing deep soft tissue infections, as well as nonsuppurative complications (strep toxic shock syndrome) [4].

Bottom Line: Scarlet Fever Clinical Pearls

- Scarlet fever is a typically benign complication of a GAS infection, usually tonsillopharyngitis. It is primarily seen in pediatric patients.
- Scarlet fever is typically suspected based on symptoms indicative of a GAS infection, absence of symptoms that would indicate a viral illness, and a characteristic bright red, sandpaper-like rash. Diagnosis is confirmed through laboratory testing.
- Once the diagnosis is confirmed, scarlet fever treatment involves an antibiotic course aimed primarily at preventing subsequent acute rheumatic fever. Other treatment goals may also include improvement of symptoms of the illness, as well as prevention of other post-GAS infection complications in the patient and patient's contacts.
- Appropriate management is contingent upon correct diagnosis and antibiotic treatment, prompt identification, and treatment of other GAS complications should they arise, as well as vigilance in screening for other disease processes, such as Kawasaki disease, which can mimic scarlet fever but would necessitate a very different management strategy.

References

1. Shulman ST, Bisno AL, Clegg HW, et al. Clinical practice guideline for the diagnosis and management of group A streptococcal pharyngitis: 2012 update by the Infectious Diseases Society of America. Clin Infect Dis. 2012;55(10):1279–82.
2. McIsaac WJ, Kellner JD, Aufricht P, Vanjaka A, Low DE. Empirical validation of guidelines for the management of pharyngitis in children and adults. JAMA. 2004;291(13):1587–95.
3. "Scarlet Fever: a group A Streptococcal infection". *Center for Disease Control and Prevention.* 19 Jan 2016.
4. Pichichero ME. "Complications of streptococcal tonsillopharyngitis". *UpToDate.* 4 Feb 2016.
5. Bisno AL, Gerber MA, Gwaltney JM Jr, Kaplan EL, Schwartz RH. Practice guidelines for the diagnosis and management of group A streptococcal pharyngitis. Infectious Diseases Society of America. Clin Infect Dis. 2002;35:113–25.
6. Meier FA, Centor RM, Graham L Jr, Dalton HP. Clinical and microbiological evidence for endemic pharyngitis among adults due to group C streptococci. Arch Intern Med. 1990;150:825–9.
7. Zabriskie JB. The role of temperate bacteriophage in the production of erythrogenic toxin by Group A *Streptococci.* J Exp Med. 1964;119(5):761–80. PMC 2137738. PMID 14157029.
8. Martin JM, Green M, Barbadora KA, Wald ER. Group A streptococci among school-aged children: clinical characteristics and the carrier state. Pediatrics. 2004;114:1212–9.

9. Kellogg JA. Suitability of throat culture procedures for detection of group A streptococci and as reference standards for evaluation of streptococcal antigen detection kits. J Clin Microbiol. 1990;28:165–9.
10. Bisno AL. Acute pharyngitis: etiology and diagnosis. Pediatrics. 1996;97:949–54.
11. Wannamaker LW. Perplexity and precision in the diagnosis of streptococcal pharyngitis. Am J Dis Child. 1972;124:352–8.
12. Gerber MA. Diagnosis of pharyngitis: methodology of throat cultures. In: Shulman ST, editor. Pharyngitis: management in an era of declining rheumatic fever. New York: Praeger; 1984. p. 61–72.
13. Schwartz RH, Gerber MA, McCoy P. Effect of atmosphere of incubation on the isolation of group A streptococci from throat cultures. J Lab Clin Med. 1985;106:88–92.
14. Centor RM, Geiger P, Waites KB. Fusobacterium necrophorum bacteremic tonsillitis: 2 cases and a review of the literature. Anaerobe. 2010;16:626–8.
15. Tanz RR, Gerber MA, Kabat W, Rippe J, Seshadri R, Shulman ST. Performance of a rapid antigen-detection test and throat culture in community pediatric offices: implications for management of pharyngitis. Pediatrics. 2009;123:437–44.
16. Gerber MA, Shulman ST. Rapid diagnosis of pharyngitis caused by group A streptococci. Clin Microbiol Rev. 2004;17:571–80.
17. Shet A, Kaplan EL. Clinical use and interpretation of group a streptococcal antibody tests: a practical approach for the pediatrician or primary care physician. Pediatr Infect Dis J. 2002;21:420–6; quiz 27–30.
18. Johnson DR, Kurlan R, Leckman J, Kaplan EL. The human immune response to streptococcal extracellular antigens: clinical, diagnostic, and potential pathogenetic implications. Clin Infect Dis. 2010;50:481–90.
19. "About Kawasaki Disease". Center for Disease Control and Prevention. 13 Dec 2013.
20. "Kawasaki Disease". PubMed Health. NHLBI Health Topics. 11 June 2014. Retrieved 26 Aug 2016.
21. Logan LK, McAuley JB, Shulman ST. Macrolide treatment failure in streptococcal pharyngitis resulting in acute rheumatic fever. Pediatrics. 2012;129:e798; originally published online February 6, 2012. https://doi.org/10.1542/peds.2011-1198.
22. McIsaac W, White D, Tannenbaum D, Low D. A clinical score to reduce unnecessary antibiotic use in patients with sore throat. Can Med Assoc J. 1998;158(1):75–83.
23. Del Mar CB, Glasziou PP, Spinks AB. Antibiotics for sore throat. Cochrane Database Syst Rev. 2006;(4):CD000023.
24. Lee GM, Wessels MR. Changing epidemiology of acute rheumatic fever in the United States. Clin Infect Dis. 2006;42(4):448–50.
25. Cunningham MW. Pathogenesis of group A streptococcal infections. Clin Microbiol Rev. 2000;13(3):470–511.

Staphylococcal Scalded Skin Syndrome

10

Louise Malburg and Garrett S. Pacheco

Background

Staphylococcus aureus is one of the most common etiologies of bacterial skin infections and may present in a variety of ways. One of the most severe manifestations is staphylococcal scalded skin syndrome (SSSS), an exotoxin-mediated disease characterized by diffuse bullae formation [1]. The incidence is estimated to be about 0.09–0.56 cases per million inhabitants in the general population [2] and has been shown to have higher incidence in summer and fall seasons [3, 4]. Historically, it has also been called Ritter's disease and pemphigus neonatorum [5]. The toxins responsible are exfoliative toxins A and B (ETA, ETB), produced by coagulase-positive *S. aureus* [2]. ETA is more common (89% of cases) than ETB, although ETB is much more virulent [2].

Initial site of infection occurs most commonly in sites of colonization, such as the nasopharynx or conjunctiva. The exotoxin produced by *S. aureus* then enters into the bloodstream and circulates, spreading diffusely to the skin. The exfoliative toxins accumulate in the skin tissue and cause breakdown of desmoglein 1 (Dsg1), which is essential to keratinocyte cell-to-cell adhesion within the superficial layers of the epidermis [2, 6, 7]. This leads to the formation of diffuse bullae and subsequent desquamation. The blisters are typically sterile as the skin findings are toxin-mediated rather than secondary to direct infection. Symptoms will continue to progress until the exotoxin has either been bound by antibodies or cleared by the kidneys. This generally lasts 24–48 h, depending on the immune status and renal function of the infected patient [2].

L. Malburg
Department of Pediatrics, University of Arizona, Tucson, AZ, USA
e-mail: Lmalburg@peds.arizona.edu

G. S. Pacheco (✉)
Departments of Emergency Medicine & Pediatrics, University of Arizona, Tucson, AZ, USA
e-mail: Gpacheco@aemrc.arizona.edu

© Springer International Publishing AG, part of Springer Nature 2018
E. Rose (ed.), *Life-Threatening Rashes*, https://doi.org/10.1007/978-3-319-75623-3_10

Although SSSS affects patients of all ages, it is most common in the pediatric population, especially in those under the age of 5 [2–4, 7, 8]. An immature renal system unable to clear the exfoliative toxin and a lack of protective antibodies against staphylococcal toxins [2–4] likely contribute to the increased risk of infection in the young. Newborns are particularly at risk and represent about 80% of SSSS cases. This is particularly true in areas where umbilical cord care with antiseptics is discouraged [9]. Older kids and adults typically have pre-formed antibodies against the staphylococcal exotoxins, making the development of SSSS less likely. However, these populations are at risk for SSSS if they are immunosuppressed due to medications or disease or in the setting of renal failure [2, 8, 9].

Classic Clinical Presentation

The time course of disease is summarized in Table 10.1. Once the triggering staphylococcal infection has been established, SSSS findings will develop in the following few days [11]. Skin findings often begin as faint but well-demarcated patches that quickly coalesce into a diffuse erythema that is significantly tender to palpation [1, 2, 12] (Fig. 10.1). Diffuse erythema may be scarlatiniform in appearance with sandpaper feel to palpation [10]. Flaccid bullae develop in the following 24–48 h with a positive Nikolsky sign (skin desquamation with gentle pressure). Rupture of the bullae reveals underlying moist, red skin with the classic "scalded" appearance (Fig. 10.2). This erythematous base then rapidly dries to create a shiny surface. Areas with creases, such as the axillae, groin, nose, and ear, are often the most noticeable areas with desquamation that mimics the appearance of tissue paper [9, 12]. While perioral lesions are common, mucous membranes are not affected (Fig. 10.3) [8]. In the newborn, the diaper area is often the first to develop these signs (Fig. 10.4). These areas will typically dry within the following 24 h. Lesions will fully heal within 7–10 days without scarring.

Table 10.1 A timeline of skin findings

Initial	Hours	24–48 h	Days 3–5	10 days
Abrupt, faint, erythematous, tender patches	Patches become well demarcated and coalesce into a confluent scarlatiniform erythema	Flaccid bullae form within the erythematous areas, beginning on the central face, axillae, groin, and neck and spreading to form diffuse, large sheets, *sparing mucous membranes*. Rupture of bullae reveals a moist, red surface that appears scalded	Within 24 h of exfoliation, areas dry with a thin, shiny crust. Fissuring occurs in perioral and periorbital skin	Skin heals without scarring

Data from Pollack [1], Handler and Schwartz [2], and Marina et al. [10]

Fig. 10.1 A school-aged female with signs of early SSSS secondary to bullous impetigo. The skin developed diffuse erythema that was tender to palpation. (Patient consent obtained. Photo credit: Elizabeth Placzek, MD.)

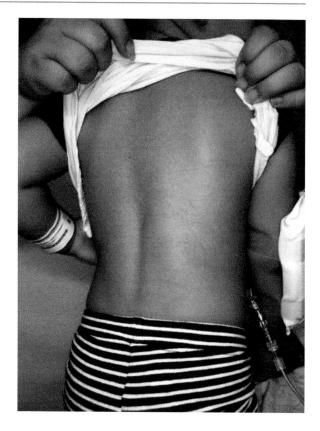

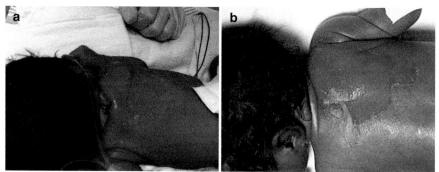

Fig. 10.2 (a) Sloughing of skin reveals moist, erythematous underlying skin that appears scalded. (b) Hours later. (From Arora et al. [13])

Atypical Presentation

The clinical presentation of SSSS may vary on a spectrum from mild to severe, depending on the strain of *S. aureus*, the amount of toxin, and the location of its release [10]. Mild cases, such as those seen in a report by Hubiche et al. [15], may

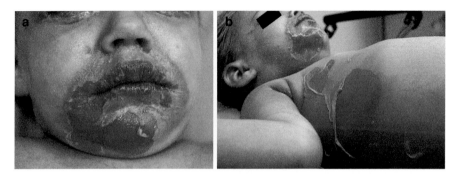

Fig. 10.3 (**a**) A school-age child with perioral SSSS skin lesions. (**b**) Significant truncal desquamation. (From Conway et al. [14])

Fig. 10.4 An infant with inguinal desquamation due to SSSS. (Photo credit: Jennifer Ballinger, MD)

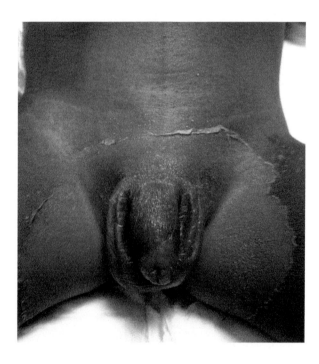

present with a mild, diffuse exanthem, followed by focal desquamation in the major skinfolds, with minimal or absent bullae formation. Additionally, some cases of SSSS may complicate other infections or conditions with cutaneous findings such as burns, graft versus host disease, and varicella (Fig. 10.5) [16–19].

Associated Systemic Symptoms

Pediatric patients often present with a short, non-specific prodrome of fever, irritability, and poor feeding, prior to onset of cutaneous manifestations [2]. Evidence of

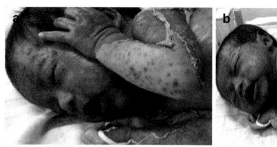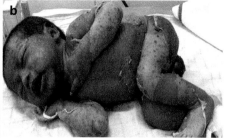

Fig. 10.5 (**a**) A neonate with varicella infection complicated by SSSS. (**b**) Irritable neonate with whole body involvement/desquamation. (From Singh et al. [16])

acute pharyngitis, conjunctivitis, or a mild upper respiratory infection have also been known to precede SSSS [11, 17]. It is suspected that upper respiratory tract infections, in particular, may alter the epithelium leading to proliferation of *S. aureus* in pediatric patients who are carriers of exfoliative toxin strains [17].

In adults, the source of infection is more varied and includes cellulitis or abscesses, septic arthritis, osteomyelitis, and endocarditis or as a complication of an invasive procedure or parenteral infection. Infection in adults is typically more severe at presentation and is commonly associated with bacteremia, shock, and a higher mortality rate. This is a stark contrast to the pediatric population, in which hypotension or signs of shock are rare on presentation and the prognosis is overall favorable with treatment [11, 20, 21].

Common Mimics and Differential Diagnosis

There are a number of rashes comparable to that of SSSS and are summarized in Table 10.2. Along the same spectrum as SSSS, is bullous impetigo, which is a milder, localized form. It most commonly affects neonates and presents with superficial bullae on the trunk and extremities (Fig. 10.6). The marked differences are the localized site, the absence of Nikolsky sign, and the presence of *S. aureus* within the bullous lesions. In few cases, bullous impetigo may progress to SSSS. For that reason, these patients should be followed closely, as the mortality of SSSS is significantly higher than the benign course of bullous impetigo [22, 23].

Other blistering conditions, such as Stevens-Johnson syndrome (SJS), toxic epidermal necrolysis (TEN), or pemphigus vulgaris, may resemble SSSS. The differentiating features of these conditions are summarized in Table 10.3.

It is important to differentiate SSSS from TEN as the treatments are markedly different. While corticosteroids may be utilized in the management of TEN, their use is contraindicated in cases of SSSS due to the potential for further immunosuppression and subsequent worsening of symptoms [11, 24]. History and physical are essential in making the diagnosis. A history of a recent new drug exposure may be suggestive of TEN [24]. There is also significant mucosal involvement in TEN, which is absent in SSSS. If there is a mixed clinical picture, frozen section histology

Table 10.2
Differential diagnosis of SSSS

Differential diagnosis
Toxic epidermal necrolysis
Erythema multiforme
Stevens-Johnsons syndrome
Pemphigus vulgaris
Pemphigus foliaceus
Toxic shock syndrome
Scarlet fever
Kawasaki disease
Coxsackie infection
Drug reaction with eosinophilia and systemic symptoms (DRESS)
Burn
Child abuse

Data from Patel and Finlay [11]

Fig. 10.6 A school-aged female with bullous impetigo. (Patient consent obtained. Photo credit: Elizabeth Placzek, MD)

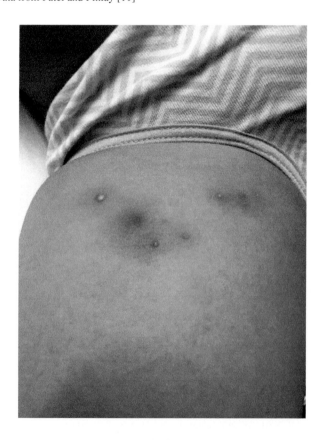

of the roof of an acute blister or a sample of sloughed skin is often all that is needed to quickly differentiate the two in an acute setting [24, 25]. TEN will show subepidermal (deeper) cleavage with evidence of necrosis, while SSSS shows a superficial epidermal break without necrosis [25, 26].

Pemphigus vulgaris is an autoimmune condition that is similar in mechanism to SSSS, as it targets desmogleins. However, the antibodies are directed against

Table 10.3 Key differentiating features of top differential diagnoses of SSSS

Disease	Clinical features	Nikolsky sign	Mucous membrane involvement	Biopsy findings	Additional characteristics
SSSS	Diffuse erythema and bullae formation with underlying scalded skin	Positive	Absent	Intraepidermal cleavage along stratum granulosum. No inflammatory or necrotic cells	
Bullous impetigo	Localized cluster of flaccid bullae containing pus that may rupture and crust	Negative	Absent	Intraepidermal cleavage along stratum granulosum, dermal inflammatory infiltrates	
Toxic epidermal necrolysis (TEN)	Rapidly progressive rash with blistering and desquamation	Positive	Present	Subepidermal cleavage, dermal inflammatory infiltrates, and necrotic keratinocytes	Often result of a severe adverse drug reaction. More common in adult population
Pemphigus Vulgaris	Painful mucosal or mucosal and skin blistering	Positive	Present	Intraepidermal cleavage along stratum granulosum, dermal inflammatory infiltrates, and positive direct immunofluorescence	More common in adult population

desmoglein 3 (Dsg3), rather than Dsg1, which is present in deeper layers of the skin and is prominent in mucous membranes. Skin biopsy shows intraepithelial cleavage in the suprabasal layers and eosinophilic inflammatory infiltrates, which are absent in SSSS [8]. Pemphigus foliaceus, on the other hand, is clinically difficult to distinguish from SSSS, as it is also common in children and affects only Dsg1, making mucosal involvement absent. Often it is only differentiated by biopsy based on the presence of dermal inflammatory infiltrates and antibodies seen on direct immunofluorescence [5, 8, 9, 11, 26].

Diagnosis is based on characteristic skin findings, histopathology on skin biopsy, and identification of the inciting staphylococcal infection [27]. This may be done by taking cultures of the nose, throat, skin, and umbilicus, as these are common commensal sites of staphylococcal growth that have been known to cause SSSS [9, 12]. In the sicker patient, there may be a more obvious source of infection, such as pneumonia, septic arthritis, abscess, or endocarditis (Fig. 10.7) [29]. Bullae of SSSS are known to be sterile. Regardless, lesional swabs should be

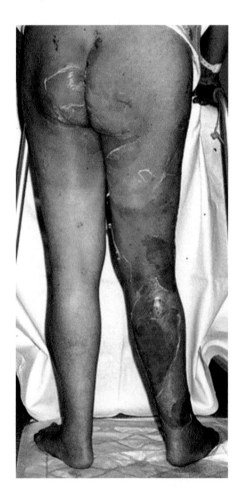

Fig. 10.7 A 63-year-old woman with SSSS affecting the buttocks and right lower extremity secondary to septic arthritis of the right knee. (From Sladden et al. [28])

obtained, as it may assist in identifying the presence of a secondary infection [29]. Blood cultures should also be obtained, though in most pediatric cases, they will remain negative [3, 29]. Blood cultures are much more likely to be positive in the adult population as there is generally a more severe infection and larger toxin burden due to immunosuppression [10, 29]. However, regardless of the patient population, a positive culture result is not required to make the diagnosis. It is also important to note that initial white blood cell counts and inflammatory markers, such as C-reactive protein (CRP), are often normal and should not provide false reassurance [30].

Though the diagnosis is typically clinical, definitive diagnosis may be made by skin biopsy, which reveals superficial intraepidermal cleavage within the stratum granulosum by acantholysis, with the roof of the bullae formed by the most superficial layer of the epidermis, the stratum corneum (Fig. 10.8). Remaining tissue will appear normal, without presence of inflammatory cells or signs of necrosis [2, 3, 12, 25, 31]. Frozen section of a blister roof may serve as rapid diagnostic tool; however, full-thickness biopsies should be obtained as well to confirm findings [24, 25, 27].

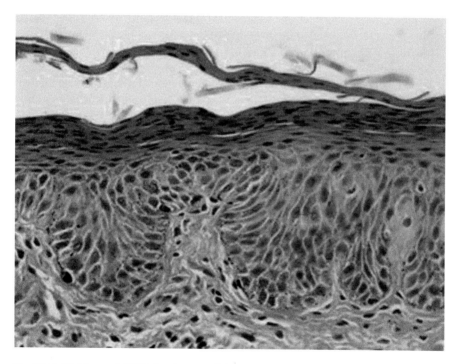

Fig. 10.8 Histology of SSSS showing superficial cleavage of the stratum granulosum. The thin layer of the stratum corneum forms the roof of the bulla (hematoxylin and eosin, original magnification ×400). (From Handler and Schwartz [2])

Recent development of more specialized testing, such as polymerase chain reaction (PCR), enzyme-linked immunosorbent assays (ELISA), and radioimmunoassays, now allows for the identification of the exfoliative toxin production in patients. However, these tests may take days to result, limiting their utility in the emergent setting. Additionally, they require sampling from the focus of infection, which is often unknown [5, 29].

Key Physical Exam Findings

Diffuse, scarlatiniform erythema with sandpaper feel to palpation and significant tenderness to palpation. Subsequent rapid development of flaccid bullae with a positive Nikolsky sign, that is most prominent in areas of skinfolds. Sloughing of the bullae reveals underlying eroded skin that is moist and brightly erythematous with a classic "scalded" appearance. There may be perioral involvement, but mucous membranes will remain unaffected [1, 2, 8–10, 12].

Management

Admission is recommended for all SSSS patients, especially in generalized cases [10]. As this condition leads to the loss of normal skin barrier, management should mimic that of a burn. Cases of severe and diffuse skin desquamation involving over 50% of body surface area should be transferred to a burn facility. Management is directed toward treating the causative staphylococcal infection and supportive care.

Parenteral anti-staphylococcal antibiotics should be administered promptly. First-line treatment is with a penicillinase-resistant synthetic penicillin, such as nafcillin or oxacillin [4]. Clindamycin may be beneficial due to its ability to inhibit bacterial toxin production [32]. However, studies of SSSS-causing bacteria have shown significant resistance rates against clindamycin, so it should not be used as monotherapy [4, 32]. Exfoliation may continue for 24–48 h despite antibiotics, until the toxin in circulation has been cleared. In an unstable, decompensating patient or if there is inadequate treatment response, vancomycin or linezolid should be given for methicillin-resistant *S. aureus* coverage [9, 29].

Supportive measures include intravenous fluids, analgesia, and nutritional support [2]. Warming methods should be utilized to preserve normal body temperature. The blisters should be left intact, if possible, to avoid further insensible losses and to minimize chance of superimposed infection on the naive skin [12]. Pressure-relieving mattresses may assist in reducing sloughing of the skin. Areas of denuded skin should be kept moist with emollients [8]. Fortunately, due to the superficiality of the condition, residual scarring is rare (Fig. 10.9) [29].

Appropriate analgesia should be provided, as the skin lesions are often painful. Acetaminophen is preferred over nonsteroidal anti-inflammatory drugs to avoid the

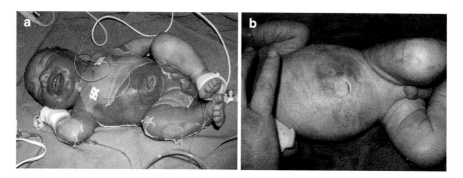

Fig. 10.9 A neonate with diffuse SSSS on day 1 of illness (**a**) versus day 7 of illness (**b**). (From Baartmans [33])

potential for renal injury and subsequent worsening of exfoliative toxin clearance [30, 34]. Patients with diffuse injury requiring regular dressing changes may require procedural sedation and/or opioids for analgesia [30].

Corticosteroids may cause worsening of SSSS and are not indicated. Treatment with fresh frozen plasma (FFP) and intravenous immunoglobulin (IVIG) have demonstrated some benefit and may be considered in refractory cases [35]. FFP is presumed to contain antibodies to the exotoxin, which could assist in curbing the exfoliative process. If no response to FFP is observed, IVIG may be considered to further attempt to neutralize circulating exotoxins [30]. Plasma exchange has also been successfully used in an adult patient who continued to have progression of skin lesions despite IVIG and ultimately improved after plasma exchange therapy [35].

Complications

The most common complications include electrolyte abnormalities, hypothermia, hypovolemia/dehydration, and secondary infection leading to cellulitis, pneumonia, and sepsis. Early diagnosis and initiation of treatment are critical to preventing serious complication and mortality [4, 7]. Mortality in children is about 4%, when substantial skin involvement is present and secondary infection develops [2, 12]. Mortality in adults is much higher, up to 40–60%, likely due the severity of staphylococcal infection as well as associated chronic underlying medical conditions particularly renal insufficiency/failure, immunosuppression, HIV/AIDS infection, or malignancy [29].

Episodes of SSSS are unlikely to recur as long as the patient develops an appropriate humoral response to the exposed exfoliative toxin. Rare cases of recurrent SSSS have been reported, mostly in premature infants with immature immune systems and therefore unable to develop an antibody response [36].

Bottom Line: Staphylococcal Scalded Skin Clinical Pearls

- SSSS is an uncommon but potentially fatal disorder mostly seen in infants and children under the age of 5 years.
- Adults have a higher mortality rates (40–60%); comorbid conditions and severe staphylococcal infections contribute.
- Caused by exfoliative toxin-producing *S. aureus* that leads to destruction of cell-to-cell connections in the most superficial layers of the epidermis.
- Starts with tender, diffuse, scarlatiniform erythema with overlying flaccid bullae that are Nikolsky sign positive.
- Rupture of bullae show moist, bright red eroded skin underneath that appears scalded.
- Absence of mucosal membrane involvement.
- Diagnosis is suspected clinically and confirmed by biopsy.
- Early treatment with penicillinase-resistant synthetic penicillin with or without clindamycin is crucial.

Resources

1. Pollack S. Staphylococcal scalded skin syndrome. Pediatr Rev. 1996;17(1):18. https://doi.org/10.1542/pir.17-1-18.
2. Handler MZ, Schwartz RA. Staphylococcal scalded skin syndrome: diagnosis and management in children and adults. J Eur Acad Dermatol Venereol. 2014;28:1418–23. https://doi.org/10.1111/jdv.12541.
3. Iwatsuki K, Yamasaki O, Morizane S, Oono T. Staphylococcal cutaneous infections: invasion, evasion and aggression. J Dermatol Sci. 2006;42(3):203–14. https://doi.org/10.1016/j.jdermsci.2006.03.011.
4. Li MY, Hua Y, Wei GH, Qiu L. Staphylococcal scalded skin syndrome in neonates: an 8-year retrospective study in a single institution. Pediatr Dermatol. 2013;31(1):43–7. https://doi.org/10.1111/pde.12114.
5. Amagai M. Desmoglein as a target in autoimmunity and infection. J Am Acad Dermatol. 2003;48(2):244–52. https://doi.org/10.1067/mjd.2003.7.
6. Amagai M, Matsuyoshi N, Wang ZH, Andl C, Stanley JR. Toxin in bullous impetigo and staphylococcal scalded-skin syndrome targets desmoglein 1. Nat Med. 2000;6(11):1275–7. https://doi.org/10.1038/81385.
7. Makhoul IR, Kassis I, Hashman N, Sujov P. Staphylococcal scalded-skin syndrome in a very low birth weight premature infant. Pediatrics. 2001;108(1) https://doi.org/10.1542/peds.108.1.e16.
8. Bukowski M, Wladyka B, Dubin G. Exfoliative toxins of Staphylococcus aureus. Toxins. 2010;2(5):1148–65. https://doi.org/10.3390/toxins2051148.
9. Mishra AK, Yadav P, Mishra AA. Systemic review on staphylococcal scalded skin syndrome (SSSS): a rare and critical disease of neonates. Open Microbiol J. 2016;10(1):150–9. https://doi.org/10.2174/1874285801610010150.
10. Marina SS, Bocheva GS, Kazanjieva JS. Severe bacterial infections of the skin: uncommon presentations. Clin Dermatol. 2005;23(6):621–9. https://doi.org/10.1016/j.clindermatol.2005.07.003.
11. Patel G, Finlay A. Staphylococcal scalded skin syndrome: diagnosis and management. Am J Clin Dermatol [serial online]. 2003;4(3):165–75. Available from: Academic Search Complete, Ipswich, MA. Accessed 10 July 2017.

12. Kouakou K, Dainguy ME, Kassi K. Staphylococcal scalded skin syndrome in neonate. Case Rep Dermatol Med. 2015;2015:1–4. https://doi.org/10.1155/2015/901968.
13. Arora P, Kalra VK, Rane S, McGrath EJ, Zegarra-Linares R, Chawla S. Staphylococcal scalded skin syndrome in a preterm newborn presenting within first 24 h of life. BMJ Case Rep. 2011;2011:bcr0820114733. https://doi.org/10.1136/bcr.08.2011.4733.
14. Conway DG, Lyon RF, Heiner JDA. Desquamating rash. Ann Emerg Med. 2013;61(1):118–29. https://doi.org/10.1016/j.annemergmed.2012.05.025.
15. Hubiche T, Bes M, Roudiere L, Langlaude F, Etienne J, Giudice PD. Mild staphylococcal scalded skin syndrome: an underdiagnosed clinical disorder. Br J Dermatol. 2011;166(1):213–5. https://doi.org/10.1111/j.1365-2133.2011.10515.x.
16. Singh SN, Tahazzul M, Singh A, Chandra S. Varicella infection in a neonate with subsequent staphylococcal scalded skin syndrome and fatal shock. Case Rep. 2012;2012(jul31 1) https://doi.org/10.1136/bcr-2012-006462.
17. Lamand V, Dauwalder O, Tristan A, et al. Epidemiological data of staphylococcal scalded skin syndrome in France from 1997 to 2007 and microbiological characteristics of Staphylococcus aureus associated strains. Clin Microbiol Infect. 2012;18(12) https://doi.org/10.1111/1469-0691.12053.
18. Thomas C, Yazdan P, Cotliar JA. Coexistence of staphylococcal scalded skin syndrome and acute graft-vs-host disease. JAMA Dermatol. 2015;151(3):343. https://doi.org/10.1001/jamadermatol.2014.2546.
19. Farroha A, Frew Q, Jabir S, Dziewulski P. Staphylococcal scalded skin syndrome due to burn wound infection. Ann Burns Fire Disasters. 2012;25(3):140–2.
20. Koufakis T, Gabranis I, Karanikas K. Staphylococcal scalded skin syndrome in an adult, immunocompetent patient. Braz J Infect Dis. 2015;19(2):228–9. https://doi.org/10.1016/j.bjid.2014.12.011.
21. Porzionato A, Aprile A. Staphylococcal scalded skin syndrome mimicking child abuse by burning. Forensic Sci Int. 2007;168(1) https://doi.org/10.1016/j.forsciint.2007.01.014.
22. Bae SH, Lee J-B, Kim S-J, Lee S-C, Won YH, Yun SJ. Case of bullous impetigo with enormous bulla developing into staphylococcal scalded skin syndrome. J Dermatol. 2015;43(4):459–60. https://doi.org/10.1111/1346-8138.13206.
23. Ugburo A, Temiye E, Ilombu C. A 12-year retrospective study of non-burn skin loss (burn-like syndromes) at a tertiary burns unit in a developing country. Burns. 2008;34(5):637–43. https://doi.org/10.1016/j.burns.2007.08.022.
24. Dobson C, King C. Adult staphylococcal scalded skin syndrome: histological pitfalls and new diagnostic perspectives. Br J Dermatol. 2003;148(5):1068–9. https://doi.org/10.1046/j.1365-2133.2003.05323.x.
25. Elston DM, Stratman EJ, Miller SJ. Skin biopsy. J Am Acad Dermatol. 2016;74(1):1–16. https://doi.org/10.1016/j.jaad.2015.06.033.
26. Stanley JR, Amagai M. Pemphigus, bullous impetigo, and the staphylococcal scalded-skin syndrome. N Engl J Med. 2006;355(17):1800–10. https://doi.org/10.1056/nejmra061111.
27. Tseng H-C, W-M W, Lin S-H. Staphylococcal scalded skin syndrome in an immunocompetent adult, clinically mimicking toxic epidermal necrolysis. J Dermatol. 2014;41(9):853–4. https://doi.org/10.1111/1346-8138.12566.
28. Sladden MJ, Mortimer NJ, Elston G, Newey M, Harman KE. Staphylococcal scalded skin syndrome as a complication of septic arthritis. Clin Exp Dermatol. 2007;32(6):754–5. https://doi.org/10.1111/j.1365-2230.2007.02483.x.
29. Ladhani S. Recent developments in staphylococcal scalded skin syndrome. Clin Microbiol Infect. 2001;7(6):301–7. https://doi.org/10.1046/j.1198-743x.2001.00258.x.
30. Blyth M, Estela C, Young AE. Severe staphylococcal scalded skin syndrome in children. Burns. 2008;34(1):98–103. https://doi.org/10.1016/j.burns.2007.02.006.
31. Gupta A, Jacobs N. Visual diagnosis. Pediatr Rev. 2013;34(3):9–12. https://doi.org/10.1542/pir.34-3-e9.
32. Braunstein I, Wanat KA, Abuabara K, Mcgowan KL, Yan AC, Treat JR. Antibiotic sensitivity and resistance patterns in pediatric staphylococcal scalded skin syndrome. Pediatr Dermatol. 2013;31(3):305–8. https://doi.org/10.1111/pde.12195.

33. Baartmans MGA. Neonate with staphylococcal scalded skin syndrome. Arch Dis Child Fetal Neonatal Ed. 2006;91(1) https://doi.org/10.1136/adc.2005.082610.
34. Dudley M, Parsh B. Recognizing staphylococcal scalded skin syndrome. Nursing. 2016;46(12):68. https://doi.org/10.1097/01.nurse.0000504683.43755.18.
35. Kato T, Fujimoto N, Nakanishi G, et al. Adult staphylococcal scalded skin syndrome successfully treated with plasma exchange. Acta Dermato Venereologica. 2015;95(5):612–3. https://doi.org/10.2340/00015555-2033.
36. Duijsters CE, Halbertsma FJ, Kornelisse RF, Arents NL, Andriessen P. Recurring staphylococcal scalded skin syndrome in a very low birth weight infant: a case report. J Med Case Reports. 2009;3:7313. https://doi.org/10.4076/1752-1947-3-7313.

Varicella and Zoster

11

Patricia Padlipsky and Kelly D. Young

Background

Varicella (chicken pox) is an acute infectious disease that causes a vesicular exanthem. It is transmitted via airborne respiratory droplets and is highly contagious with an attack rate up to 90% [1]. In temperate climates, it is seen most commonly in winter and early spring. It is caused by the varicella-zoster virus (VZV), also known as human herpesvirus 3, and affects only humans [2]. After initial infection, VZV remains latent in sensory ganglion neurons and can reactivate years to decades later as herpes zoster, commonly referred to as shingles. Zoster, unlike varicella, has no seasonal variation [3–5].

Prior to the introduction of the varicella vaccine in 1995, there were four million cases, over 11,000 hospitalizations, and 100–150 deaths per year in the United States, the majority of which occurred in children [6]. Implementation of the one-dose routine varicella vaccination program in 1996 resulted in a 90% decline in varicella incidence, and adding a second dose in 2006 resulted in an additional 85% decline in disease [6, 7]. As of 2015, 83% of 13–17-year-olds have received two doses of varicella vaccine [8].

Varicella incidence is currently 13–16 cases per 1000 population per year, peaking in preschool and elementary age children; > 90% cases occur before adolescence. Approximately 5 per 1000 varicella patients are hospitalized, and the

P. Padlipsky (✉)
David Geffen School of Medicine at UCLA, Los Angeles, CA, USA

Harbor-UCLA Medical Center, Department of Emergency Medicine, Torrance, CA, USA
e-mail: padlipsky@emedharbor.edu

K. D. Young
Health Sciences Clinical Professor of Emergency Medicine, David Geffen School
of Medicine at UCLA, Los Angeles, CA, USA

Harbor-UCLA Medical Center, Department of Emergency Medicine, Torrance, CA, USA
e-mail: kyoung@emedharbor.edu

© Springer International Publishing AG, part of Springer Nature 2018
E. Rose (ed.), *Life-Threatening Rashes*, https://doi.org/10.1007/978-3-319-75623-3_11

mortality rate is 2–3 per 100,000 [9]. Although certain groups (< 1 year or > 15 years old, immunocompromised, pregnant women) are at increased risk of severe varicella and/or complications, most varicella-related deaths occur among previously healthy persons eligible for vaccination [10]. As the majority of children are vaccinated, many varicella cases are occurring in immunized people as breakthrough disease. Primary varicella infection leads to lifetime immunity; a second episode of chicken pox occurs rarely (1 in 500), usually in an immunocompromised host, particularly those with impaired cell-mediated immunity [5].

There are over one million episodes of zoster in the United States annually, and the lifetime risk is 32%; risk is increased with advanced age and immunocompromise, particularly loss of cell-mediated immunity, and in those who had varicella at <18 months of age [4, 11]. Zoster vaccine has been recommended for adults ≥60 years since 2008 [12]. As of 2015, only 31% of adults ≥60 years old have received the zoster vaccine [13]. Although zoster incidence and number of ED visits for zoster has increased in the last several decades, incidence was increasing prior to the introduction of varicella vaccine, and available data indicate that zoster risk is lower after immunization compared to after wild-type varicella infection [5]. Zoster is typically seen in patients over age 50 years; the rate in children aged 10–14 years is one-fifth to one-tenth the rate in patients aged 55–65 years [14].

Classic Clinical Presentation

Varicella (Chicken Pox)

A mild prodrome of fever, malaise, and sometimes abdominal pain may occur 1–2 days prior to rash onset, particularly in adolescents and adults. A generalized, pruritic rash typically starts on the face and scalp, progresses to the trunk, and then quickly involves the extremities. The rash is concentrated centrally, with more lesions on the face and trunk and fewer on the extremities. Two or more successive crops of 1–4 mm-diameter lesions that begin as macules and papules, rapidly progressing to fluid-filled vesicles over 24–48 h, result in various stages of lesions (papule, vesicles, crust) seen all at once (Figs. 11.1 and 11.2). Vesicles develop on an erythematous base, giving the classic "dew drop on a rose petal" appearance (Fig. 11.3). Vesicles crust over and fall off over the next 1–2 weeks, often leaving hypo- or hyperpigmentation and sometimes scarring. Most patients develop 200–500 lesions, although breakthrough varicella in immunized patients may result in an attenuated disease course with fewer than 50 lesions (Fig. 11.4). Lesions commonly occur on mucous membranes, particularly the mouth, conjunctiva, and vagina; palms and soles are usually spared [1, 2, 4] (Fig. 11.5).

Herpes Zoster (Shingles)

Herpes zoster (aka shingles) results from reactivation of VZV, with spread from a single nerve ganglion to the neural tissue of the affected segment and the corresponding cutaneous dermatome [11, 14]. Approximately 70–80% of patients with herpes zoster will have prodromal pain or tingling in the dermatome prior to the appearance

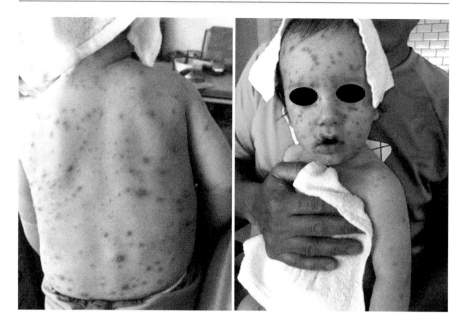

Figs. 11.1 and 11.2 Young child with varicella lesions in different stages. (Courtesy of Michaela Cribb)

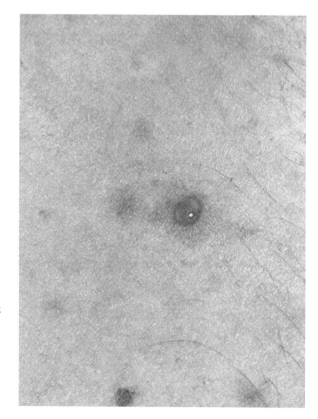

Fig. 11.3 Classic "dew drop on a rose petal" appearance of a chicken pox blister. (By F malan (Own work) [CC BY-SA 3.0 (https://creativecommons. org/licenses/by-sa/3.0) or GFDL. (http://www.gnu. org/copyleft/fdl.html)], via Wikimedia Commons)

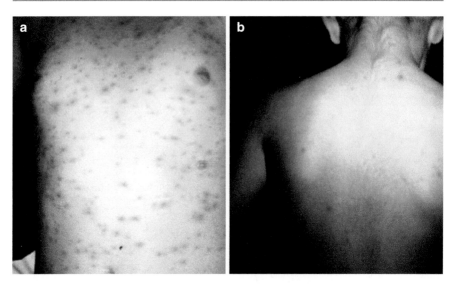

Fig. 11.4 Classic varicella vs. attenuated in an immunized child. (Used with permission from Wutzler et al. [15])

Fig. 11.5 Mucosal involvement with chicken pox. (Courtesy of CDC Public Health Figure Library [Public Domain])

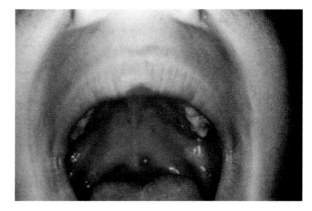

of skin lesions, typically lasting 2–3 days but often over a week. Pain may be constant or intermittent and sometimes occurs only when the affected area is touched. Pain quality differs for each patient but is often described as tingling, burning, stabbing, shooting, or throbbing. Prior to the appearance of the rash, it is not uncommon for the patient to undergo workup for other etiologies of discomfort [14, 16].

A transient erythematous macular phase to the skin rash is often unnoticed, followed by rapid appearance of grouped clusters of papules, which develop into vesicles within 1–2 days (Fig. 11.6). Lesions in various stages (papules, vesicles, crusts) may be present all at once. In an immunocompetent patient, usually only a single dermatome is affected, and the rash does not cross the midline, although sometimes 2–3 adjacent unilateral dermatomes may be affected. New vesicles

Fig. 11.6 Shingles on day 1. (Courtesy: Public domain via Wikimedia Commons)

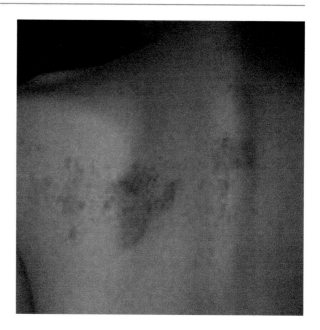

Fig. 11.7 Day 3 – shingles with lesions in various stages; affecting one dermatome; may vary from mild to extensive disease. (By melvil (Own work) [CC BY-SA 4.0 (https:// creativecommons.org/ licenses/by-sa/4.0)], via Wikimedia Commons)

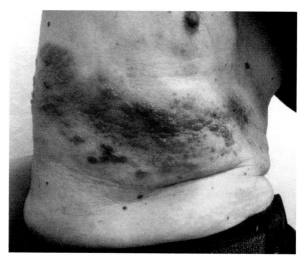

continue to appear for 3–4 days and then often become pustules 1 week after rash onset, followed in 3–5 days by ulceration and crusting (Fig. 11.7). Similar to varicella, lesions are contagious until crusted over. The rash may continue to be painful or may be itchy. Mucous membrane lesions usually do not form vesicles and crusts but instead are shallow erythematous ulcers that may go entirely unnoticed [14]. Crusts usually resolve in 3–4 weeks, but scarring and hypo- or hyperpigmentation may persist for months to years [2, 11, 14, 16].

Atypical Presentation

Varicella (Chicken Pox)

It is rare to have asymptomatic cases of primary varicella. However, breakthrough varicella in vaccinated individuals, defined as wild-type disease occurring >42 days after vaccination, often presents as a milder form of the disease with <50 lesions and no systemic symptoms, although 25–30% of cases are *not* milder than classic disease (Fig. 11.4). The rash may be mainly maculopapular rather than vesicular. The disease is of shorter duration, but the patient is still contagious [2, 4]. Neonates born to mothers with onset of varicella rash from 5 days before to 2 days after birth (due to lack of maternal antibody formation and passage to the neonate prior to birth), or to mothers with active varicella and no evidence of prior immunity, are at high risk for more severe, disseminated disease. The usual interval from mother's rash to onset in the neonate is 9–15 days [2, 4]. Rarely, varicella may be bullous, hemorrhagic, or gangrenous in appearance (Fig. 11.8).

Herpes Zoster (Shingles)

Zoster sine herpete is an atypical presentation with dermatomal pain but no rash. Diagnosis is difficult, and there are few reported cases, possibly due to underdiagnosis [11]. *Bilateral zoster is another uncommon atypical presentation, occurring either as two widely separated affected bilateral dermatomes, or in a belt-like distribution crossing midline* [11]. VZV reactivation from the trigeminal ganglion into the central nervous system can cause a focal encephalitis that mimics low-grade glioma on imaging [11]. Zoster may present with atypical appearance of lesions such as clusters, erosions and hemorrhagic appearance (Figs. 11.9, 11.10, and 11.11).

Associated Systemic Symptoms

Varicella (Chicken Pox)

Malaise, fever, abdominal pain, pharyngitis, and headache prior to the onset of the typical rash are particularly common in adolescents and adults. Children usually develop the rash first, but then may also have mild systemic symptoms, and often have fever for 2–3 days [2, 4].

Herpes Zoster (Shingles)

Associated systemic symptoms, such as fever, headache, malaise, photophobia, or fatigue, are less common than with primary varicella and are seen in fewer than 20% of zoster patients [14, 16].

Fig. 11.8 Bullous
varicella. (Courtesy of
Stanley Inkelis, MD)

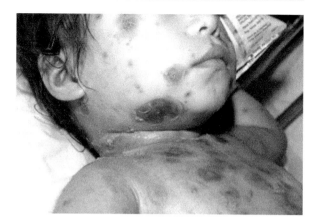

Time Course of Disease

Varicella (Chicken Pox)

Patients are contagious from 1 to 2 days before the onset of the rash until all lesions have crusted, usually 5–7 days after onset. After exposure, the incubation period is typically 14–16 days, with a range of 10–21 days, and can be shorter in immunocompromised patients [2, 4]. A nonspecific prodrome may occur 1–2 days before the onset of the rash, or rash may be the first presenting symptom. Successive crops [2–4] of lesions break out over the next 5 days or so, with each crop progressing from macule to papule to vesicle over 24–48 h. Lesions then crust over and fall off in the next 1–2 weeks [1, 2, 4].

Herpes Zoster (Shingles)

Zoster occurs at any time from reactivation of latent VZV virus in a nerve ganglion, often years after the original varicella infection or vaccination. Pain may precede rash development by a few days to a week [14]. Once the rash begins, papules develop into vesicles over 1–2 days, and new lesions appear for 3–4 days, followed by pustule formation, ulceration, and crusting. Resolution of crusts occurs in 3–4 weeks in uncomplicated zoster [14].

Common Mimics and Differential Diagnosis

There are a number of rashes and infectious diseases that can mimic varicella (Table 11.1). The natural distribution and the classic appearance of varicella lesions, along with the patient's exposure history and vaccine status, aid in differentiating varicella from other conditions (Figs. 11.12, 11.13, 11.14, and 11.15).

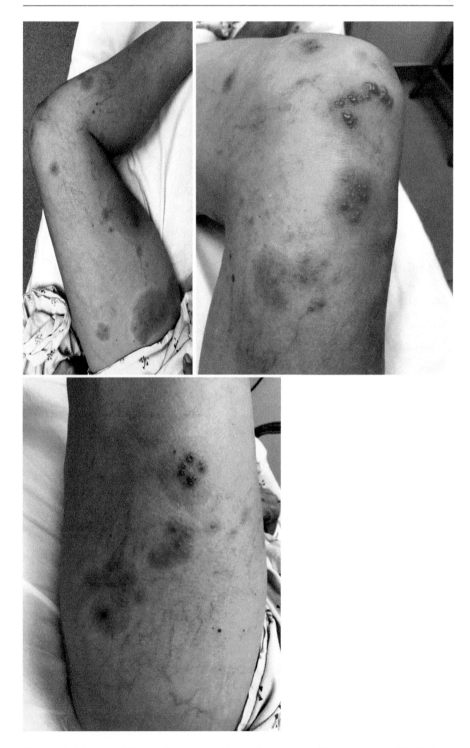

Figs. 11.9, 11.10, and 11.11 Clustered and hemorrhagic zoster. (Photo courtesy of Emily Rose MD)

Table 11.1 Differential diagnosis of varicella and zoster [17, 18]

Condition	Differentiating features
Disseminated herpes simplex virus	Immunocompromised patient or neonate; hemorrhagic vesicles, crusts, erosions, and ulcers, not in crops
Eczema herpeticum (Fig. 11.15)	Patient has h/o eczema, crops of vesicles rapidly progress to hemorrhagic vesicles, and crusted lesions are localized to areas of eczema
Smallpox (Fig. 11.12)	Distribution more on face and extremities vs varicella face and trunk, palms and soles affected, slower progression from macule to crust, lesions all in the same stage, lesions often umbilicated
Coxsackie virus	Lesions often localized to the mouth, hands, feet, and buttocks, although Coxsackie A6 may be more widespread; lesions not in crops and do not crust
Poxviruses	Exposure to infected animal, lesions all in the same stage, and often umbilicated similar to smallpox
Molluscum (Fig. 11.13)	Localized, not widespread lesions, small umbilicated papules, not vesicles or crusts, not in crops, no associated fever, not dermatomal
Stevens-Johnson syndrome	Purpura and blisters; sloughing of the skin; oral mucosa always involved; palms and soles may be involved; positive Nikolsky sign
Bullous impetigo	Vesicles progress to large bullae that rupture and erode, not in crops, localized often on extremities or trunk, not dermatomal
Bullous flea bite reaction	Localized but not dermatomal, body parts exposed to insects (often legs)
Scabies (Fig. 11.14)	Burrows instead of vesicles, favors finger and toe webs, belt line, intertriginous folds, affected close contacts, no associated fever
Viral exanthem	No progression to vesicles (early varicella prior to vesicle formation may be mistaken for nonspecific viral exanthema)
Guttate psoriasis	Scaly papules, do not progress to vesicles or crusts, no associated fever, not in crops or different stages
Incontinentia pigmenti	Neonate with early vesicular stage may be confused for varicella, linear vesicles, and plaques following Blaschko's lines
Poison ivy/oak	Linear vesicles may be mistaken for zoster; history of exposure to poison ivy/oak; itchiness more prominent than pain

Key Physical Exam Findings and Diagnostic Features

Varicella and zoster are primarily clinical diagnoses, made based on classic presentation and physical exam features (Table 11.2).

Diagnosis

Diagnosis of varicella and zoster is usually clinical based on classic presentation and findings. Confirmation of the diagnosis in atypical or uncertain cases, in particular with breakthrough varicella, is typically done by polymerase chain reaction (PCR) testing of the contents of a skin vesicle or swab of a crust. Direct fluorescent antibody (DFA) testing and Tzanck smear of vesicle contents can also be used but are less sensitive. Serology can be used to verify previous exposure and presence of protective antibodies, and acute and convalescent IgG titers may be used to verify acute disease (IgM is unreliable if negative but indicates acute disease if detected) [2, 9].

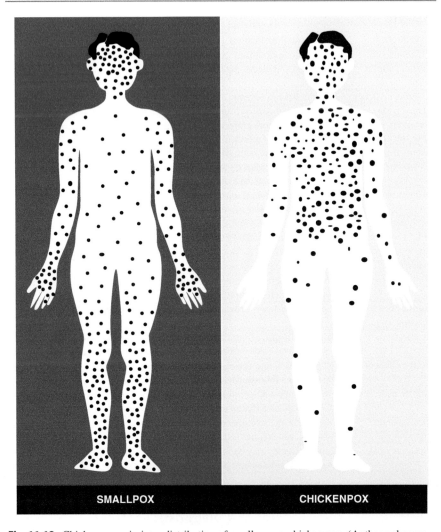

Fig. 11.12 Chicken pox mimics – distribution of smallpox vs. chicken pox. (Author unknown [public domain], via Wikimedia Commons)

Fig. 11.13 Molluscum contagiosum – chicken pox look-alike. (By Dave Bray, MD, Walter Reed Army Medical Center [public domain], via Wikimedia Commons)

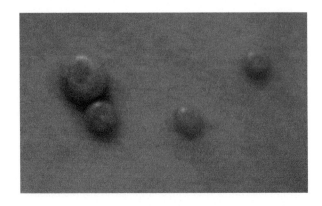

Fig. 11.14 Scabies mimicking chicken pox. (Courtesy: Stanley Inkelis, MD)

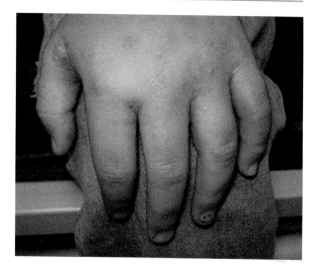

Fig. 11.15 Eczema herpeticum: varicella look-alike. (Created by Samuel Freire da Silva, M.D. in homage to The Master And Professor Delso Bringel Calheiros. Figure obtained from Dermatology Atlas http://www.atlasdermatologico.com.br/disease.jsf?diseaseId=117)

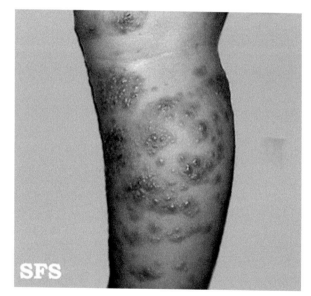

Management

Varicella (Chicken Pox)

Varicella in immunocompetent, healthy children, including infants outside the neo-natal age range is self-limited. Symptomatic care with antipyretics for fever is indi-cated. Acetaminophen is the antipyretic of choice, as aspirin should not be given due to the risk of Reye's syndrome, and NSAIDs may increase the risk of associated bacterial necrotizing skin and soft tissue infection. Pruritus can be managed with topical antipruritic lotions, colloidal oatmeal baths, cool wet compresses, and oral

Table 11.2 Varicella and zoster key diagnostic features [1, 2, 4, 9, 14, 17]

Rash	Location/ distribution	Lesions	Associated symptoms (may precede rash)	Epidemiology
Varicella (chicken pox)	Starts on the face/ scalp, spreads to trunk and then extremities, spares palms and soles, may have mucosal lesions	Crops of lesions progress from papules to vesicles to crusts; lesions in different stages; "dewdrop on a rose petal" appearance	Fever, malaise, pruritus	Most common in children aged 1–9 years; peak in winter to early spring
Zoster (shingles)	Unilateral dermatomal distribution, often on the trunk	Grouped papules rapidly progress to vesicles and then crusts	Pain	Most common in ≥50 years old; no seasonal variation

Table 11.3 Medications for varicella and zoster [2, 14, 17]

Medication	Dose
Acyclovir oral for varicella or zoster	For ≥2 years old: ≤ 40 kg, 80 mg/kg/day in 4 divided doses × 5 days (maximum 3200 mg/day); > 40 kg, 800 mg QID × 5–7 days
Acyclovir IV for varicella or zoster	10 mg/kg or 500 mg/m² TID × 7–10 days
Valacyclovir oral for varicella or zoster	For ≥2 years old: 20 mg/kg TID × 5 days (maximum 1 gm/dose)
Famciclovir oral for zoster in adults	500 mg PO TID × 7 days
VariZIG for varicella postexposure prophylaxis	62.5 units (1/2 vial) IM for ≤2 kg, 125 units (1 vial) IM for 2.1–10 kg, 250 units (2 vials) IM for 10.1–20 kg, 375 units (3 vials) IM for 20.1–30 kg, 500 units (4 vials) IM for 30.1–40 kg, 625 units (5 vials) IM for >40 kg
IVIG for varicella postexposure prophylaxis	400 mg/kg IV once

antihistamines. Children's nails should be cut short to prevent excoriation which may increase scarring and/or result in bacterial superinfection [1, 17]. Oral mucosal lesions may result in decreased oral intake and dehydration; patients may benefit from analgesia and may require IV rehydration. Patients with active varicella are highly contagious and must be kept in airborne precautions/respiratory isolation.

Moderate-risk patients including unvaccinated patients >12 years old, those on chronic salicylate therapy or any steroid therapy (including short courses and inhaled or nebulized), and those with chronic dermatologic or pulmonary disorders should receive oral acyclovir or valacyclovir, particularly if medication can be started within 24 h of rash onset (Table 11.3) [2, 17]. However, medication is unlikely to be beneficial in immunocompetent individuals beyond 72 h after rash onset. High-risk patients such as immunocompromised patients (including those on high-dose corticosteroid therapy), pregnant women, and neonates should receive IV acyclovir and be admitted to an inpatient room with respiratory isolation capabilities (Table 11.3) [2, 9, 17].

Postexposure prophylaxis with VariZIG varicella-specific immune globulin should be provided within 10 days of significant varicella exposure for high-risk unvaccinated patients without evidence of prior immunity: immunocompromised, pregnant women, neonates with maternal onset of varicella from 5 days before to 2 days after birth, hospitalized preterm infants <28 weeks gestation or > 28 weeks gestation, and no maternal varicella immunity (Table 11.3). Some experts also recommend any neonate with varicella up to age 2 weeks born to a mother without evidence of immunity receive VariZIG [2]. If VariZIG is unavailable, IVIG may be used. If neither VariZIG nor IVIG are available or for unvaccinated exposed patients unable to be vaccinated, oral acyclovir or valacyclovir 7-day course may be given [2]. Healthy immunocompetent unvaccinated exposed patients should receive their first dose of varicella vaccine, preferably within 3 days of exposure but up to 5 days after exposure, with a follow-up second dose at the appropriate interval [2].

Herpes Zoster (Shingles)

Oral antiviral medications (acyclovir, valacyclovir, or famciclovir) are indicated for immunocompromised patients, patients with moderate to severe disease or non-trunk involvement, and those ≥50 years old, preferably within 72 h of rash onset (Table 11.3) [11, 14]. Immunocompromised patients should be treated with IV acyclovir. Symptomatic treatment with analgesics to manage pain is usually needed, and opiates may be required to provide adequate pain control. Patients with active lesions are contagious and should be appropriately maintained in contact isolation with lesions covered.

Complications

Varicella (Chicken Pox)

Varicella in the healthy immunocompetent host is usually a mild self-limited disease; however complications can occur (Table 11.4). Groups at increased risk for severe disease and complications include neonates and infants <1 year old, adolescents, adults, immunocompromised patients (HIV/AIDS, leukemia, and other malignancies, immunosuppressive therapies including corticosteroids, transplant recipients), and pregnant women [1, 2, 4, 9]. The most common complications of primary varicella include bacterial skin superinfections, pneumonia, and cerebellar ataxia (Fig. 11.16). Varicella has historically been the most common etiology of

Table 11.4 Complications of varicella and zoster [1, 2, 4, 9, 11, 14, 16]

System / Location	Complications
Varicella	
Cutaneous	Bacterial superinfection of skin: group A streptococcal infection may lead to necrotizing infection (Fig. 11.16), toxic shock, death
	Hemorrhagic varicella more common in immunocompromised
	Eczema herpeticum in patient with history of eczema (even if no active eczema at the time of varicella infection)
	Post-inflammatory hypo- and hyperpigmentation and scarring
Pulmonary	Pneumonia (1 per 400 cases), more common in <1 year old
Central nervous system	Cerebellar ataxia (1 per 4000 cases), aseptic meningitis, encephalitis (1.8 per 10,000 cases), stroke, rare Guillain-Barre syndrome, transverse myelitis
Ophthalmic	Eczema herpeticum and lesions near the eye can cause vision-threatening keratitis
Gastrointestinal	Mild hepatitis and elevated liver function tests common
	Pancreatitis rare
Hematologic	Mild neutropenia and thrombocytopenia can occur 1–2 weeks after initial infection
	Rare purpura fulminans, disseminated intravascular coagulation, Henoch-Schönlein purpura
Congenital varicella	Risk 0.4–2% in fetuses exposed between 8 and 20 weeks gestation (rare cases at exposure up to 28 weeks gestation): limb hypoplasia, skin scarring, chorioretinitis and cataracts, central nervous system abnormalities
Multiple	Reye's syndrome: associated with salicylate use, encephalopathy and hepatitis, high fatality rate
Rare other organ systems	Uveitis, iritis, arthritis, orchitis, nephritis
Zoster	
Pain	Postherpetic neuralgia: neuropathic pain lasting longer 30 days
Cutaneous	Bacterial superinfection; scarring
Central nervous system	Aseptic meningitis, encephalitis, stroke, transverse myelitis, sensorineural hearing loss, delayed contralateral hemiparesis, cranial and peripheral motor neuropathies
Ophthalmic	Keratitis with potential vision loss. Retinitis, rapidly progressive herpetic retinal necrosis (RPHRN)
Ramsay-Hunt syndrome (geniculate ganglion zoster)	Peripheral facial nerve palsy, vesicles in ear canal or in the mouth, tinnitus, vertigo, nystagmus, hearing loss, nausea and vomiting, unilateral loss of taste to anterior 2/3 of the tongue
Bell's palsy	Cranial nerve VII involvement, Ramsay-Hunt without the rash, may be difficult to distinguish from other causes of Bell's palsy
Sacral zoster	S2–S4 dermatomes, associated with urinary retention/ neurogenic bladder

Fig. 11.16 Varicella
pneumonia. (Courtesy:
CDC/Joel D. Meyers, M.D.
[Public domain] CDC
Public Health Figure
Library)

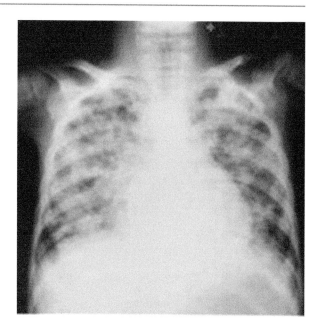

acute cerebellar ataxia in children and has been a common culprit in inducing arte-
riopathies associated with pediatric stroke. Decreased oral intake due to painful
mouth lesions can lead to dehydration.

Zoster (Shingles)

Postherpetic neuralgia (PHN) is one of the most feared complications of zoster,
occurring in 8–70% of patients [16]. PHN increases with increasing age and can
severely impact quality of life. Treatments include analgesics, gabapentin, lidocaine
patches, pregabalin, and nortriptyline. Postherpetic itch can also persist after rash
healing [14]. Zoster occurring around the eye may cause vision-threatening keratitis, anterior uveitis, iritis, and other ophthalmologic complications; urgent consultation with an ophthalmologist is indicated. Vesicles on the side or tip of the nose
("Hutchinson's sign") are associated with zoster ophthalmicus as the nasociliary
branch of the trigeminal nerve innervates both these parts of the nose and the globe.
Ocular fluorescein staining to evaluate for herpetic dendrites as well as ophthalmology follow-up is indicated in every case of zoster occurring near the eye or involving the nasociliary branch of the trigeminal nerve. Other central and peripheral
nervous system complications often depend on the location of the nerve ganglion
with reactivated virus (Table 11.4) (Fig. 11.17).

Fig. 11.17 Varicella necrotizing fasciitis. (Courtesy: Stanley Inkelis, M.D.)

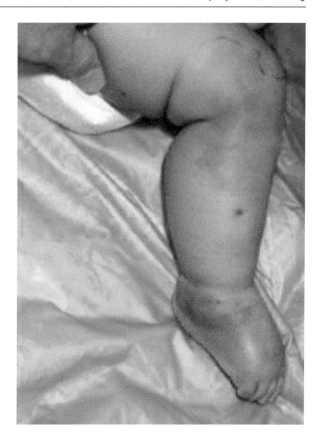

Bottom Line: Clinical Pearls

Varicella (Chicken Pox)

Primary varicella is much less commonly seen since routine immunization began in 1996, and clinicians are more likely to see breakthrough varicella, a milder manifestation with <50 lesions. High clinical suspicion must be maintained when seeing a patient with successive crops of pruritic lesions (papules, vesicles, and crusts) in different stages all at once. Neonates, adolescents and adults, pregnant women, and immunocompromised patients are at high risk and should be treated with antiviral medication. Beware of common complications such as dehydration, bacterial skin superinfections, pneumonia, and central nervous system complications. Varicella is highly contagious, and patients should be isolated as soon as the diagnosis is suspected.

Zoster (Shingles)
Zoster is reactivation of VZV in a nerve ganglion of a patient that has had wild-type varicella or varicella vaccine in the past. It is much more common in patients ≥50 years old. Grouped papules, vesicles, and crusts occur in a dermatomal distribution, typically on the trunk. Pain is a hallmark symptom and may precede the rash. Moderate-high-risk patients should be treated with antivirals, and all patients need analgesics.

References

1. Heininger U, Seward JF. Varicella. Lancet. 2006;368:1365–76.
2. American Academy of Pediatrics. Varicella-Zoster virus infections. In: Kimberlin DW, Brady MT, Jackson MA, Long SS, editors. Red Book®: 2015 report of the committee on infectious diseases: American Academy of Pediatrics. Elk Grove Village, IL. 2015. p. 846–60.
3. Gilden DH, Kleinschmidt-DeMasters BK, LaGuardia JJ, Mahalingam R, Cohrs RJ. Neurologic complications of the reactivation of varicella-zoster virus. N Engl J Med. 2000;342:635–45.
4. Centers for Disease Control and Prevention. Epidemiology and prevention of vaccine-preventable diseases. In: Hamborsky J, Kroger A, Wolfe S, editors. Chapter 22 Varicella. 13th ed. Washington, DC: Public Health Foundation; 2015, accessed on line at URL https://www.cdc.gov/vaccines/pubs/pinkbook/varicella.html on 7/25/2017.
5. Hambleton S, Gershon AA. Preventing varicella-zoster disease. Clin Microbiol Rev. 2005;18(1):70–80.
6. Lopez AS, Zhang J, Marin M. Epidemiology of varicella during the 2-dose varicella vaccination program – United States 2005–2014. MMWR Morb Mortal Wkly Rep. 2016;65(34):902–5.
7. American Academy of Pediatrics Committee on Infectious Diseases. Prevention of varicella: recommendations for use of varicella vaccines in children, including a recommendation for a routine 2-dose varicella immunization schedule. Pediatrics. 2007;120:221–31.
8. Reagan-Steiner S, Yankey D, Jeyarajah J, Elam-Evans LD, Curtis CR, MacNeil J, Markowitz LE, Singleton JA. National, regional, state, and selected local area vaccination coverage among adolescents aged 13–17 years – United States, 2015. MMWR Morb Mortal Wkly Rep. 2016;65(33):850–8.
9. Gershon AA, Breuer J, Cohen JI, Cohrs RJ, Gershon MD, Gilden D, Grose C, Hambleton S, Kennedy PG, Oxman MN, Seward JF, Yamanishi K. Varicella zoster virus infection. Nat Rev Dis Primers. 2015;1:15016.
10. Nguyen HQ, Jumaan AO, Seward JF. Decline in mortality due to varicella after implementation of varicella vaccination in the United States. N Engl J Med. 2005;352(5):450–8.
11. Dayan RR, Peleg R. Herpes zoster – typical and atypical presentations. Postgrad Med. 2017;129(6):567–71.
12. Dommasch ED, Joyce CJ, Mostaghimi A. Trends in nationwide herpes zoster emergency department utilization from 2006 to 2013. JAMA Dermatol. 2017;153(9):874–81.
13. Williams WW, Lu PJ, O'Halloran A, Kim DK, Grohskopf LA, Pilishvili T, Skoff TH, Nelson NP, Harpaz R, Markowitz LE, Rodriguez-Lainz A, Fiebelkorn AP. Surveillance of vaccination coverage among adult populations – United States, 2015. MMWR Surveill Summ. 2017;66(11):1–28.

14. Dworkin RH, Johnson RW, Breuer J, Gnann JW, Levin MJ, Backonja M, Betts RF, et al. Recommendations for the management of herpes zoster. Clin Infect Dis. 2007;44(Suppl 1):S1–26.
15. Wutzler P, Knuf M, Liese J. Varicella: efficacy of two-dose vaccination in childhood. Dtsch Arztebl Int. 2008;105(33):567–72.
16. Gnann JW Jr, Whitley RJ. Clinical practice. Herpes zoster. N Engl J Med. 2002;347:340–6.
17. Habif TP. Clinical dermatology: a color guide to diagnosis and therapy. St. Louis, Missouri. 6th ed: Elsevier Inc; 2016.
18. Goldsmith LA, editor. VisualDx. Rochester: VisualDx; 2016. URL: https://www.visualdx.com/visualdx/7/

Omphalitis

12

Ghazala Q. Sharieff

Background

Omphalitis is an acute infection of the umbilical stump and has an overall incidence ranging from 0.2 to 0.7% in industrialized countries [1] and up to 21% of live births in developing countries.

Although omphalitis typically presents as a superficial cellulitis, it can potentially involve the entire abdominal wall and lead to severe systemic illness with associated myonecrosis or necrotizing fasciitis. Omphalitis may extend into the portal vein resulting in portal vein thrombosis, liver abscess, or septic emboli. While it is known to be a disease of the newborn, cases have been reported into the adult years. In full-term infants, the mean age at onset is 5–9 days of life, whereas in preterm infants, the mean age at onset is 3–5 days of life [2].

The umbilical cord becomes ischemic as the umbilical stump dries and falls off. Particularly with dry cord care, local inflammation and irritation may normally occur (see Figs. 12.1 and 12.2). Bacteria have the potential to invade the umbilical stump, leading to omphalitis. The infection can spread along the umbilical artery, umbilical veins, abdominal wall lymphatics, and blood vessels and contiguously to the surrounding areas resulting in a potentially life-threatening infection.

Common Mimics and Differential Diagnosis

The differential diagnoses of omphalitis include the following conditions and associated findings:

G. Q. Sharieff
University of California, San Diego, CA, USA

Scripps Health, San Diego, CA, USA

Fig. 12.1 Local skin irritation from a hard, dry cord rubbing when constricted by clothing. This erythema resolved after removing the constriction. Additionally, the erythema is removed from the base of the cord which is reassuring that the erythema is not secondary to omphalitis. (Photo used with permission from Janelle Aby, MD)

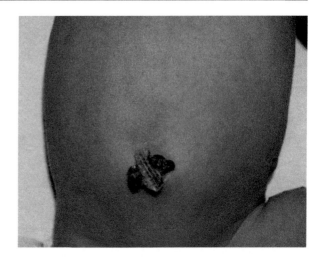

Fig. 12.2 Periumbilical erythema in an infant with dry cord care who did not have omphalitis. This rim of erythema is theorized to be secondary to normal WBC infiltration that occurs with cord separation. This erythema should be monitored for signs of progression to omphalitis and reassessed after removing the diaper and constrictive clothing. (Photo used with permission from Janelle Aby, MD)

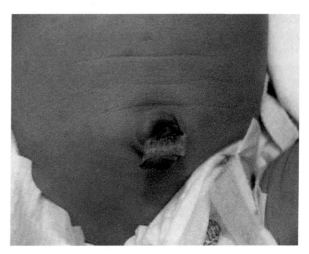

- Normal periumbilical skin irritation (see Figs. 12.1 and 12.2).
- Umbilical granuloma
- Patent vitellointestinal duct remnants, which present as cystic swelling or fistulous opening with feculent discharge matter
- Patent urachus, which is a fistulous opening with urinary drainage
- Necrotizing enterocolitis (which presents typically with abdominal distention, bilious vomiting, bloody stools, and fever)

Key Physical Examination and History Findings

As with any history in newborns, the following should be obtained as they may be of assistance in the diagnosis:

1. Was the delivery complicated by premature or prolonged rupture of the membranes or amnionitis? These incidents can lead to anaerobic infection particularly with *B. fragilis*.
2. Is there any discharge, tenderness, or erythema around the umbilicus?
3. How is the newborn feeding?
4. Is there a fever?
5. If there is erythema on the abdominal wall, how rapidly has it progressed? *Erythema extending from the umbilicus to the abdominal wall is a key feature distinguishing omphalitis from more benign conditions.* Progressive extension of erythema is a diagnostic feature of omphalitis.

Signs of sepsis or other systemic disease are nonspecific and include the following:

- Fever (temperature > 38 °C), hypothermia (temperature < 36 °C), or temperature instability.
- Tachycardia (pulse >180 beats per minute [bpm]), hypotension (systolic blood pressure < 60 mm Hg in full-term infants), or delayed capillary refill (<2–3 s)
- Hypoxia, apnea, tachypnea (respirations >60/min), nasal flaring, grunting, or intercostal or subcostal retractions
- Poor feeding, vomiting, distended abdomen, or absent bowel sounds
- Jaundice, petechiae, or cyanosis
- Irritability, lethargy, weak suck reflex, hypotonia, or hypertonia

Causes

Omphalitis may be a polymicrobial infection typically caused by a mixture of aerobic and anaerobic organisms. *Staphylococcus aureus*, group A streptococcus, *Escherichia coli*, *Klebsiella pneumoniae*, and *Proteus mirabilis* are the most commonly implicated organisms [3]. *Pseudomonas* species have been implicated in rapidly spreading and invasive disease. *Bacteroides fragilis*, *Clostridium perfringens*, and *Peptostreptococcus* are the most common anaerobic causative agents resulting in up to one third of cases. The prognosis of newborns with uncomplicated omphalitis associated with cellulitis of the anterior abdominal wall is favorable. However, in a study by Sawin et al. [4], the mortality rate among all infants with omphalitis, including those who develop complications, was estimated to range between 7% and 15%. The mortality rate is significantly higher (38–87%) after the development of necrotizing fasciitis or myonecrosis.

Associated risk factors include the following:

- Low birth weight (<2500 g)
- Prior umbilical catheterization
- Septic delivery (as suggested by premature rupture of membranes, nonsterile delivery, or maternal infection)
- Prolonged rupture of membranes

Omphalitis occasionally manifests from an underlying immunologic disorder. Leukocyte adhesion deficiency (LAD) [5–7] is a rare immunologic disorder with an autosomal recessive pattern of inheritance. These infants typically present with leukocytosis, a history of recurrent infections, and delayed separation of the umbilical cord:

Omphalitis may also be the initial manifestation of neonatal alloimmune or congenital neutropenia in the neonate [8]. Neonatal alloimmune neutropenia is a disease similar to Rh hemolytic disease and is to maternal sensitization to fetal neutrophils with antigens that are different than the mother's. Maternal immunoglobulin G antibodies cross the placenta and result in an immune-mediated neutropenia that can be severe and lasts up to 6 months. Affected infants also may present with other skin infections, meningitis, pneumonia, or sepsis.

In rare cases, an anatomic abnormality such as a patent urachus, patent omphalomesenteric duct, or urachal cyst may be present [9, 10].

Management

The initial management includes performing a sepsis evaluation of the neonate which can include a complete blood count, blood culture, C-reactive protein, urinalysis and culture, wound culture if there is associated drainage, and a lumbar puncture. All patients with omphalitis should be admitted for antimicrobial therapy and possible surgical debridement in complex cases. Blood products (e.g., packed RBCs, platelets, fresh frozen plasma) and other medications (e.g., inotropic agents, sodium bicarbonate) may be required for supportive care. Ultrasound, CT, or MRI can help delineate the extent of tissue plane involvement. However, if the infant is critically ill, these studies should not delay surgical intervention. Surgical consultation is warranted in ill-appearing infants, infants with rapid spreading of erythema, or those with portal venous or intramural bowel gas. Of note, these patients can initially appear quite benign with some minimal periumbilical abdominal wall erythema and rapidly progress to being critically ill (see Figs. 12.3 and 12.4). Early and complete surgical debridement of the affected tissue and muscle is important to avoid disease progression.

The role of hyperbaric oxygen in treatment of patients with anaerobic necrotizing fasciitis and myonecrosis is controversial because no prospective controlled data are available, and therefore surgical consultation for critically ill infants is the priority.

Antimicrobial Therapy

Parenteral antibiotics are indicated to target both gram-positive and gram-negative organisms. A combination of an antistaphylococcal penicillin, vancomycin, and an aminoglycoside antibiotic is recommended. Omphalitis complicated by necrotizing fasciitis or myonecrosis should include an antimicrobial regimen which targets

Fig. 12.3 Image of an infant with omphalitis who died several days after admission. (Photo courtesy of Nobuaki Inoue, MD, MPH)

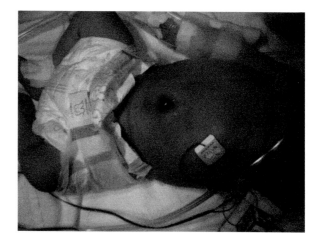

Fig. 12.4 An infant with omphalitis demonstrating rapid progression of erythema. The inner circle was marked <12 h after onset of erythema. The second marking was several hours after the first. (Photo by JoDee Anderson, MD. Used with permission from https://med.stanford. edu/newborns/professional-education/photo-gallery/ umbilical-cord. html#omphalitis)

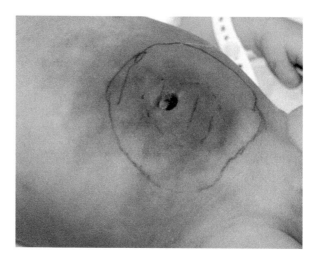

anaerobic organisms in addition to gram-positive and gram-negative organisms. Metronidazole or clindamycin is commonly used. However, local antibiotic susceptibility patterns should be taken into account when choosing an effective antibiotic regimen.

Antibiotics

Gentamicin

Aminoglycoside antibiotic for gram-negative coverage. Used in combination both with an agent against gram-positive organisms and with an agent that covers anaerobes. The dose is 5 mg/kg IV/IO daily.

Clindamycin

A lincosamide class antibiotic used for treatment of serious skin and soft tissue staphylococcal infections and infections caused by anaerobic bacteria. This antibiotic inhibits bacterial protein synthesis and decreases toxin production in necrotizing infections. Also effective against aerobic and anaerobic streptococci (except enterococci). The dose is 20–40 mg/kg/day IV divided q6–8 h.

Metronidazole IV

Anaerobic antibiotic that also has amebicide and antiprotozoal actions. The dose is 1.5 mg/kg/dose IV/IO, every 12 h.

Ampicillin

Broad-spectrum penicillin. Interferes with bacterial cell wall synthesis during active replication, causing bactericidal activity against susceptible organisms. Bactericidal for organisms, such as GBS, *Listeria*, non-penicillinase-producing staphylococci, some strains of *Haemophilus influenzae*, and meningococci. The dose is 50 mg/kg/dose IV/IO, every 6 h.

Vancomycin

Bactericidal agent against most aerobic and anaerobic gram-positive cocci and bacilli. Especially important in the treatment of MRSA. Recommended therapy when coagulase-negative staphylococcal sepsis is suspected. The first dose is 15–20 mg/kg IV.

Complications

Complications of omphalitis include sepsis; necrotizing fasciitis; myonecrosis; septic embolization, particularly endocarditis and liver abscess formation; and abdominal complications such as spontaneous evisceration, peritonitis, bowel obstruction, abdominal or retroperitoneal abscess, and death [11–15].

Sepsis is the most common complication of omphalitis and occurs in 13% of infants with omphalitis. Disseminated intravascular coagulation (DIC) and multiple organ failure may ensue.

Necrotizing fasciitis may be present in 8–16% of cases of neonatal omphalitis and is associated with a rapid spread of infection involving the abdominal wall involvement which may extend to the perineum. Causative agents include group A *Streptococcus*, *S. aureus*, and *Clostridium* species.

Myonecrosis may occur in the presence of necrotic tissue, poor blood supply, foreign material, and established infection by aerobic bacteria such as staphylococci or streptococci.

Septic embolization arises from infected umbilical vessels; it may lead to metastatic foci in various organs, including the heart, liver, lungs, pancreas, kidneys, and skin.

Long-term complications of omphalitis include nonneoplastic cavernous transformation of the portal vein, portal vein thrombosis, extrahepatic portal hypertension, and biliary obstruction.

Prevention

Recent post delivery trends have moved to dry cord care, without routine application of topical antiseptic agents. This recommendation has been adopted by the American Academy of Pediatrics (AAP) and the World Health Organization (WHO). However, dry cord care may not be appropriate in all environments particularly if the delivery occurs in a non-hygienic area. The WHO recommends topical application of chlorhexidine to the umbilical cord stump during the first week of life for neonates born at home in high neonatal mortality settings (i.e., those with at least 30 neonatal deaths per 1000 live births) [15]. Meta-analysis of topical application of chlorhexidine to the umbilical cord of children born in underdeveloped countries under non-hygienic conditions revealed that this intervention significantly reduced the incidence of omphalitis, as well as overall neonatal mortality. Furthermore, a Cochrane review of 12 trials revealed that there was high-quality evidence that chlorhexidine skin or cord care in the community setting led to a 50% reduction in the incidence of omphalitis and a 12% reduction in neonatal mortality [16]. There was no difference noted for neonatal mortality or the risk of infections in the hospital setting for the utilization of maternal vaginal chlorhexidine washes when compared to customary care.

> **Bottom Line: Clinical Pearls**
> Umbilical inflammation with erythema extending to the abdominal wall should be presumed to be omphalitis and monitored for progression. All patients with suspected omphalitis should be admitted for further observation despite how benign their initial appearance may be. These patients can suddenly deteriorate, hence the need for close observation and intravenous antibiotic administration. Surgical intervention may be required.

Acknowledgment The author would like to thank Aleena Shad, research assistant, for her help with this chapter.

References

1. Gallagher PG, Shah SS. Omphalitis: overview Available at http://emedicine.medscape.com/article/975422-overview. 2008.
2. Ameh EA, Nmadu PT. Major complications of omphalitis in neonates and infants. Pediatr Surg Int. 2002;18:413–6.
3. Brook I. Microbiology of necrotizing fasciitis associated with omphalitis in the newborn infant. J Perinatol. 1998;18(1):28–30.
4. Sawin RS, Schaller RT, Tapper D, et al. Early recognition of neonatal abdominal wall necrotizing fasciitis. Am J Surg. 1994;167(5):481–4.
5. van Vliet DN, Brandsma AE, Hartwig NG. Leukocyte-adhesion deficiency: a rare disorder of inflammation. Ned Tijdschr Geneeskd. 2004;148(50):2496–500.
6. Alizadeh P, Rahbarimanesh AA, Bahram MG, Salmasian H. Leukocyte adhesion deficiency type 1 presenting as leukemoid reaction. Indian J Pediatr. 2007;74(12):1121–3.
7. Parvaneh N, Mamishi S, Rezaei A, et al. Characterization of 11 new cases of leukocyte adhesion deficiency type 1 with seven novel mutations in the ITGB2 gene. J Clin Immunol. 2010;30(5):756–60.
8. Donadieu J, Fenneteau O, Beaupain B, Mahlaoui N, Chantelot CB. Congenital neutropenia: diagnosis, molecular bases and patient management. Orphanet J Rare Dis. 2011;6:26.
9. Razvi S, Murphy R, Shlasko E, Cunningham-Rundles C. Delayed separation of the umbilical cord attributable to urachal anomalies. Pediatrics. 2001;108(2):493–4.
10. Masuko T, Nakayama H, Aoki N, Kusafuka T, Takayama T. Staged approach to the urachal cyst with infected omphalitis. Int Surg. 2006;91(1):52–6. Weber DM, Freeman NV, Elhag KM. Periumbilical necrotizing fasciitis in the newborn. Eur J Pediatr Surg 2001. 11(2):86–91
11. Nazir Z. Necrotizing fasciitis in neonates. Pediatr Surg Int. 2005;21(8):641–4.
12. Bingol-Kologlu M, Yildiz RV, Alper B, et al. Necrotizing fasciitis in children: diagnostic and therapeutic aspects. J Pediatr Surg. 2007;42(11):1892–7.
13. Orloff MJ, Orloff MS, Girard B, Orloff SL. Bleeding esophagogastric varices from extrahepatic portal hypertension: 40 years' experience with portal-systemic shunt. J Am Coll Surg. 2002;194(6):717–28; discussion 728–30
14. Feo CF, Dessanti A, Franco B, et al. Retroperitoneal abscess and omphalitis in young infants. Acta Paediatr. 2003;92(1):122–5.
15. WHO. Guidelines on maternal, newborn, child and adolescent health: recommendations on newborn health. Available at http://www.who.int/maternal_child_adolescent/documents/guidelines-recommendations-newborn-health.pdf. Accessed: 5/2/2017.
16. Sinha A, Sazawal S, Pradhan A, Ramji S, Opiyo N. Chlorhexidine skin or cord care for prevention of mortality and infections in neonatesCochrane Database Syst Rev. 2015 3:CD007835.

Human Immunodeficiency Virus-Associated Rashes

13

Elizabeth Crow and Ilene Claudius

Introduction

Dermatology plays a critical role in the care of patients with HIV. Nearly every patient will develop at least one cutaneous manifestation of HIV during the course of his or her illness. These rashes range from isolated dermatologic conditions to severe systemic disease. An abbreviated list of the cutaneous conditions associated with HIV can be found in Table 13.1. While some of these rashes are limited to patients with HIV, many are also seen in the general population but tend to present more severely or atypically in patients with significant immunocompromise. A selection of the most common and most classic HIV-associated rashes is discussed in this chapter.

Primary HIV

Background

With 40,000–50,000 new cases per year in the past decade, it is not uncommon for primary HIV infection to present to EDs and primary care offices [1, 2]. While some patients show no symptoms of primary infection, as many as 40–90% of patients present with an acute viral illness [3]. Despite frequently presenting to the ED, the majority of primary HIV cases are not diagnosed during the acute illness. This high rate of missed

E. Crow
Los Angeles County Medical Center, Department of Emergency Medicine,
Los Angeles, CA, USA

I. Claudius (✉)
Harbor-UCLA Medical Center,
Los Angeles, CA, USA

© Springer International Publishing AG, part of Springer Nature 2018
E. Rose (ed.), *Life-Threatening Rashes*, https://doi.org/10.1007/978-3-319-75623-3_13

Table 13.1 Selection of dermatologic conditions associated with HIV

Atopic dermatitis	Ecthyma	Psoriasis
Bacillary angiomatosis	Herpes simplex infections	Reiter's syndrome
Basal cell carcinoma	Herpes zoster infections	Scrofula
Bullous impetigo	Hypersensitivity reactions	Seborrheic dermatitis
Candidal infections	Ichthyosis	Sporotrichosis
Condyloma acuminata	Kaposi sarcoma	Squamous cell carcinoma
Cryptococcosis	Molluscum contagiosum	Syphilis
Cutaneous *Aspergillus*	Oral hairy leukoplakia	Tinea infections
Disseminated histoplasmosis	Papular pruritic eruption	Xerosis
Drug reactions	Prurigo nodularis	

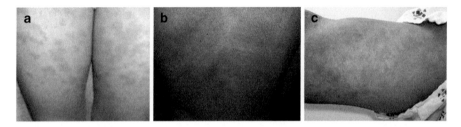

Fig. 13.1 (**a**) Primary HIV rash. (Source: Deznet.com(http://www.denznet.com/wp-content/uploads/2011/02/hiv-rash-picture-150x150.jpg)). (**b**) Primary HIV rash on the back. Used with permission from VisualDx. (**c**) Primary HIV rash on the leg. Used with permission from VisualDx

diagnoses is in part due to the vague and nonspecific nature of symptoms. While not always present, rash has been shown to be one of the more common symptoms in the syndrome of acute HIV infection [4, 5]. Evidence suggests that patients are at highest infectivity during acute infection, making recognizing primary HIV syndrome not only critical for individual patients but also of great public health importance [6].

Classic Clinical Presentation

The rash of acute HIV infection is typically a generalized, erythematous, or red maculopapular eruption most common on the neck and upper trunk. Frequently, extension of the rash can be seen on the face and extremities, including palms and soles. These flat or slightly raised lesions range from 5 to 10 mm and are generally nontender and rarely pruritic. Many patients will also develop painful, round- or oval-shaped shallow ulcers of the mucous membranes including the oral cavity, genitals, and anus [7, 8] (Fig. 13.1).

Atypical Presentation

While rare, both pustular and urticarial variants of the primary HIV rash have been described in the literature [9, 10].

Associated Systemic Symptoms

The majority of patients with symptomatic primary HIV infection will report constitutional symptoms including fever, fatigue, and myalgias. The next most common symptoms are pharyngitis and the maculopapular rash. When present, nontender adenopathy can be localized to the head, neck, and axillae or can be generalized. Gastrointestinal symptoms including nausea, vomiting, diarrhea, and anorexia are frequently noted as well. Varied neurological symptoms have been reported ranging from headache and photophobia to aseptic meningitis, encephalitis, or acute peripheral neuritis [9, 11, 12].

Time Course of Disease

Primary HIV syndrome typically presents 2–4 weeks after initial HIV exposure. Rash develops 48–72 h after illness begins and lasts 5–8 days [7]. The duration of illness varies from days to months; however, symptoms generally resolve within 7–10 days without intervention [1, 4]. Highly sensitive antigen/antibody immunoassays are used for HIV screening and will typically become positive within 2–3 weeks from exposure. This time frame allows for diagnosis during the acute viral syndrome in most, but not all cases.

Common Mimics and Differential Diagnosis

Other viral illnesses including infectious mononucleosis, rubella, roseola, and hepatitis A and B share a similar viral syndrome with primary HIV. Cases that demonstrate extension of the maculopapular rash onto the palms and soles may resemble secondary syphilis or disseminated gonococcal infection.

Key Physical Exam Findings

1. Fever.
2. Maculopapular rash typically on the neck and upper trunk.
3. Ulcerations of mucous membranes.
4. Pharyngitis.
5. Nontender adenopathy.

Management

Antiretroviral therapy (ART) involves a combination of multiple therapies targeted at different mechanisms of HIV virus proliferation and action. To ensure adequate therapy, proper ART therapy should be selected based on viral genotyping and resistance patterns. The risks and benefits of initiating ART should be weighed as noncompliance to medication for even brief periods of time can lead to significant drug resistance. Patients with significant opportunistic infections should delay initiation of ART to avoid immune reconstitution inflammatory syndrome (IRIS). Patients with new HIV diagnoses should also be provided psychological support and counseling.

Complications

While the acute illness of primary HIV is self-limited, failure to diagnose and initiate treatment leads to progression of the illness. Patient with undiagnosed or untreated HIV will inevitably develop immunocompromise and eventually progress to AIDS.

Bottom Line: Primary HIV Clinical Pearls

1. Primary HIV infection presents as a viral syndrome which frequently involves a generalized rash.
2. Acute viral illness is self-limited.
3. Consider HIV testing in acute viral illness in at-risk populations.

Eosinophilic Folliculitis

Background

HIV-associated eosinophilic folliculitis (EF) is a common dermatologic condition in the HIV population characterized by pustular lesions and severe pruritis. EF is considered a subtype of Ofuji's disease, a similar condition occurring in healthy patients, particularly in Japan. While EF is considered common in HIV patients, with one study reporting an incidence of 9%, the pathogenesis is not fully understood [13]. Current theories involve infection with various pathogens including the *Demodex* mite, *pityrosporum* yeast or bacteria as well as an autoimmune response to the skin and sebaceous gland antigens.

Classic Clinical Presentation

HIV-associated EF initially presents with pustules on the scalp, face, neck, and upper trunk. Due to intractable pruritis, however, these classically described pustules are rarely seen, and patients more commonly present with excoriated lesions. These lesions may exhibit crusting or hyperpigmentation and are typically 2–3 mm in size [14]. Biopsy is recommended, as it is often impossible to distinguish HIV-associated EF from other etiologies of folliculitis without histologic examination. Other considerations are listed in Table 13.2 (Fig. 13.2).

Table 13.2 Differential diagnosis of EF

Vesicular or pustular	Acne vulgaris
	Impetigo
	Dermatitis herpetiformis
	Bacterial, fungal, or steroid-incued folliculitis
Pruritic	Scabies
	Atopic dermatitis
	Urticarial
	Pruritic popular eruption

Fig. 13.2 Excoriated eosinophilic folliculitis lesions. (Source: Wikidoc (www.wikidoc.org))

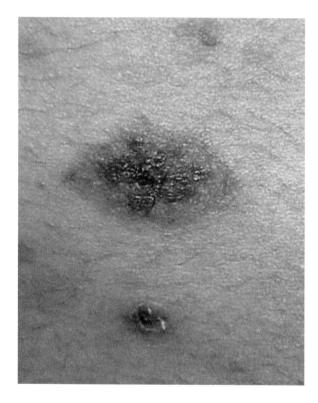

Atypical Presentation

EF in HIV patients rarely presents with lesions in the lower body; therefore, other diagnoses should be considered in patients demonstrating generalized or lower trunk or extremity symptoms [14].

Associated Systemic Symptoms

HIV-associated EF does not present with systemic symptoms [14]. Given that the condition is correlated with worsening degree of immunocompromise, patients may exhibit signs or symptoms of unrelated AIDS-defining conditions or opportunistic infections. Despite the name, only 25–50% of patients present with peripheral eosinophilia or elevated IgE; therefore, laboratory testing for this purpose is not recommended [15].

Time Course of Disease

While HIV-associated EF can occur at any stage, the vast majority of cases present in advanced HIV. Studies demonstrate EF most commonly occurs with CD4 counts below 250 [15–18].

Common Mimics and Differential Diagnosis

The differential diagnosis of HIV-associated EF includes dermatologic conditions that present with pustules or vesicles, such as acne vulgaris, impetigo, dermatitis herpetiformis, or other etiologies of folliculitis including bacterial, fungal, and steroid-induced. Other common EF mimics are those conditions that cause severe pruritis such as scabies, atopic dermatitis, urticaria, and pruritic papular eruption.

Key Physical Exam Findings

1. Excoriated lesions on the scalp, face, neck, and upper trunk.
2. Rarely the initial pustules will be seen prior to excoriation.
3. Intense pruritis.

Management

Due to the correlation with downtrending CD4 counts, the first-line management of HIV-associated EF is initiation of ART. However, worsening symptoms during early ART have been reported and are believed to be associated with immune reconstitution inflammatory syndrome (IRIS) [18]. In patients who demonstrate increased severity with ART or do not respond, topical steroids are generally used next. Other treatment options include topical tacrolimus, oral metronidazole, or itraconazole. Phototherapy with UVB has been shown to be highly effective in severe cases [19–22]. Antihistamines such as cetirizine are often used to treat severe pruritis. Unlike in other forms of EF, indomethacin has been shown to be ineffective in HIV-associated EF and is not recommended [19].

Complications

Like any open wound, the excoriated pustules of EF can become superinfected with various bacterial, viral, and fungal pathogens. Bacterial infections can lead to bacteremia and sepsis if not treated appropriately.

> **Bottom Line: Eosinophilic Folliculitis Clinical Pearls**
> 1. Intensely pruritic pustules or excoriated lesions on the scalp, face, and upper trunk.
> 2. HIV-associated EF presents in advanced HIV, generally with CD4 counts <250.
> 3. First-line treatment is ART.
> 4. Other treatments include topical immunomodulators as well as antihistamines, antibiotics, antifungal medications, and UVB phototherapy.

Crusted Scabies

Background

Crusted scabies, previously known as Norwegian scabies, is a severe form of scabies seen in the immunocompromised, including HIV patients. Compromised immunity allows for widespread proliferation of the *Sarcoptes scabiei* mite and tissue destruction. This severe form of scabies is highly contagious and transmitted through skin-to-skin contact as well as contact with clothing or bedding containing the mites.

Classic Clinical Presentation

As the name suggests, crusted scabies presents with well-demarcated hyperkeratotic plaques that appear as thick crusts on the skin. The thickened lesions can be white, gray, or yellow with erythematous bases. Crusts contain thousands to millions of mites. Unlike typical scabies, crusted scabies classically presents with minimal pruritis and can develop slowly over weeks. Like classic scabies, crusted scabies is commonly located on the extremities and in flexural surfaces; however, severe cases can involve the entire body including the scalp and nails. Like most opportunistic conditions, the severity of crusted scabies correlates with the degree of host immunocompromise [23–25].

Atypical Presentation

Several cases of bullous scabies or crusted scabies with exophytic, warty lesions have been documented. Significant infestations in the subungual spaces may also occur. On rare occasion, severe pruritis may occur (Fig. 13.3).

Associated Systemic Symptoms

Fissures within plaques may cause bleeding and pain as well as provide a point of entry for infection. Many patients also have accompanying lymphadenopathy at the

Fig. 13.3 Severe,
untreated crusted scabies
in AIDS patient. (Source:
Wikemedia Commons
(https://commons.
wikimedia.org))

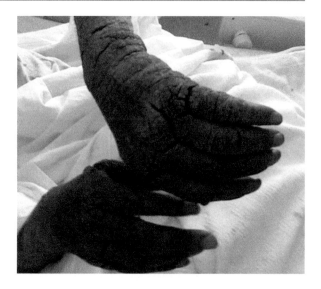

Fig. 13.3 Severe,
untreated crusted scabies
in AIDS patient. (Source:
Wikemedia Commons
(https://commons.
wikimedia.org))

time of presentation. More than half of patients will demonstrate eosinophilia on laboratory evaluation [26].

Time Course of Disease

The incubation period after infestation with the scabies mite is 3–6 weeks. In cases of reinfestation, the onset of symptoms can occur much more rapidly, on the order of days [27]. Given that lesions are often asymptomatic, patients with crusted scabies typically have a more indolent course and present for treatment later than those with typical scabies. Patients with severe immunocompromise are most commonly affected, frequently those with CD4 counts below 100 [28].

Common Mimics and Differential Diagnosis

The flaky or scaly appearance of hyperkeratosis in crusted scabies can resemble eczema, psoriasis, or seborrheic dermatitis. When crusted scabies becomes widespread, it can mimic erythroderma. Other dermatologic conditions in the differential diagnosis include pityriasis rubra pilaris, Darier's disease, and lichen planus.

Key Physical Exam Findings

1. White, gray, or yellow plaques of hyperkeratosis.
2. Erythematous base remains when plaques are removed.
3. Skin base may show mild bleeding when plaques are removed.

Table 13.3 Treatment of crusted scabies	Crusted scabies treatment
	Isolate the patient
	Wash all clothing and bedding in hot water
	Treat pruritis with antihistamines
	Treat pain with proper analgesia
	Oral ivermectin is usually required for true crusted scabies
	Given antibiotics for any evidence of bacterial superinfection or sepsis

Management

The initial management of crusted scabies involves strict patient isolation as the heavy mite burden makes the patient highly contagious. Clothing and bedding should be washed in hot water to kill mites and prevent reinfestation. While topical therapies such as benzyl benzoate or permethrin are generally sufficient in classic scabies, thickened and crusted skin in crusted scabies can prevent adequate penetration of these medications. Most cases require the addition of systemic treatment with oral ivermectin, often with multiple doses [29]. Patient may also require symptomatic treatment with antihistamines for pruritis and analgesics for any associated pain. Table 13.3 lists treatment options.

Complications

The feared complicated of crusted scabies is superinfection as this can rapidly lead to sepsis and shock in the immunocompromised host. Bacterial superinfection most commonly occurs with *Staphylococcus aureus* or other skin flora [30]. Cases of fungal and viral superinfection including herpes have been cited in the literature as well.

> **Bottom Line: Crusted Scabies Clinical Pearls**
> 1. Caused by the same mite as typical scabies, *Sarcoptes scabiei*.
> 2. Highly contagious and requires isolation and meticulous laundering of clothing and bedding.
> 3. Often requires both oral and topical treatment for sufficient penetration.
> 4. Can be complicated by bacterial superinfection.

Kaposi Sarcoma

Background

Kaposi sarcoma is a vascular neoplasm seen rarely outside of patients with AIDS. It is the most common HIV-associated malignancy and is aggressive and disseminated in AIDS patients [31]. Although incidence of AIDS-associated KS has steadily declined with improvements in antiretroviral therapy, in the United States, it is diagnosed in about six people per million per year [2]. The pathogenesis of Kaposi sarcoma requires infection with human herpesvirus 8 (HHV8), which is transmitted via multiple routes including sexual transmission. Primary infection is asymptomatic, and coinfection rates in patients with HIV are high.

Classic Clinical Presentation

Cutaneous Kaposi sarcoma initially presents as painless, nonpruritic round, or oval shaped lesions with erythematous or rust coloration. The early sarcomas may be flat or slightly raised and typically progress to red, brown, or violaceous patches or plaques. AIDS-associated Kaposi sarcoma is most commonly found on the head, neck, and upper trunk; however, it may present anywhere on the body, including mucus membranes. KS presents as oral lesions in 15–20% with a predilection for the hard palate and tongue. In contrast to other subtypes of KS, AIDS-associated Kaposi often presents as multiple lesions simultaneously representing multifocal disease rather than metastasis. Most KS lesions are asymptomatic, although larger sarcomas can result in significant edema and pain.

Atypical Presentation

Less commonly, lesions can advance to large exophytic tumors, or the typical deep red or purple coloration can be disguised by erosions, crusting, hyperkeratosis, or ulceration. Case reports exist describing Kaposi sarcoma in nearly every organ system including the heart, liver, bone marrow, pancreas, conjunctiva, and testes. Atypical presentations of Kaposi sarcoma become more common with worsening degree of immunocompromise.

Associated Systemic Symptoms

Some patients will present with constitutional symptoms including weight loss, fevers, and pain. Generalized lymphadenopathy frequently exists early in the disease.

The majority of cases of KS will have extracutaneous involvement, most commonly in the gastrointestinal and respiratory tracts. Presenting signs and symptoms of extracutaneous tumors vary depending on the organ systems involved. Gastrointestinal tumors may present with abdominal pain, nausea, vomiting, diarrhea, upper or lower GI bleeding, anemia, bowel obstruction, or malabsorption. Dyspnea, chest pain, and hemoptysis are common symptoms in patients with respiratory tract tumors. While these are the more common signs and symptoms, a wide array of presentations are possible and depend greatly on the location of internal organ tumors.

Time Course of Disease

AIDS-associated KS can develop at any stage of HIV infection, but incidence generally increases with degree of immunocompromise. The majority of cases are diagnosed at CD4 counts below 200 with mean CD4 in the 50s. The extent of disease and aggressiveness of tumors are also correlated with worsening CD4 counts [32].

Common Mimics and Differential Diagnosis

Kaposi sarcomas of the skin can be mistaken for other vascular lesions including hemangiomas, pyogenic granulomas, or bacillary angiomatosis. The typical pigmentation can mimic ecchymoses. Ulcerations and erosions of cutaneous KS can appear similar to granulation tissue.

Key Physical Exam Findings

1. Early lesions are usually painless, nonpruritic round- or oval-shaped lesions with erythematous or rust coloration.
2. Later lesions appear as red, brown, or violaceous patches or plaques.
3. Sarcomas often present in oral cavity including the hard palate, gingiva, and tongue.
4. Generalized lymphadenopathy is common.

Management

The primary treatment in AIDS-associated Kaposi sarcoma is combined antiretroviral therapy (CRT), as improvement in immunocompromise can often halt progression of lesions or even resolve tumors. Small cutaneous sarcomas may be treated with topical or local therapies although these treatments alone will not prevent formation of new lesions. These treatments include topical tretinoin therapies, cryotherapy, surgical excision, intralesional chemotherapy, and local radiation. Widespread cutaneous or internal involvement is often managed with systemic chemotherapy or immunotherapy medications.

Complications (Mortality/Prognosis)

The prognosis of AIDS-associated Kaposi sarcoma has improved drastically since the early AIDS era. Five-year mortality in the 1990s was estimated at 10%; however, advances in both detection and therapies have increased survival to 72% at 5 years [33].

Bottom Line: Kaposi Sarcoma Clinical Pearls
1. Most common HIV-associated malignancy.
2. Pathogenesis requires coinfection with HHV8.
3. Red, brown, or violaceous patches or plaques on the skin or mucus membranes.
4. Most common extracutaneous sites are GI and respiratory tracts.
5. Primary treatment is CRT (Fig. 13.4).

Fig. 13.4 Kaposi sarcoma. (Source: Wikidoc (www. wikidoc.org))

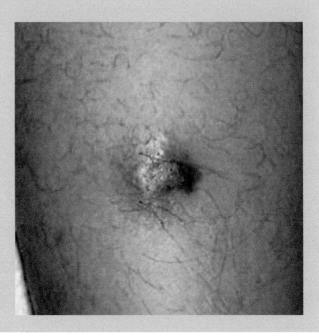

Molluscum Contagiosum

Molluscum contagiosum (MC) is a generally benign skin condition caused by a poxvirus. The virus is ubiquitous and transmitted via skin-to-skin contact or fomites. Typical MC is most common in children or sexually active young adults where it presents as a mild and usually self-limited disease. However, MC is also frequently seen in the immunocompromised. The prevalence of HIV-associated MC was estimated at 5–18% in the 1980s; however, infection rates have declined with advances in the management of HIV [34–37]. In the HIV population, MC may become disseminated and disfiguring.

Typical MC presents with pink or flesh-colored, umbilicated papules ranging from 2 to 5 mm in size. Lesions tend to occur on the trunk, axillae, and groin; however, they generally spare the palms. In HIV, these papules are more likely to present on the face than in immunocompetent patients [38]. Case reports of giant lesions greater than 1 cm have been reported in the literature in patients with severe AIDS [38, 39] (Fig. 13.5).

Fig. 13.5 Molluscum contagiosum. (Source: Wikidoc (www.wikidoc. org))

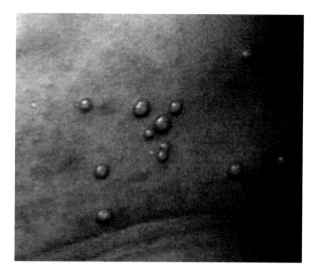

The diagnosis of MC is usually clinical and based on appearance of lesions, although biopsy may be required in atypical cases. A wide range of treatment options exist including cryotherapy, curettage, and various topical agents such as retinoids, salicylic acid, imiquimod, or cantharidin. However, HIV-associated MC is extremely resistant to typical therapy but can improve and even resolve with ART [40].

Seborrheic Dermatitis

Seborrheic dermatitis is among the most common skin disorders associated with HIV. In milder forms, the condition is also seen in the general population in a bimodal distribution with peaks in infancy and in the third and fourth decades of life. The prevalence of seborrheic dermatitis is greater than 35% in early HIV and is therefore a common presenting symptom of HIV infection [41]. The condition tends to be more common and more severe as the HIV progresses to AIDS [41–45].

Clinically, seborrheic dermatitis can range from mild dandruff to a severe dermatologic condition. Mild lesions will have erythematous patches with poorly defined borders covered in white or yellow scaling. These patches are classically described as moist or greasy. The most severe cases will exhibit papules and plaques of scales on brightly erythematous bases. The most common locations for seborrheic dermatitis include the scalp, hairline, eyebrows, nasolabial folds, postauricular region, external auditory meatus, beard, trunk, and perineum. Blepharitis is also common. In cases of severe immunocompromise, however, the extremities and genitals are frequently involved as well. The diagnosis is made clinically based on physical characteristics and distribution (Fig. 13.6).

Seborrheic dermatitis is a chronic and relapsing condition making it difficult to treat. Furthermore, cases associated with HIV are typically more resistant to standard treatments. First-line therapies include topical corticosteroids, antifungals, or anti-inflammatory medications. Oral antifungals such as itraconazole are often used in difficult-to-treat cases [46]. Like many skin conditions associated with HIV, seborrheic dermatitis has been shown to improve with antiretroviral therapy [47].

Herpes Zoster and Secondary Syphilis

There are a great number of dermatologic conditions associated with HIV. Two other important rashes in the HIV population are discussed in other chapters of this text. For a complete discussion of herpes zoster and syphilis, please see Chaps. 11 and 14 respectively (Fig. 13.7).

Fig. 13.6 Auricular seborrheic dermatitis. (Source: Wikidoc (www. wikidoc.org))

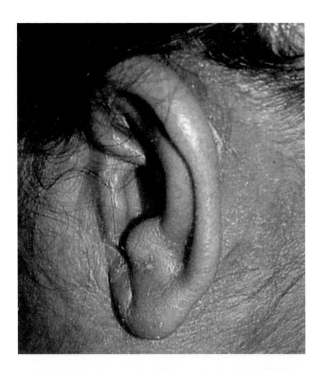

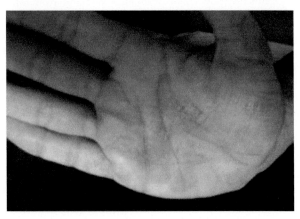

Fig. 13.7 Secondary syphilis. (Source: David Stone, M.D.)

References

1. Centers for Disease Control and Prevention. HIV surveillance report, 2015; vol. 27. http://www.cdc.gov/hiv/library/reports/hiv-surveillance.html. Published November 2016. Accessed Feb 2017.
2. Prejean J, Song R, Hernandez A, Ziebell R, Green T, Walker F, et al. Estimated HIV incidence in the United States, 2006-2009. PLoS One. 2011;6:e17502. https://doi.org/10.1371/journal.pone.0017502.
3. Schacker T, Collier AC, Hughes J, Shea T, Corey L. Clinical and epidemiologic features of primary HIV infection. Ann Intern Med. 1996;125:257–64.
4. Hecht FM, Busch MP, Rawal B, Webb M, Rosenberg E, Swanson M, et al. Use of laboratory tests and clinical symptoms for identification of primary HIV infection. AIDS. 2002;16:1119–29.
5. Bollinger RC, Brookmeyer RS, Mehendale SM, Paranjape RS, Shepherd ME, Gadkari DA, et al. Risk factors and clinical presentation of acute primary HIV infection in India. JAMA. 1997;278:2085–9.
6. Pilcher CD, Tien HC, Eron JJ, Vernazza PL, Leu S-Y, Stewart PW, et al. Brief but efficient: acute HIV infection and the sexual transmission of HIV. J Infect Dis. 2004;189:1785–92. https://doi.org/10.1086/386333.
7. Lapins J, Gaines H, Lindbäck S, Lidbrink P, Emtestam L. Skin and mucosal characteristics of symptomatic primary HIV-1 infection. AIDS Patient Care STDs. 1997;11:67–70. https://doi.org/10.1089/apc.1997.11.67.
8. Rabeneck L, Popovic M, Gartner S, McLean DM, McLeod WA, Read E, et al. Acute HIV infection presenting with painful swallowing and esophageal ulcers. JAMA. 1990;263:2318–22.
9. Calabrese LH, Proffitt MR, Levin KH, Yen-Lieberman B, Starkey C. Acute infection with the human immunodeficiency virus (HIV) associated with acute brachial neuritis and exanthematous rash. Ann Intern Med. 1987;107:849–51.
10. Ho DD, Sarngadharan MG, Resnick L, Dimarzoveronese F, Rota TR, Hirsch MS. Primary human T-lymphotropic virus type III infection. Ann Intern Med. 1985;103:880–3.
11. Hellmuth J, Fletcher JLK, Valcour V, Kroon E, Ananworanich J, Intasan J, et al. Neurologic signs and symptoms frequently manifest in acute HIV infection. Neurology. 2016;87:148–54. https://doi.org/10.1212/WNL.0000000000002837.
12. Braun DL, Kouyos RD, Balmer B, Grube C, Weber R, Günthard HF. Frequency and spectrum of unexpected clinical manifestations of primary HIV-1 infection. Clin Infect Dis. 2015;61:1013–21. https://doi.org/10.1093/cid/civ398.
13. Uthayakumar S, Nandwani R, Drinkwater T, Nayagam AT, Darley CR. The prevalence of skin disease in HIV infection and its relationship to the degree of immunosuppression. Br J Dermatol. 1997;137:595–8.
14. Simpson-Dent S, Fearfield LA, Staughton RC. HIV associated eosinophilic folliculitis – differential diagnosis and management. Sex Transm Infect. 1999;75:291–3. https://doi.org/10.1136/sti.75.5.291.
15. Fearfield LA, Rowe A, Francis N, Bunker CB, Staughton RC. Itchy folliculitis and human immunodeficiency virus infection: clinicopathological and immunological features, pathogenesis and treatment. Br J Dermatol. 1999;141:3–11.
16. Rosenthal D, LeBoit PE, Klumpp L, Berger TG. Human immunodeficiency virus-associated eosinophilic folliculitis. A unique dermatosis associated with advanced human immunodeficiency virus infection. Arch Dermatol. 1991;127:206–9.
17. Soeprono FF, Schinella RA. Eosinophilic pustular folliculitis in patients with acquired immunodeficiency syndrome. Report of three cases. J Am Acad Dermatol. 1986;14:1020–2.
18. Rajendran PM, Dolev JC, Heaphy MR, Maurer T. Eosinophilic folliculitis: before and after the introduction of antiretroviral therapy. Arch Dermatol. 2005;141:1227–31. https://doi.org/10.1001/archderm.141.10.1227.
19. Ellis E, Scheinfeld N. Eosinophilic pustular folliculitis: a comprehensive review of treatment options. Am J Clin Dermatol. 2004;5:189–97.

20. Buchness MR, Lim HW, Hatcher VA, Sanchez M, Soter NA. Eosinophilic pustular folliculitis in the acquired immunodeficiency syndrome. Treatment with ultraviolet B phototherapy. N Engl J Med. 1988;318:1183–6. https://doi.org/10.1056/NEJM198805053181807.

21. Misago N, Narisawa Y, Matsubara S, Hayashi S. HIV-associated eosinophilic pustular folliculitis: successful treatment of a Japanese patient with UVB phototherapy. J Dermatol. 1998;25:178–84. https://doi.org/10.1111/j.1346-8138.1998.tb02376.x.

22. Porneuf M, Guillot B, Barneon G, Guilhou JJ. Eosinophilic pustular folliculitis responding to UVB therapy. J Am Acad Dermatol. 1993;29 (259–60.

23. Rau RC, Baird IM. Crusted scabies in a patient with acquired immunodeficiency syndrome. J Am Acad Dermatol. 1986;15:1058–9.

24. Glover A, Young L, Goltz AW. Norwegian scabies in acquired immunodeficiency syndrome: report of a case resulting in death from associated sepsis. J Am Acad Dermatol. 1987;16 (396–9.

25. Drabick JJ, Lupton GP, Tompkins K. Crusted scabies in human immunodeficiency virus infection. J Am Acad Dermatol. 1987;17:142.

26. Arlian LG, Morgan MS, Estes SA, Walton SF, Kemp DJ, Currie BJ. Circulating IgE in patients with ordinary and crusted scabies. 2004; https://doi.org/10.1603/0022-2585-41.1.74.

27. Karthikeyan K. Crusted scabies. Indian J Dermatol Venereol Leprol. 2009;75:340–7. https://doi.org/10.4103/0378-6323.53128.

28. Josephine M, Issac E, George A, Ngole M, Albert S-E. Patterns of skin manifestations and their relationships with CD4 counts among HIV/AIDS patients in Cameroon. Int J Dermatol. 2006;45:280–4. https://doi.org/10.1111/j.1365-4632.2004.02529.x.

29. Roberts LJ, Huffam SE, Walton SF, Currie BJ. Crusted scabies: clinical and immunological findings in seventy-eight patients and a review of the literature. J Infect. 2005;50:375–81. https://doi.org/10.1016/j.jinf.2004.08.033.

30. Lin S, Farber J, Lado L. A case report of crusted scabies with methicillin-resistant Staphylococcus Aureus bacteremia. J Am Geriatr Soc. 2009;57:1713–4. https://doi.org/10.1111/j.1532-5415.2009.02412.x.

31. Friedman-Kien AE. Disseminated Kaposi's sarcoma syndrome in young homosexual men. J Am Acad Dermatol. 1981;5:468–71. https://doi.org/10.1016/S0190-9622(81)80010-2.

32. Goldstein B, Berman B, Sukenik E, Frankel SJ. Correlation of skin disorders with CD4 lymphocyte counts in patients with HIV/AIDS. J Am Acad Dermatol. 1997;36:262–4.

33. S.A. Cancer, Cancer Facts & Figures 2012, 2012.

34. Coldiron BM, Bergstresser PR. Prevalence and clinical spectrum of skin disease in patients infected with human immunodeficiency virus. Arch Dermatol. 1989;125:357–61.

35. Goodman DS, Teplitz ED, Wishner A, Klein RS, Burk PG, Hershenbaum E. Prevalence of cutaneous disease in patients with acquired immunodeficiency syndrome (AIDS) or AIDS-related complex. J Am Acad Dermatol. 1987;17:210–20.

36. Hira SK, Wadhawan D, Kamanga J, Kavindele D, Macuacua R, Patil PS, et al. Cutaneous manifestations of human immunodeficiency virus in Lusaka, Zambia. J Am Acad Dermatol. 1988;19:451–7.

37. Matis WL, Triana A, Shapiro R, Eldred L, Polk BF, Hood AF. Dermatologic findings associated with human immunodeficiency virus infection. J Am Acad Dermatol. 1987;17:746–51.

38. Schwartz JJ, Myskowski PL. Molluscum contagiosum in patients with human immunodeficiency virus infection. A review of twenty-seven patients. J Am Acad Dermatol. 1992;27:583–8.

39. Schwartz JJ, Myskowski PL. Hiv-related MoUuscum contagiosum presenting as a cutaneous horn. Int J Dermatol. 1992;31:142–4. https://doi.org/10.1111/j.1365-4362.1992.tb03258.x.

40. Hicks CB, Myers SA, Giner J. Resolution of intractable molluscum contagiosum in a human immunodeficiency virus-infected patient after institution of antiretroviral therapy with ritonavir. Clin Infect Dis. 1997;24:1023–5.

41. Berger RS, Stoner MF, Hobbs ER, Hayes TJ, Boswell RN. Cutaneous manifestations of early human immunodeficiency virus exposure. J Am Acad Dermatol. 1988;19 (298–303.

42. Soeprono FF, Schinella RA, Cockerell CJ, Comite SL. Seborrheic-like dermatitis of acquired immunodeficiency syndrome. A clinicopathologic study. J Am Acad Dermatol. 1986;14:242–8.

43. Muñoz-Pérez MA, Rodriguez-Pichardo A, Camacho F, Colmenero MA. Dermatological findings correlated with CD4 lymphocyte counts in a prospective 3 year study of 1161 patients with human immunodeficiency virus disease predominantly acquired through intravenous drug abuse. Br J Dermatol. 1998;139:33–9.
44. Mallal SA. The Western Australian HIV cohort study, Perth, Australia. J Acquir Immune Defic Syndr Hum Retrovirol. 1998;17(Suppl 1):S23–7.
45. Mathes BM, Douglass MC. Seborrheic dermatitis in patients with acquired immunodeficiency syndrome. J Am Acad Dermatol. 1985;13:947–51.
46. Gupta AK, Richardson M, Paquet M. Systematic review of oral treatments for seborrheic dermatitis. J Eur Acad Dermatol Venereol. 2014;28:16–26. https://doi.org/10.1111/jdv.12197.
47. Dunic I, Vesic S, Jevtovic DJ. Oral candidiasis and seborrheic dermatitis in HIV-infected patients on highly active antiretroviral therapy. HIV Med. 2004;5:50–4.

Syphilis

14

Molly Hartrich and Taku Taira

Background

Syphilis is a sexually transmitted disease caused by the spirochete *Treponema pallidum*. Transmission occurs either through direct contact with the infected site or vertically from the mother to fetus. Syphilis has both a variety of cutaneous and systemic presentations that overlap with many other diseases. The protean nature of syphilis is further compounded by the waxing and waning incidence of the disease. An additional challenge is the varied presentations of syphilis.

The incidence of syphilis peaked in the 1940s followed by a steady decline that reached a nadir in the year 2000. However, since this nadir, there has been a steady resurgence [1]. Traditionally, syphilis was evenly distributed between men and women in their 20s. With the increased incidence, demographics have shifted, and now the majority of syphilis infections are seen in 30–40-year-old [7] men who have sex with men (MSM) clustered in large urban areas [2], worldwide, with resurgences being reported in countries as diverse as Russia [3], China [4], the UK [5], and Canada [6].

Despite having an effective treatment, syphilis continues to be a great source of both direct and indirect morbidity and mortality. Worldwide, syphilis continues to be a leading cause of stillbirth and perinatal mortality [8]. The impact of syphilis is further magnified by its ability to both enhance the transmission of HIV and increase the severity of the disease.

M. Hartrich (✉) · T. Taira
Department of Emergency Medicine, University of Southern California,
Los Angeles, CA, USA
e-mail: takutair@usc.edu

© Springer International Publishing AG, part of Springer Nature 2018
E. Rose (ed.), *Life-Threatening Rashes*, https://doi.org/10.1007/978-3-319-75623-3_14

Classic Clinical Presentation

The clinical manifestations of syphilis can be broadly separated into an early and late phase. Early phase syphilis consists of primary, secondary, and early latent stage (see Table 14.1). This stage stretches from weeks to several months after infection. The "late phase" includes the latent phase, tertiary, and neurosyphilis. This stage typically presents years after the initial infection [23, 24]. The early and late phases are separated by the latent phase where the patient has seropositivity without any manifestations of the disease.

The dermatological presentations are seen primarily in the early stage, while the late stages are either asymptomatic or manifest through organ systems, particularly the CNS. Although most untreated patients will reliably progress through the early stages of disease, there is variability in who will progress through the later stages as well as the varied manifestations of late disease. The exception to this pattern is in patients with HIV, as the stages of the disease tend to overlap [59].

Classic Presentation of Early Syphilis

Primary Syphilis

Primary syphilis is characterized by the classic chancre (see Fig. 14.1). The primary chancre begins as a papule and then evolves into a 1–2 cm indurated, non-exudative ulcer with a clean base which is often associated with nonsuppurative, non-tender regional lymphadenopathy. The ulcer is classically painless, which helps to differentiate a syphilitic chancre from other clinical mimics.

The initial chancre of primary syphilis typically presents at several weeks after inoculation. However it may appear as early as 1 week and as late as 3 months after inoculation [9]. Because they are painless and innocuous and resolve spontaneously

Table 14.1 Time course of the disease

Stage	Time from exposure	Time to resolution	Clinical features
Primary	2–3 weeks	4–12 weeks	Well-circumscribed, non-tender, hard-based ulcer (chancre) with a nonpurulent clean base Associated regional lymphadenopathy
Secondary	4–8 weeks after a primary lesion [37]	1–6 months	Diffuse immune rash involving the palms and the soles Associated with systemic symptoms of malaise, myalgias, headaches, fevers Associated with diffuse lymphadenopathy
Tertiary	Years		Gummas Cardiovascular involvement
Neuro−/ocular/otic involvement	Variable		Uveitis Cranial nerve paresis Sensorineural deficits

in 2–8 weeks, patients will commonly be unaware of the lesion. This is underscored by the fact that only 30–40% of disease is diagnosed at this stage [10, 11].

Primary syphilis occurs at the site of the initial infection. Classically, these lesions are seen on the genitals (Fig. 14.1). In men, the chancre is typically seen on the glans, the coronal sulcus, and the foreskin, while in women, the chancre is typically seen on the labia and fourchette [11]. In women, the primary chancre can be seen both externally and on internal surfaces such as the cervix (Fig. 14.2). The rates of chancres on the cervix have been reported to be as high as 44% in infected women [11].

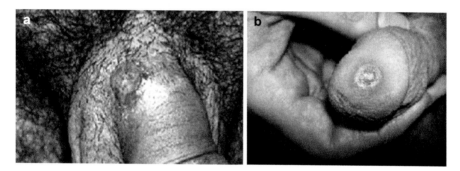

Fig. 14.1 Chancres of primary syphilis on male genitalia [26]

Fig. 14.2 Chancre of primary syphilis on the cervix https://www.huidziekten.nl/zakboek/dermatosen/stxt/SOASyphilis.htm

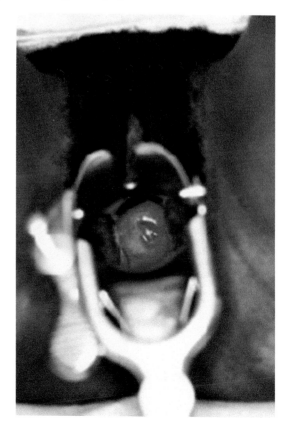

Chancres are also found surrounding the anus and the mouth. Lesions around the mouth include the oral mucosa, lips, and tongue (Fig. 14.3) [12–16]. Because the chancre occurs at the site of inoculation, chancres have also been described in a variety of locations including fingers (Fig. 14.4), nipples, arms, eyelid, and toes [11].

Fig. 14.3 Pseudotumoral chancre on the tongue [38]

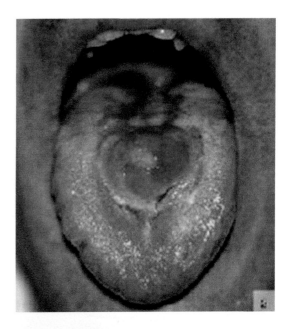

Fig. 14.4 Chancre of primary syphilis on finger [26]

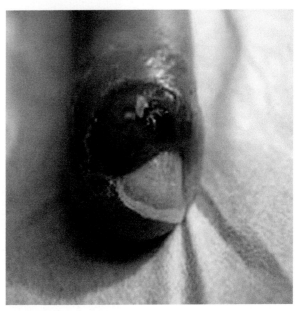

Secondary Syphilis

Cutaneous manifestations of secondary syphilis are highly variable. The classic rash typically presents 2–8 weeks after the resolution of the primary lesion and lasts for 4–12 weeks [11, 17, 18] if untreated. Approximately 80% of patients with secondary syphilis have a rash. The maculopapular rash is discrete with red, brown, or even violaceous lesions that range from 3 to 10 mm. It typically starts on the trunk and may spread acrally to involve the palms and soles (Figs. 14.5 and 14.6). It is typically non-pruritic, diffuse, and symmetric. Palmoplantar involvement is often

Figs. 14.5 and 14.6 Classic plantar rash of secondary syphilis as well as diffuse rash of secondary syphilis across trunk https://www. huidziekten.nl/zakboek/ dermatosen/stxt/ SOASyphilis.htm)

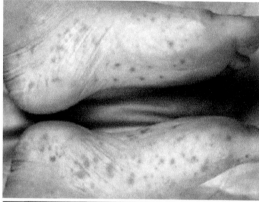
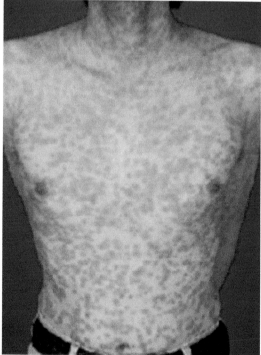

followed by desquamation [19], and while palmoplantar involvement is the classic finding, it only occurs in approximately 70% of cases of secondary syphilis [11], and its absence cannot be used to rule out the disease. When it does involve the palms and soles, it helps distinguish it from other extensive maculopapular rashes such as guttate psoriasis or pityriasis rosea [17]. Diseases including Rocky Mountain spotted fever, atypical measles, and meningococcemia are associated with palmo-plantar rash with systemic symptoms; however, these patients are typically much more severely ill at presentation [21].

Fifty percent of patients will have mucosal involvement [11], and these mucous patches typically present with multiple, oval-shaped shallow ulcers on the tongue, gingival or buccal mucosa, palate, or pharynx. They may also occur on the moist surface of the genitalia and intertriginous areas. When mucous patches enlarge and coalesce, they can cause papillary excrescences called condyloma lata. Because of both the appearance and the location of condyloma lata, they can often be mistaken for genital warts/condyloma accuminata, but unlike condyloma accuminata, hair growth is not impeded in condyloma lata [22]. Like the ulcers of primary syphilis, both mucous patches and condyloma lata are dense with spirochetes and are highly infectious. In addition, spirochetes can invade the hair follicles, can cause a patchy alopecia with a typical "moth eaten" appearance, and may cause thinning of eye-brows, eyelashes, and beard [20, 21].

Latent Phase

The key feature of latent syphilis is seropositive testing in the absence of clinical manifestations or symptoms.

Tertiary Syphilis

There are three typical manifestations of tertiary syphilis: neurosyphilis, cardiovas-cular syphilis, and benign tertiary or gummatous syphilis.

Neurosyphilis
There are four subcategories of neurosyphilis. Meningovascular syphilis clinically resembles cerebrovascular accidents secondary to the endarteritis cause by spiro-chete. Syphilitic meningitis manifests similarly to other forms of aseptic meningitis with headache, meningismus, nausea, vomiting, and seizure. Patients may also have cranial nerve abnormalities including acoustic and vestibular symptoms given the preferential basilar inflammation of CNS syphilis infection. Parenchymal disease varies widely and may include fibrosis and atrophy of tissue manifesting in progres-sive paresis, tabes dorsalis, dementia, delirium, psychosis, delusions, difficulty with speech, and Argyll Robertson pupil. Finally, gummas have been observed in the brain parenchyma mimicking neoplasms or other space-occupying lesions similar to toxoplasmosis in HIV-infected patients.

Fig. 14.7 Gummatous
Syphilis [25]

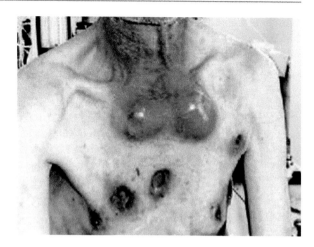

Cardiovascular Syphilis

The endarteritis caused by *T. pallidum* affects the aortic vasa vasorum leading eventually to aneurysm, most often of the proximal thoracic aorta and arch. Involvement of abdominal aorta is very rare. Aortic insufficiency is seen; however, these aneurysms rarely dissect [20] and are often only discovered when they become so large, compressive, or erosive that symptoms arise. Uncommonly, coronary ostia are involved leading to ischemic heart disease.

Gummatous Syphilis

Gummas are painless, firm nodules ranging from millimeters to large, tumorlike masses. Gummas preferentially manifest on the skin and mucous membranes but are also seen in the skeletal system and virtually any organ [20, 21]. They will often involute leaving punched out ulcers which resemble pyoderma gangrenosum [25] and leave areas severely scarred. Gummas are benign; however, when they involute they cause significant tissue damage, as seen in the saddle nose deformity, or mass effect depending on size. These lesions rapidly resolve with penicillin (Fig. 14.7).

CNS/Ocular/Otic Involvement

Neurosyphilis is defined by involvement of the brain parenchyma. It may consist of progressive paresis, tabes dorsalis, dementia, delirium, psychosis, delusions, difficulty with speech, and Argyll Robertson pupil. While the neuropsychiatric manifestations of tertiary syphilis occur years after the initial infection, they do not encompass all of the CNS manifestations from syphilis.

Though neurosyphilis has classically categorized as a tertiary form of syphilis, CNS symptoms may develop at any stage. CSF irregularities are common in secondary syphilis with T. *pallidum* isolated from at least 40% of CSF samples of patients in the early stage [21]. During the spirochetemia or secondary syphilis, there can be meningeal, nervous, otic, and ocular involvement. These can in turn present as meningitis [11, 20, 21], cranial nerve abnormalities, particularly of cranial nerves II, III, VI, VII, and VIII [26] along with gradual or sudden onset tinnitus or sensorineural deafness [20, 27]. Ocular involvement can present as anterior and posterior uveitis, interstitial keratitis, and optic neuritis [11, 19, 21, 28–30].

These presentations not only overlap with a wide range of diseases; they can often present after the resolution of the rash of secondary syphilis [21]. Both ocular and CNS involvement are commonly grouped together. In these situations, the infection is in a sequestered site with poor antibiotic penetrance. As a result they require a more aggressive treatment with a longer course of IV penicillin. In the case of penicillin allergy, patients require ICU admission for desensitization.

Congenital Syphilis

Congenital syphilis (CS) refers to the vertical transmission of syphilis from the mother to child. It is a serious infection with varying manifestations. *T. pallidum* transmission may occur via infected lesions at the time of delivery or in utero. Transplacental infections may result in stillbirth, hydrops fetalis, intrauterine growth retardation, and preterm or asymptomatic birth [31]. While transmission may occur at any disease stage, 60–100% of transmissions occur in the primary and secondary stages, and infection rates drop to 8–40% in the latent stages [21].

"Snuffles" or neonatal rhinitis, often bloody, is commonly the earliest sign of CS and is soon followed by a diffuse maculopapular rash which eventually desquamates (Figs. 14.8 and 14.9) particularly on the palms, soles, periorally, and around the anus. Alopecia also develops in the newborn with CS especially of the eyebrows, and the hair is particularly brittle. Lesions that look similar to the mucous patches of secondary syphilis may develop around mucocutaneous areas but then become deeply fissured and hemorrhagic [20]. These lesions and the nasal secretions are highly infectious [31]. Aside from cutaneous manifestations, as in the adult, CS has a myriad of manifestations at multiple organ levels. Hepatic disease in the syphilis-infected neonate is a significant cause of morbidity and mortality. Hepatosplenomegaly can be seen as well as osteochondritis and perichondritis which later leads to the classic findings of anterior tibial bowing or saber shins and saddle nose deformity as well as frontal bossing [31]. Neurologic manifestations in congenital infection manifest as eighth nerve deafness, meningitis with signs of increased ICP, hydrocephalus, strokes, and loss of developmental milestones [32].

Associated Symptoms

The associated systemic symptoms are typically seen during secondary syphilis. In secondary syphilis, there is a hematogenous dissemination of spirochetes. This spirochetemia is associated with a host of non-specific constitutional symptoms including lymphadenopathy (in particular, epitrochlear lymph nodes), myalgias, fevers, malaise, and headache. This spirochetemia can in turn lead to infection and inflammation in any organ system [1]. Bony and articular syphilis may manifest as osteitis,

Figs. 14.8 and 14.9 Desquamating rash of congenital syphilis. Courtesy of Dr Stanford T. Shulman, MD Virginia H. Rogers Professor of Pediatric Infectious Diseases Northwestern University Feinberg School of Medicine Ann & Robert H. Lurie Children's Hospital of Chicago

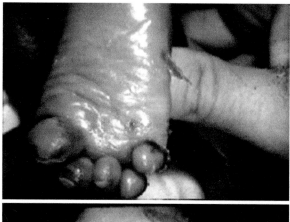
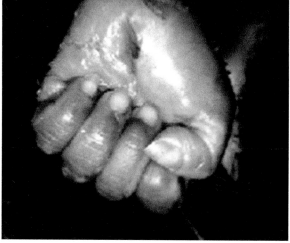

bursitis, and arthritis [33]. Syphilitic hepatitis causes hepatomegaly with elevated alkaline phosphatase, mildly elevated aminotransferases with normal bilirubin, portal inflammation, caseating granulomas, and cholestasis [34]. Renal involvement can result in glomerulonephritis and nephritic syndromes [35]. Gastric involvement results in gastritis with nausea, vomiting, and abdominal pain [36]. Infiltration and ulceration by spirochetes may be so significant; this presentation may be mistaken for lymphoma.

Atypical Presentation

The chancre of primary syphilis is usually solitary. However, in immunocompromised patients, there can be multiple primary chancres [37]. These multiple chancres may take longer than the typical 2–8 weeks to resolve without treatment. Rarely, a large primary chancre can be seen on the dorsum of the tongue. These pseudotumoral chancres [38] (Fig. 14.3) can easily be confused for a mass.

Although secondary syphilis is traditionally associated with the classic diffuse maculopapular and palmar/plantar rash, secondary syphilis can have a wide range of presentations. Split papules, another mucous membrane manifestation of secondary syphilis, look very similar to angular cheilitis. Infection of the fingernails can lead to transverse grooves and pitting of the nails as well as syphilitic paronychia and onycholysis [11, 27, 39].

The atypical cutaneous manifestations of secondary syphilis are numerous and are more commonly seen in immunocompromised individuals, particularly with HIV coinfection (see Chap. 13). Atypical cutaneous manifestations include annular, nodular, noduloulcerative, pustular, framboesiform, photodistributed papulosquamous (SLE)-like, chancriform, corymbose, malignant, and lichen planus-type lesions [38, 39, 41], each of which has common mimics (see Tables 14.2a and 14.2b for common syphilis mimics).

Nodular secondary syphilis may present as a localized or generalized eruption of erythematous or violaceous plaques or nodules. There is sparing of the palms, soles, and mucous surfaces. It may present as either an arciform pattern or as a solitary lesion. These typically present on the scalp, tongue, or lip. Some presentations of nodular syphilis are covered with a diffuse scale which can appear similar to a psoriatic eruption, and heavy disease burden of the face results in leonine faces which can be mistaken for leprosy [38, 39].

Annular secondary syphilis also has a variable phenotype ranging from delicate, lacy slightly raised lesions to thick verrucous, violaceous plaques (Fig. 14.10) and is typically found on the scalp, palms, soles, and intertriginous areas. Involvement of the scalp may cause scarring and alopecia [38, 39].

Table 14.2a Clinical mimics of syphilis

Palmar rashes [60]	Genital ulcers [11, 61]	Oral ulcers [62]
Rocky Mountain spotted fever	Herpes	Aphthous ulcer
Meningococcemia	Chancroid	Acute necrotizing ulcerative gingivitis
Hand-foot-and-mouth disease	Behcet's syndrome	Varicella
Kawasaki disease	Systemic lupus erythematosus	Hand-foot-and-mouth disease
Measles	Rheumatoid arthritis	Herpangina
Toxic shock syndrome	Genital tuberculosis	Human immunodeficiency virus
Bacterial endocarditis (Janeway lesions/Osler nodes)	Lymphogranuloma venereum	Epstein-Barr virus
	Granuloma inguinale (donovanosis) caused by *Klebsiella granulomatis*	Tuberculosis
	Epstein-Barr virus/ *Cytomegalovirus*	Blasto/crypto/histo
	Herpes zoster	Trauma/chemical/ irradiation/burn

Adapted from Refs. [38, 39]

Table 14.2b Clinical mimics of atypical cutaneous findings in syphilis [38, 39]

Atypical cutaneous manifestations of secondary syphilis	Clinical mimics
Nodular syphilis	Lepromatous leprosy, lymphoma, lymphoproliferative disease, tuberculosis, sarcoidosis, histiocytosis, fungal reactions, leukemia cutis, granular cell tumors, adnexal tumors, scleromyxedema
Annular syphilis	Lichen planus, sarcoidosis, scabies, granuloma annulare, subacute cutaneous lupus erythematosus, erythema annulare centrifugum
Frambesiform syphilis	Common warts, pinta, endemic syphilis
Pustular syphilis	Folliculitis, abscess, papulopustular rosacea, ecthyma, pyoderma gangrenosum, Behcet disease, steroid acne
Malignant syphilis (noduloulcerative syphilis)	Ecthyma, ecthyma gangrenosum, vasculitis, atypical mycobacterial infection, fungal infection, pyoderma gangrenous, anthrax, blastomycosis-like pyoderma

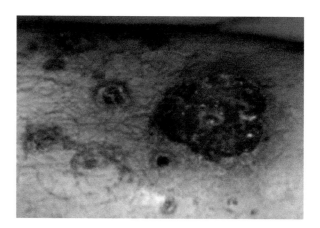

Fig. 14.10 Annular Syphilis [38]

Frambesiform secondary syphilis, after the French "raspberry," is also very rarely seen and refers to vegetating, hypertrophic keratitis lesion which appears moist and has a variable distribution on the body but has a predilection for the face and scalp particularly the personal region and, like many other manifestations of secondary syphilis, may be seen on the palms. They have a high serous content and tend to have an offensive odor [38–40].

Pustular syphilis is the most rare form of secondary syphilis. Typically the pustule begins as a scale-covered vesicle which eventually becomes fluctuant and ruptures leaving a punched-out ulcer surrounded by an inflammatory ring. These lesions may be found anywhere but have a predilection for the face especially the nose and may also be seen in a plantopalmar distrubution and on the genitals [27, 38–40]. The literature also notes that this form of secondary syphilis may herald the development of lues maligna praecox (Fig. 14.11).

Fig. 14.11 Pustular
syphilis [38]

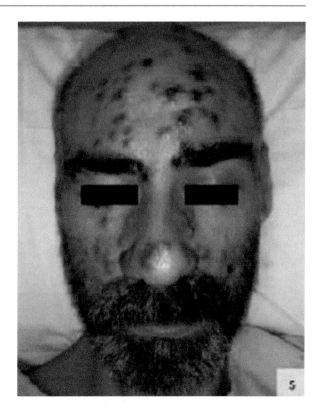

Lues maligna (noduloulcerative secondary syphilis) aka malignant syphilis is a rare
form of secondary syphilis, increasingly seen in HIV coinfection. It was described long
before the HIV pandemic in malnourished individuals, those in poor health, and alco-
holics. Currently, those with HIV/AIDS are 60 times more likely to present with this
form of syphilis [30]. Lues maligna is characterized by severe prodromal symptoms
followed by irregularly distributed lesions that are in various stages of development and
may look like the primary chancre. These lesions eventually progress to necrotic ulcers
on the forehead, trunk, and extremities (Figs. 14.12 and 14.13) and can progress so
rapidly; it is termed malignant syphilis. The characteristic palmar-plantar rash of other
forms of secondary syphilis is frequently absent in noduloulcerative syphilis. Another
characteristic of malignant syphilis is rapid resolution of lesions with appropriate therapy but greater incidence of severe Jarisch-Herxheimer reactions [39].

Diagnostic Testing

Traditionally, the definitive diagnosis of syphilis was made by the identification of
the *T. pallidum* using dark-field microscopy from samples taken from chancres or
condyloma. However dark-field microscopy is no longer readily available and has
limited ability to diagnose later disease.

Fig. 14.12 Lues Maligna [63]

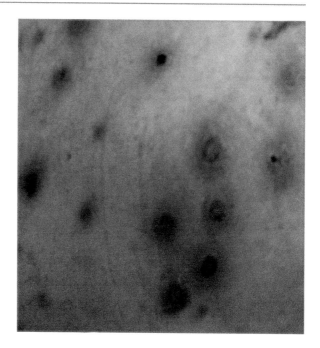

Fig. 14.13 Lues Maligna https://www.huidziekten. nl/zakboek/dermatosen/ stxt/SOASyphilis.htm

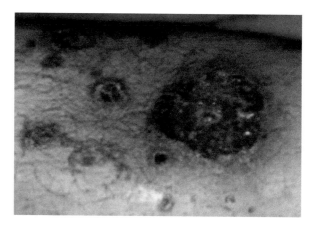

Currently the mainstay of diagnostic testing in syphilis is serological testing. Serological tests can be broadly split into treponemal and non-treponemal tests (see Table 14.3) [18]. The definitive diagnosis of syphilis requires both a treponemal and a non-treponemal test. The use of a single test can lead to both false positives and false negatives. In the traditional diagnostic algorithm, the non-treponemal test was considered the screening test, and the treponemal test was considered the confirmatory test. However with the advent of automated EIA/CIA (enzyme and chemiluminescence immunoassays), many labs are adopting a "reverse screening" process, where the EIA/CIA is used as the initial test, followed by a non-treponemal test.

Table 14.3 Diagnostic testing for syphilis

Non-treponemal tests	RPR VDRL	Positive 1–3 weeks after the primary lesion Considered a screening test in patients without known history of infection [32] Typically has a characteristic rise and fall with the course of disease Better for the evaluation of the response to treatment Can be negative in both early and late disease In some patients, the levels never become nonreactive despite treatment (serofast reaction)
Treponemal tests	EIA/CIA FTA-ABS (fluorescent treponemal antibody test) TP-PA (*T. Pallidum* hemagglutination) Various immunoassays	Typically used to confirm a non-treponemal test Slightly more sensitive in early primary syphilis Will remain positive in late disease Typically stay positive even after adequate treatment With automated EIA/CIA (automated enzyme and chemiluminescence immunoassays) some labs are screening with the EIA/CIA and confirming with the non-treponemal assay (see CDC table below)
CSF testing For neurosyphilis	CSF VDRL CSF-FT-ABS CSF cell count	CSF-VDRL is highly specific for neurosyphilis CSF-FT-ABS more sensitive for neurosyphilis It is unclear what course of action should be taken in a patient with + CSF testing without symptoms suggestive of neurosyphilis

Patients with discordant results between the EIA/CIA and the non-treponemal test are treated according to the results of the traditional treponemal tests (FTA-ABS or TP-PA) [42].

Non-treponemal Testing

The non-treponemal tests include the RPR and the VDRL. These tests are fairly rapid and characteristically rise and fall in untreated disease. The levels change with disease activity and can be used to both diagnose syphilis and monitor the response to treatment. The sensitivity in primary syphilis has been reported to be as low as 59% but approaches nearly 100% in secondary syphilis [11]. These tests are frequently falsely positive in many unrelated conditions [43] (see Table 14.4).

Treponemal Tests

Treponemal tests typically are used to confirm the diagnosis of syphilis. They are more sensitive for early disease but continue to stay elevated despite treatment and cannot be used to monitor response to treatment. Infection with another non-pallidum treponemal species can result in a false-positive test.

Patients with presentations concerning for CNS, meningeal, or ocular/otic involvement should undergo a lumbar puncture. In addition to the standard cell count, protein, glucose, and culture, the CSF samples should also be tested for CSF VDRL. Because the CSF VDRL is very highly specific but less sensitive, the more

Table 14.4 Causes of false-positive non-treponemal testing

Chronic infections	Leprosy
	HIV
	Malaria
	Tuberculosis
Autoimmune conditions	Lupus
	Polyarteritis nodosa
	ITP
Debilitated states	Chronic malnutrition
	Malignancy
	Cirrhosis
	IV drug use
	Old age
Infectious	Non-pallidum treponemal infections
	Spirochetal infections
	Vaccinations
Other	Persistent positive testing (serofast reaction)
	Pregnancy

Adapted from Ref. [43]

sensitive CSF FT-ABS should be sent to confirm the diagnosis if there is a high suspicion for neurological involvement [18, 44]. A lumbar puncture is considered positive for evidence of CNS involvement if there is a CSF WBC >5 cells/microliter, and/or a positive CSF VDRL, and/or a positive FT-ABS. There are no current recommendations for the treatment and management of a patient with a positive CSF-VDRL in a patient without neurological symptoms [18]. Additionally, patients with HIV and a very high titer (>1:32) should be evaluated for neurological involvement, even in the absence of neurological symptoms.

All testing should be interpreted in the context of a careful history. Important parts of the medical history include previous exposure and/or treatment of syphilis, response/resolution after treatment, exposure to non-pallidum treponemal species, comorbid conditions known to cause false-positive testing (see Table 14.4), as well as a detailed sexual history including timing and routes of exposure. All of the tests remain reliable in patients with HIV.

Additional/Adjunctive Testing

All patients who have a suspicion for syphilis should be tested for concurrent HIV infection due to the high coinfection rate. The coinfection can be as high as 16–28% with rates as high as 86% in MSM populations [21, 45–47]. This is due to the fact that syphilis enhances the transmission of HIV. Of additional concern is that infection with syphilis can worsen the severity of HIV disease by increasing HIV replication and lowering CD4 counts [48]. See Chap. 13 for more information on HIV and syphilis coinfection.

All patients who receive treatment should also have follow-up to monitor response to treatment. Typically patients have follow-up titers at 6 and 12 months.

The non-treponemal tests should have a fourfold decrease within 6–12 months. Persistent symptoms and inadequate decline or rising titers are suggestive of treatment failure or reinfection [18].

Management

Penicillin G is the treatment of choice for all forms and stages of syphilis. Only the length of treatment increases with the later stages of the disease (see Table 14.5). However it is important to note that the dosage, frequency, length of treatment, and route of administration change when there is evidence of infection in sequestered sites such as in CNS, ocular structures, or otic structures. This change in management underscores the importance in identifying CNS, ocular, and otic infections.

Penicillin Allergy

Due to the superiority of treatment of penicillin and concerns about the efficacy of alternative treatments, the expert recommendation is to consider either performing penicillin skin testing or admission for PCN desensitization before considering an alternative regimen [18, 21, 49, 50, 53]. There is weak evidence to support alternative options including ceftriaxone, doxycycline, tetracycline, and azithromycin, but none has very strong evidence of clinical efficacy (see Table 14.6). Further complicating matters are the steady worldwide rise in antibiotic resistance to azithromycin. This is especially true among MSM and HIV+ patients where azithromycin is no longer a recommended treatment [8].

Additionally clinicians should consider the patient's ability/willingness to be compliant with a lengthy and complicated PO regimen and their ability to access

Table 14.5 Treatment regimens for syphilis

Stage of disease	Treatment regimen
Primary syphilis, Secondary syphilis, and Early latent syphilis	Adult: Benzathine penicillin G 2.4 million units IM × 1 Child: Benzathine penicillin G 50,000 units/kg IM × 1 (up to the adult dose)
Late latent syphilis, Latent syphilis of unknown duration, Tertiary syphilis, and Retreatment	Adult: Benzathine penicillin G 2.4 million units IM × 3 doses spaced 1 week apart Child: Benzathine penicillin G 50,000 units/kg IM × 3 spaced 1 week apart (up to the adult dose)
Neuro−/ocular/otic syphilis	Aqueous crystalline penicillin G 18–24 million units per day, administered as 3–4 million units IV every 4 h or continuous infusion, for 10–14 days If there is no question about compliance: Procaine penicillin G 2.4 million units IM once daily plus probenecid 500 mg orally four times a day, both for 10–14 days

Adapted from Ref. [31]

Table 14.6 Alternative treatments for syphilis in the penicillin-allergic patient

Doxycycline 100 mg, PO BID × 14 days [45]
Tetracycline 500 mg po 4 × day 14 days [46]
Second line
Ceftriaxone 1–2 g / day im/iv for 10–14 days
(poor quality data supports the use in primary and secondary syphilis only)
Third line [31]
Azithromycin 2 g PO ×1 [47, 48]
(this regimen should only be used if there is a contraindication to both penicillin and doxycycline. This regimen should be only be used in populations with excellent follow-up and low rates of resistance. Thus should be avoided in MSM and HIV-positive patients and contraindicated in pregnant patients) [31]

care for repeat serological testing before starting an alternative treatment. In general experts continue to advocate for treatment with penicillin unless absolutely contraindicated.

There are *no* approved alternatives to the treatment of syphilis in pregnant women. Penicillin G is the only antibiotic with known efficacy for preventing maternal-fetal transmission and treating fetal infection [51, 54]. Therefore, all pregnant women with penicillin allergies must be admitted for desensitization and receive subsequent treatment with penicillin. Additionally pregnant women who miss any dose of therapy must repeat the full course of therapy [52, 55].

CNS/otic/ophthalmic syphilis infections should also be treated with IV penicillin to ensure cure in the infection of a "sequestered" site. Penicillin-allergic patients should also be admitted to the ICU for penicillin desensitization [56–58].

Jarisch-Herxheimer Reaction

The Jarisch-Herxheimer reaction commonly occurs with treatment of syphilis and can mimic sepsis or anaphylaxis with fevers, rigors, hypotension, flushing, myalgias, and headache. These systemic symptoms are a reaction to the large-scale death of the spirochetes. It typically occurs within 24 h of starting the treatment but has been described as early as 2 h after treatment. It is seen most commonly after the treatment of early syphilis.

The treatment for this is largely supportive. Although this reaction is generally not dangerous, there have been some case reports of early labor and fetal distress secondary to the Jarisch-Herxheimer reaction [43], but this should not be considered a contraindication for the treatment of a pregnant patient.

Partner Treatment

Transmission only occurs when there are mucocutaneous manifestations. Thus sexual transmission does not occur in late secondary and tertiary syphilis and is only indicated in early syphilis (see Table 14.7).

Table 14.7 Treatment of sexual contacts of patients with syphilis [18]

Sexual contact within the last 90 days	Sexual contacts of patients infected with early syphilis should be treated presumptively, even if diagnostic nesting is negative
Sexual contact greater than 90 days ago	If testing is not readily available or if follow-up is uncertain, sexual contacts should be treated empirically for early syphilis If diagnostic testing is available, treatment should be based on the results of the testing

Bottom Line: Clinical Pearls

- Syphilis has many atypical cutaneous presentations.
- Chancres are painless and develop at the site of inoculation and may be present anywhere on the body weeks to months after exposure.
- A diffuse rash involving the palms and soles occurs in 70% of patients with secondary syphilis. Half of patients will also have mucosal involvement.
- Syphilis typically has a latent period where the patient is asymptomatic but serologic positive.
- Tertiary syphilis includes numerous complications including neurologic and cardiac sequelae.
- In an immunocompromised patients, the stages of syphilis can overlap instead of being sequential [61].
- Diagnosis is by screening with non-treponemal testing (VDRL and RPR) and confirmed with treponemal testing (such as FTA-ABS).
- The preferred treatment for all cases of syphilis is penicillin. The dosing and route vary with the stage. Tertiary syphilis requires IV penicillin.
- All pregnant women must be treated with IV penicillin to prevent complications of congenital syphilis.

References

1. Centers for Disease Control and Prevention (CDC). Primary and secondary syphilis—United States, 2003-2004. JAMA. 2006;295:1890–1. https://doi.org/10.1001/jama.295.16.1890.
2. Peterman TA, Heffelfinger JD, Swint EB, Groseclose SL. The changing epidemiology of syphilis. Sex Transm Dis. 2005;32(10 Suppl):S4–10.
3. Barton J, Braxton J, Davis DW, et al. Centers for Disease Control and Prevention. Sexually Transmitted Disease Surveillance 2015. Atlanta: U.S. Department of Health and Human Services; 2016.
4. Karapetyan AF, Sokolovsky YV, Araviyskaya ER, et al. Syphilis among intravenous drug-using population: epidemiological situation in St Petersburg, Russia. Int J STD AIDS. 2016;13:618–23. https://doi.org/10.1258/09564620260216326.
5. Chen Z-Q, Zhang G-C, Gong X-D, et al. Syphilis in China: results of a national surveillance programme. Lancet. 2007;369:132–8.
6. Simms I, Fenton KA, Ashton M, et al. The re-emergence of syphilis in the United Kingdom: the new epidemic phases. Sex Transm Dis. 2005;32:220.

7. Martin IE, Tsang RSW, Sutherland K, et al. Molecular characterization of syphilis in patients in Canada: azithromycin resistance and detection of Treponema pallidum DNA in whole-blood samples versus ulcerative swabs. J Clin Microbiol. 2009;47:1668–73. https://doi.org/10.1128/JCM.02392-08.

8. Stamm LV. Global challenge of antibiotic-resistant Treponema pallidum. Antimicrob Agents Chemother. 2010;54:583–9. https://doi.org/10.1128/AAC.01095-09.

9. Lautenschlager S. Cutaneous manifestations of syphilis: recognition and management. Am J Clin Dermatol. 2006;7:291–304.

10. Lynn WA, Lightman S. Syphilis and HIV: a dangerous combination. Lancet Infect Dis. 2004;4:456–66. https://doi.org/10.1016/S1473-3099(04)01061-8.

11. Lautenschlager S. Cutaneous manifestations of syphilis. Am J Clin Dermatol. 2006;7:291.

12. Chapel TA, Prasad P, Chapel J, Lekas N. Extragenital syphilitic chancres. J Am Acad Dermatol. 1985;13:582–4. https://doi.org/10.1016/S0190-9622(85)70200-9.

13. Schofer H. Syphilis Klinik der Treponema-pallidum-Infektion. Der Hautarzt. 2004.

14. Haustein UF, Pfeil B, Zschiesche A. Analyse der von 1983–1991 an der Universitäts-Hautklinik Leipzig beobachteten Syphilisfälle. Der Hautarzt. 1993.

15. Alam F, Argiriadou AS, Hodgson TA, Kumar N, Porter SR. Primary syphilis remains a cause of oral ulceration. Br Dent J. 2000;189(7):352–4.

16. Arunkumar S, Prasad S, Loganathan B, et al. Extragenital chancre of the tongue. Int J STD AIDS. 2016;8:655–6. https://doi.org/10.1258/0956462971918814.

17. Sanchez MR. Syphilis. In: Freedberg IM, Eisen AZ, Wolff K, Austen KF, Goldsmith LA, Katz SI, editors. Fitzpatricks dermatology in general medicine. 6th ed. New York: McGraw-Hill; 2003. p. 2163–88.

18. Workowski KA, Berman SM. Centers for Disease Control and Prevention sexually transmitted diseases treatment guidelines. Clin Infect Dis. 2007;44(Suppl 3):S73–6. https://doi.org/10.1086/511430.

19. Singh AE, Romanowski B. Syphilis: review with emphasis on clinical, epidemiologic, and some biologic features. Clin Microbiol Rev. 1999;12:187–209.

20. Radolf JD, Tramont EC, Salazar JC. 239 – Syphilis (Treponema pallidum). In: Mandell, Douglas, and Bennett's principles and practice of infectious diseases. 8th ed. Philadelphia: Elsevier/Saunders; 2015. p. 2684–709.e5. https://doi.org/10.1016/B978-0-323-40161-6.00239-4.

21. Augenbraun M. 24 syphilis and the nonvenereal treponematoses. 2003; https://doi.org/10.2310/7900.1234.

22. de Vries HJC. Skin as an indicator for sexually transmitted infections. Clin Dermatol. 2014;32:196–208. https://doi.org/10.1016/j.clindermatol.2013.08.003.

23. Centers for Disease Control and Prevention. Recommendations for public health surveillance of syphilis in the United States. Atlanta: US Department of Health and Human Services; 2003.

24. World Health Organization. Guidelines for the management of sexually transmitted infections. World Health Organization. 2003. ISBN: 9241546263.

25. Chudomirova K, Chapkanov A, Abadjieva T, Popov S. Gummatous cutaneous syphilis. Sex Transm Dis. 2009;36:239–40. https://doi.org/10.1097/OLQ.0b013e3181917202.

26. Cohen SE, Klausner JD, Engelman J, Philip S. Syphilis in the modern era: an update for physicians. Infect Dis Clin North Am. 2013;27:705–22. https://doi.org/10.1016/j.idc.2013.08.005.

27. Dourmishev LA, Dourmishev AL. Syphilis: uncommon presentations in adults. Clin Dermatol. 2005;23:555–64. https://doi.org/10.1016/j.clindermatol.2005.01.015.

28. Tait IA. Uveitis due to secondary syphilis. Sex Transm Infect. 1983;59:397.

29. Sivaram M, Radcliffe KW. Acute visual loss as a presenting manifestation of syphilis. Int J STD AIDS. 2007;18(6):429–30.

30. Eandi CM, Neri P, Adelman RA, Yannuzzi LA, Cunningham ET Jr, Group ISS. Acute syphilitic posterior placoid chorioretinitis: report of a case series and comprehensive review of the literature. Retina. 2012;32(9):1915–41.

31. Diseases AAOPCOI (2015) Red Book.

32. Shah S. Pediatric practice infectious diseases: McGraw Hill Professional; New York, NY. 2008.
33. Tight RR, Warner JF. Skeletal involvement in secondary syphilis detected by bone scanning. JAMA. 1976;235:2326.
34. Campisi D, Whitcomb C. Liver disease in early syphilis. Arch Intern Med. 1979;139:365.
35. Bhorade MS, Carag HB, Lee HJ, Potter EV. Nephropathy of secondary syphilis: a clinical and pathological spectrum. JAMA. 1971;216(7):1159–66.
36. Winters HA, Notar-Francesco V, Bromberg K, Rawstrom SA, Vetrano J, Prego V, et al. Gastric Syphilis: Five Recent Cases and a Review of the Literature. Ann Intern Med. 1992;116:314–319. https://doi.org/10.7326/0003-4819-116-4-314.
37. Watts PJ, Greenberg HL, Khachemoune A. Unusual primary syphilis: presentation of a likely case with a review of the stages of acquired syphilis, its differential diagnoses, management, and current recommendations. Int J Dermatol. 2016;55:714–28. https://doi.org/10.1111/ijd.13206.
38. Lleó MI, Escribano PC, Prieto BM. Atypical cutaneous manifestations in syphilis. Actas Dermo-Sifiliográficas (English Edition). 2016;107:275–83. https://doi.org/10.1016/j.adengl.2016.02.002.
39. Balagula Y, Mattei PL, Wisco OJ, et al. The great imitator revisited: the spectrum of atypical cutaneous manifestations of secondary syphilis. Int J Dermatol. 2014;53:1434–41. https://doi.org/10.1111/ijd.12518.
40. Baughn RE, Musher DM. Secondary syphilitic lesions. Clin Microbiol Rev. 2005;18:205–16. https://doi.org/10.1128/CMR.18.1.205-216.2005.
41. Kelly JD, LeLeux TM, Citron DR, et al. Ulceronodular syphilis (lues maligna praecox) in a person newly diagnosed with HIV infection. BMJ Case Rep. 2011;2011:bcr1220103670. https://doi.org/10.1136/bcr.12.2010.3670.
42. Centers for Disease Control and Prevention (CDC). Discordant results from reverse sequence syphilis screening – five laboratories, United States, 2006-2010. MMWR Morb Mortal Wkly Rep. 2011;60:133–7.
43. Nandwani R, Evans DT. Are you sure it's syphilis? A review of false positive serology. Int J STD AIDS. 1995;6(4):241–8. https://doi.org/10.1177/095646249500600404.
44. Libois AS, De Wit SP, Poll BND, et al. HIV and syphilis: when to perform a lumbar puncture. Sex Transm Dis. 2007;34:141–4. https://doi.org/10.1097/01.olq.0000230481.28936.e5.
45. Ciesielski CA. Sexually transmitted diseases in men who have sex with men: an epidemiologic review. Curr Infect Dis Rep. 2003;5:145.
46. Su JR, Weinstock H (2011) Epidemiology of co-infection with HIV and syphilis in 34 states, United States—2009. In: Proceedings of the 2011 national HIV prevention ….
47. Centers for Disease Control and Prevention (CDC). Notes from the field: repeat syphilis infection and HIV coinfection among men who have sex with men – Baltimore, Maryland, 2010-2011. MMWR Morb Mortal Wkly Rep. 2013;62:649–50.
48. Shockman S, Buescher LS, Stone SP. Syphilis in the United States. Clin Dermatol. 2014;32:213–8. https://doi.org/10.1016/j.clindermatol.2013.08.005.
49. Zeltser R, Kurban AK. Syphilis. Clin Dermatol. 2004;22:461–8. https://doi.org/10.1016/j.clindermatol.2004.07.009.
50. Gadde J, Spence M, Wheeler B, Adkinson NF. Clinical experience with penicillin skin testing in a large inner-city STD clinic. JAMA. 1993;270:2456–63. https://doi.org/10.1001/jama.1993.03510200062033.
51. Alexander JM, Sheffield JS, Sanchez PJ. Efficacy of treatment for syphilis in pregnancy. Obstet Gynecol. 1999;93:5. https://doi.org/10.1016/S0029-7844(98)00338-X.
52. Nathan L, Bawdon RE, Sidawi JE, et al. Penicillin levels following the administration of benzathine penicillin G in pregnancy. Obstet Gynecol. 1993;82:338–42.
53. Sammet S, Draenert R. Case report of three consecutive lues maligna infections in an HIV-infected patient. Int J STD AIDS. 2017;28:523–5. https://doi.org/10.1177/0956462416674102.

54. Hook EW, Baker-Zander SA, Moskovitz BL, et al. Ceftriaxone therapy for asymptomatic neurosyphilis. Case report and Western blot analysis of serum and cerebrospinal fluid IgG response to therapy. Sex Transm Dis. 1986;13:185–8.
55. Hook EW, Roddy RE, Handsfield HH. Ceftriaxone therapy for incubating and early syphilis. J Infect Dis. 1988;158:881.
56. Ghanem KG, Erbelding EJ, Cheng WW, Rompalo AM. Doxycycline compared with benzathine penicillin for the treatment of early syphilis. Clin Infect Dis. 2006;42:e45–9. https://doi.org/10.1086/500406.
57. Wong T, Singh AE, De P. Primary syphilis: serological treatment response to doxycycline/tetracycline versus benzathine penicillin. Am J Med. 2008;121:903–8. https://doi.org/10.1016/j.amjmed.2008.04.042.
58. Riedner G, Rusizoka M, Todd J, et al. Single-dose azithromycin versus penicillin G benzathine for the treatment of early syphilis. N Engl J Med. 2005;353:1236–44. https://doi.org/10.1056/NEJMoa044284.
59. Rompalo AM, Joesoef MR, O'donnell JA, et al. Clinical manifestations of early syphilis by HIV status and gender: results of the syphilis and HIV study. Sex Transm Dis. 2001;28(3):158–65.
60. Ely JW, Stone MS. The generalized rash: part II. Diagnostic approach. Am Fam Physician. 2010;15(81.), 6th ser):735–9.
61. Augenbraun MH. Diseases of the reproductive organs and sexually transmitted diseases: genital skin and mucous membrane lesions. In: Mandell GL, Bennett JE, Dolin R, editors. Mandell, Douglas, and Bennett's principles and practice of infectious diseases. 7th ed. Philadelphia: Churchill Livingstone; 2009. p. 475–1484.
62. Scully C. Chapter 14: Soreness and ulcers. In: Oral and maxillofacial medicine : the basis of diagnosis and treatment. 2nd ed. Edinburgh: Churchill Livingstone; 2008. p. 131–9.
63. Gevorgyan O, Owen B, Balavenkataraman A, Weinstein M. A nodular-ulcerative form of secondary syphilis in AIDS. Proc (Bayl Univ Med Cent). 2017;30(1):80–2.

Meningococcemia

15

Danielle Wickman and Jan M. Shoenberger

Background

Neisseria meningitidis is an obligate human bacterial pathogen and must cause disease to be transmitted from one host to another. Meningococci are gram-negative, diplococci that can be encapsulated or unencapsulated. Meningococcemia is an infection caused by *N. meningitidis*, which has 13 clinically significant serogroups that are distinguishable by the structure of their capsular polysaccharides [1]. *N. meningitidis* is the leading cause of bacterial meningitis in children and young adults in the United States, with an overall mortality rate of 13%, and it is the second most common cause of community-acquired adult bacterial meningitis [2]. Worldwide, it also is known to cause outbreaks of epidemic meningitis and rapidly progressive fatal shock.

Classic Clinical Presentation

Four clinical syndromes are associated with meningococcal disease: (1) meningitis without shock (the most common presentation of invasive meningococcal disease); (2) fulminant meningococcal septicemia (fever, rash, hypotension, meningitis); (3) fever, rash, and hypotension but no clinical evidence of meningitis; and [3, 4] (4) chronic meningococcemia (rare).

D. Wickman · J. M. Shoenberger (✉)
Department of Emergency Medicine, Los Angeles County + USC Medical Center, Keck School of Medicine of the University of Southern California, Los Angeles, CA, USA
e-mail: shoenber@usc.edu

© Springer International Publishing AG, part of Springer Nature 2018
E. Rose (ed.), *Life-Threatening Rashes*, https://doi.org/10.1007/978-3-319-75623-3_15

Typical Presentation

Signs/symptoms:

- The disease often starts with a mild upper respiratory tract infection.
- Sudden onset fever, nausea, vomiting, headache, decreased ability to concentrate, myalgias (typically more painful than those in influenza).
- Up to a third of patients present without clinically apparent meningitis present with persistent hypotension in the setting of a fever and a rash [4].

Age Distribution:

- Two peak ages: infancy and late adolescence [4].

Time Course:

- Incubation: 1–14 days [4].
- Symptoms develop usually within 2 weeks of exposure and can rapidly progress over 6–24 h [2].

Rash:

- The classic non-blanching petechial rash appears as discrete lesions 1–2 mm in diameter, most frequently on the trunk and lower portions of the body but can be seen all over the body. The mucous membranes of the soft palate, ocular, and conjunctiva must be carefully examined for signs of hemorrhage. Over 50% of patients will have petechiae upon presentation. The petechiae of meningococcemia are usually larger and bluer than pinpoint petechiae caused by thrombocytopenia [4]. Petechiae can coalesce into larger purpuric and ecchymotic lesions.
- Mucosal petechiae may appear first, followed by skin petechiae that may become confluent as microvascular thrombosis progresses [3].
- Although skin findings in acute meningococcal infections are characteristically petechial, transient macular or papular lesions (Fig. 15.1) which can resemble those seen in viral exanthems, may be evident [3]. The petechiae are small and irregular with a "smudged" appearance. Although most often located on the extremities and trunk, lesions can also be found on the head, palms, soles, and mucous membranes.
- Skin findings in fulminant meningococcal septicemia can appear as extensive hemorrhagic lesions with central necrosis. Bullae can develop. Mucous membrane hemorrhages can be seen. Gangrenous hemorrhagic areas (indistinguishable from purpura fulminans) can appear in severe meningococcemia, often with disseminated intravascular coagulopathy (DIC) (Figs. 15.2 and 15.3).
- Skin lesions and bacteremia are rarely seen with meningococcal pneumonia.

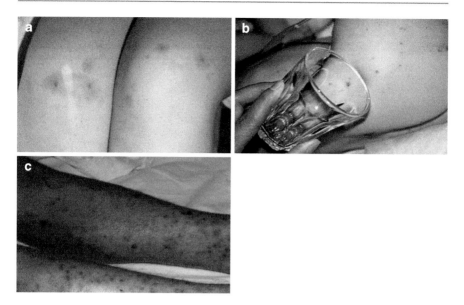

Fig. 15.1 Macular (**a**) and non-blanching petechial (**b**, **c**) rashes in meningococcemia. (Reproduced with permission from Ref. [4])

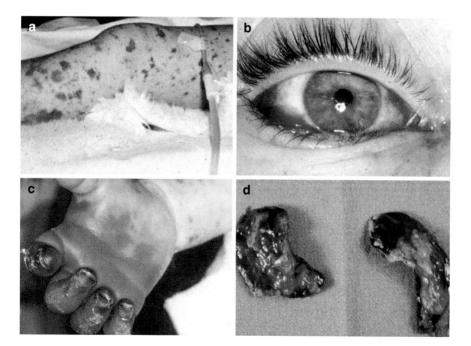

Fig. 15.2 Fulminant meningococcal septicemia. Skin with ecchymoses (**a**), conjunctival hemorrhage (**b**), thrombosis and gangrene of the fingers in a child who survived fulminant meningococcal septicemia (**c**), hemorrhagic adrenals in fulminant meningococcal septicemia (**d**). (Reproduced with permission from Ref. [4])

Fig. 15.3 Purpura
fulminans. (Photo credit:
Garrett Sterling, MD)

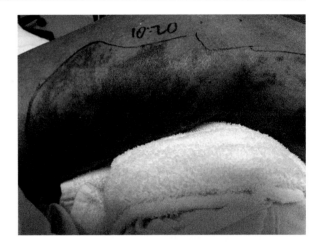

- Petechiae may be absent in up to 20% of children with meningococcemia. Peripheral circulatory failure is common in meningococcal sepsis, and ventricular dysfunction with elevated central venous pressure (CVP) is also seen in severe disease. Waterhouse-Friderichsen syndrome results from adrenal hemorrhage with resultant corticosteroid deficiency and causes circulatory collapse (Fig. 15.2) [3].
- Petechiae directly correlate with the degree of thrombocytopenia and serve as an important indicator of potential for bleeding secondary to DIC [2].

Atypical Presentation

Extrameningeal manifestations of meningococcal disease have been well described in the literature but are clinically rare [5–8]. Table 15.1 includes some of these possible clinical presentations. A myriad of atypical presentations have been reported including abdominal pain and meningococcal peritonitis [9–15]. Patients have presented with acute focal right lower quadrant pain which clinically mimicked appendicitis. Lower extremity myalgia is also a well described presenting complaint [12].

Most patients with atypical presentations subsequently grow gram-negative cocci on blood cultures [8], and some patients eventually develop the classic skin findings. Of note, some patients appear to have an attenuated course and do not manifest any skin changes or constitutional symptoms classically seen with meningococcemia. However, atypical presentations are not protective for a more severe course as subsequent disseminated intravascular coagulopathy and purpura fulminans may also occur [15].

Table 15.1 Meningococcemia presentations

Meningitis
Fulminant meningococcal septicemia
Persistent hypotension with rash and fever but no meningeal signs
Extrameningeal (e.g., pneumonia, epiglottitis, conjunctivitis, pericarditis, arthritis)

Table 15.2 Systemic symptoms of meningococcal infection

URI symptoms (nonspecific prodrome with cough, headache, sore throat)
Fever
Headache
Nausea, vomiting
Photophobia
Lethargy
Neck stiffness
Petechial rash
Hypotension
Disseminated intravascular coagulation (DIC)
Multiple organ failure

Associated Systemic Symptoms

The associated systemic symptoms range from URI-type symptoms to hypotension and DIC. Table 15.2 highlights some of the systemic symptoms that may be seen in the typical spectrum of meningococcal infection.

Time Course of Disease

Symptoms began within 2 weeks after exposure to an infected host. Initial symptoms include nonspecific symptoms such as cough, runny nose, and fever and may look like a typical viral infection. Symptoms can rapidly progress over 6–24 h to include rash, headache, photophobia, and systemic signs of infection (meningitis and/or septicemia).

Early recognition and treatment are critical since effective antibiotics immediately stop the proliferation of the bacteria. All meningococci in cerebrospinal fluid (CSF) are killed within 3–4 h after intravenous treatment with appropriate antibiotics. The case fatality rate is approximately 10% in developed nations (with treatment), and if untreated, the mortality rate is 70–90%.

Common Mimics and Differential Diagnosis

The differential diagnosis can include a variety of viral exanthems which can present with rash, fever, and headache. Rubella can look very similar on initial presentation as can various enteroviral infections. Other considerations include acute bacteremia and endocarditis, cutaneous necrotizing vasculitis, Rocky Mountain spotted fever (RMSF), toxic shock syndrome, purpura fulminans (Fig. 15.3), and leptospirosis.

Key Physical Exam Findings

Key physical exam findings include fever, headache, meningeal signs, and non-blanching rash. More than 60% of patients will present with meningitis without shock. As many as 30% of patients present without distinct signs of meningitis but will have hypotension, fever, and rash. A less common presentation will be severe, persistent shock without distinct signs of meningitis (fulminant meningococcal septicemia). Overall, most patients will present with fever (often high), but occasionally patients will have hypothermia which most often occurs in the setting of sepsis.

The rash is classically petechial and can be seen on the skin and, at times, the mucous membranes, including the sclera. The extremities are the most common regions involved. In fulminant disease, extensive hemorrhagic lesions may be seen. Purpura fulminans is associated with consumptive coagulopathy and is visualized as purpuric patches with sharply marginated borders, progressing to necrosis and eschar formation. Autoamputation is also a potential complication. Checking for meningeal signs including jolt accentuation test, nuchal rigidity, and Kernig and Brudzinski signs is advised; however, studies have shown that these physical exam findings are poor predictors for meningitis [16].

Diagnosis

- The gold standard for the identification of meningococcal infection is the bacteriologic isolation of *N. meningitidis* from sterile body fluids such as blood, cerebrospinal fluid (CSF), synovial fluid, pleural fluid, and pericardial fluid or skin biopsy.

Treatment

- Prompt antimicrobial treatment and aggressive septic shock management are the cornerstones of treatment. *Empiric antimicrobial treatment should be initiated immediately if diagnosis is suspected.*
- IV ceftriaxone or cefotaxime (can also be given IM if IV access is difficult or delayed).
- Treat sepsis and septic shock as appropriate including aggressive fluid resuscitation and vasopressor support, if necessary. Children should initially receive 20 cc/kg of fluid over 5–10 min and 60 cc/kg within 15 min with persistent hypotension. Adults should be given 20 cc/kg with escalation to further boluses as indicated.

- Treat adrenal insufficiency with corticosteroids. Patients with fulminant meningo-coccal septicemia often develop adrenal hemorrhage and may need corticosteroid support. Adrenal insufficiency should be suspected and treated in fluid-refractory shock.
  - Dexamethasone reduces morbidity in pneumococcal and *Haemophilus influenza b* meningitis. However, there is no evidence from randomized controlled trials that dexamethasone reduces death caused by cerebral edema or sequelae such as deafness in meningococcal meningitis [17, 18].
- Chemoprophylaxis of close contacts of those with invasive disease (including health-care workers directly involved in their care and exposed to respiratory secretions) may be accomplished with rifampin, ciprofloxacin, or ceftriaxone.

Complications

Meningococcal infection is fatal in approximately 10% of cases. There are both systemic and neurologic complications from bacterial meningitis. Systemic complications include: septic shock, disseminated intravascular coagulation, Waterhouse-Friderichsen syndrome, acute respiratory distress syndrome (ARDS), septic/reactive arthritis, and limb necrosis which may necessitate skin grafting. Neurologic complications are variable and can include seizures, sensorineural hearing loss, focal neurologic deficits, and intellectual disability.

> **Bottom Line: Clinical Pearls**
> Meningococcus is a life-threatening infection that has a significant mortality rate even with early recognition and initiation of treatment. This pathogen infects young, otherwise healthy people and is rapidly progressive. Symptoms are initially typically subtle and mimic benign viral infections. This diagnosis must be considered in every febrile patient with a rash, and return precautions for "viral syndromes" should include instruction to return for evaluation if a rash develops. Always reassess a patient prior to discharge if a rash develops or there is change in vital signs.

Essentials of the Clinical Presentation of Meningococcemia

- Fever
- Non-blanching petechial rash
- Headache +/− meningeal signs
- Mucous membrane petechiae
- Hypotension
- Shock

References

1. Takada S, Fujiwara S, Inoue T, et al. Meningococcemia in adults: a review of the literature. Intern Med. 2016;55(6):567–72.
2. Durand ML, Calderwood SB, Weber DJ, et al. Acute bacterial meningitis in adults. A review of 493 episodes. N Engl J Med. 1993;328(1):21–8.
3. Cohen MS, Rutala WA, Weber DJ. Chapter 180. Gram-negative coccal and bacillary infections. In: Fitzpatrick's dermatology in general medicine, 8th ed. (Goldsmith LA, Katz SI, Gilchrest BA, Paller AS, Leffell DJ, Wolff K. eds) McGraw-Hill, New York, 2012. http://accessmedicine.mhmedical.com/content.aspx?bookid=392&sectionid=41138907. Accessed 24 June 2017.
4. Stephens DS, Greenwood B, Brandtzaeg P. Epidemic meningitis, meningococcemia and *Neisseria meningitidis*. Lancet. 2007;369(9580):2196–210.
5. Kelly SJ, Robertson RW. *Neisseria meningitidis* peritonitis. ANZ J Surg. 2004;74(3):182–3.
6. Schaad UB. Arthritis in disease due to Neisseria meningitidis. Rev Infect Dis. 1980;2(6):880–8.
7. Wolf RE, Birbara CA. Meningococcal infections at an army training center. Am J Med. 1968;44(2):243–55.
8. Austin RP, Field AG, Beer WM. Right lower quadrant abdominal pain, fever, and hypotension: an atypical presentation of meningococcemia. Am J Emerg Med. 2015;33(11):1713.e3–4.
9. Wendlandt D, King B, Ziebell C, et al. Atypical presentation of fatal meningococcemia: peritonitis and paradoxical centrifugal purpura fulminans of late onset. Am J Emerg Med. 2011;29(8):960.e3–5.
10. Seaton RA, Nathwani D, Dick J, et al. Acute meningococcaemia complicated by late onset gastrointestinal vasculitis. J Infect. 2000;41(2):190–1.
11. Odegaard A. Unusual manifestations of meningococcal infection. A review. NIPH Ann. 1983;6(1):59–63.
12. Buckmaster ND, Boyce N. Two unusual presentations of *Neisseria meningitides* infection. Med J Aust. 1993;158(4):286.
13. Lannon DA, Smyth YM, Waldron R. Acute abdomen' with a rash. Int J Clin Pract. 2000;54(7):470–1.
14. Schmid ML. Acute abdomen as an atypical presentation of meningococcal septicaemia. Scand J Infect Dis. 1998;30(6):629–30.
15. Carpenter RR, Petersdorf RG. The clinical spectrum of bacterial meningitis. Am J Med. 1962;33:262–75.
16. Nakao JH, Jafri FN, Shah K, et al. Jolt accentuation of headache and other clinical signs: poor-predictors of meningitis in adults. Am J Emerg Med. 2014;32(1):24.8.
17. Gupta S, Tuladhar AB. Does early administration of dexamethasone improve neurological outcome in children with meningococcal meningitis? Arch Dis Child. 2004;89:82–3.
18. De Gans J, van de Beek D, et al. Dexamethasone in adults with bacterial meningitis. N Engl J Med. 2002;347(20):1549–56.

RMSF and Serious Tick-Borne Illnesses (Lyme, Ehrlichiosis, Babesiosis and Tick Paralysis)

Maureen McCollough

Background

Tick-borne illnesses plague large parts of North America especially in the warm summer months when vector burden is higher and exposure is more frequent due to outdoor activities. Rocky Mountain spotted fever (RMSF) along with other serious tick-borne illnesses found in the United States (US) such as Lyme disease, ehrlichiosis, babesiosis, and tick paralysis will be the focus of this chapter.

Tick-borne diseases include rickettsiae organisms such as intracellular gram-negative coccobacilli (e.g., *Rickettsia*, *Ehrlichia*, and *Anaplasma*), spirochetes (e.g., *Borrelia*), other bacteria (e.g., *Francisella tularensis*), protozoa (e.g., *Babesia*), and viruses.

Tick paralysis, or *tick toxicosis*, is unique to the "tick-borne illnesses"; in the fact it is not caused by an infectious organism. Tick paralysis is caused by a neurotoxin that is produced in the tick's salivary gland. Once the tick is fully engorged and still attached to the host, the tick transmits the toxin to its host.

The life cycle of tick-borne disease organisms includes ticks as the "vector" and vertebrates such as dogs, deer, or mice as "hosts." Humans are considered "accidental hosts" [1].

Table 16.1 shows organism, vector, and geographic distribution of Rocky Mountain spotted fever and other selected serious tick-borne illnesses.

According to the Centers for Disease Control and Prevention (CDC), tick-borne rickettsial diseases are on the increase in the United States (US) and continue to cause morbidity and mortality despite the availability of effective antibiotics [1].

M. McCollough
David Geffen School of Medicine at UCLA, Department of Emergency Medicine,
Los Angeles, CA, USA

Oliveview-UCLA Medical Center, Sylmar, CA, USA

© Springer International Publishing AG, part of Springer Nature 2018
E. Rose (ed.), *Life-Threatening Rashes*, https://doi.org/10.1007/978-3-319-75623-3_16

Table 16.1 Serious tick-borne illnesses demographics in the United States

Disease	Organism	US vector	US location (predominant)
RMSF *R. Rickettsii*	Spirochete *Rickettsia rickettsia*	*Dermacentor variabilis* (American dog tick) most commonly (Fig. 16.1 dog tick)	Most prevalent in southeastern and south Central United States
Lyme disease	Bacteria *Borrelia burgdorferi*	*Ixodes ricinus*	Northeastern and upper Midwestern states; some presence in Pacific Northwest
Ehrlichiosis, *E. chaffeensis*	Bacteria *Ehrlichia chaffeensis*	Lone star tick (*Amblyomma americanum*)	Southeastern United States, also Midwest and New England states
Babesiosis	Protozoa *Babesia*	*Ixodes* species	Northeast and Midwest areas
Tick paralysis	Toxin (not organism)	*Dermacentor andersoni* and *variabilis* (wood tick) most common	Pacific Northwest

Ten percent of children living in the Southeastern region of the United States have been found to be seropositive for prior rickettsial infections [2]. The lower incidence of clinically apparent cases is likely due to rickettsial infections with unknown or subclinical findings.

Increase in tick replication and increase in human outdoor activities in the warmer months result in a predominance of tick-borne infections occurring from April to October. Colder months are not immune with the CDC reporting 3% of RMSF and 3% of ehrlichiosis cases occurring in 2000–2007 from December to February. Almost 10% of RMSF cases in New York, New Jersey, and Pennsylvania occur in these winter months [3, 4].

Tick-borne infections are often not considered when the patient or parent of a child does not reveal or is unaware of exposure. Especially in summer months when tick illnesses are more prevalent, a thorough clinical history should include questions regarding tick exposure, work or recreational exposure to tick-infested areas, travel to areas where tick illness is endemic, and similar illness in family members, coworkers, or pet dogs [1]. Dogs can act as a transport for ticks into human dwellings and can transfer ticks directly to humans during human-dog interactions such as petting or bathing. A history of recent tick removal from a family pet might be useful in evaluating the potential for human tick exposure. Pets are susceptible to the same tick-borne illnesses as humans such as *R. rickettsia*, *E. chaffeensis*, *E. ewingii*, and *A. phagocytophilum*.

Ticks are small especially early on in their life cycle (nymphs are 1–2 mm) and will often attach themselves, usually painlessly, to less visible areas such as the hair or groin (Fig. 16.1). Ticks may remain on the skin feeding for several days without being noticed by the host. Data shows at least one-third of seropositive RMSF or ehrlichiosis patients do not remember being bitten [1, 5]. Patients may attribute a bite to other insects such as mosquitos, spiders, chiggers, or fleas which may be

Fig. 16.1 Dog tick
Dermacentor variabilis.
(Image appears with
permission from Centers
for Disease Control and
Prevention (CDC))

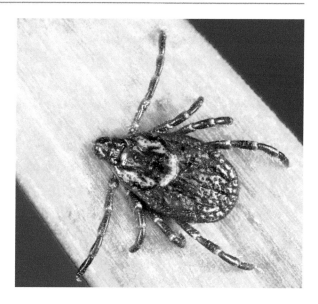

indistinguishable from a tick bite. Transmission of the tick-borne infection from the tick to the host occurs while the tick is feeding and has been attached to the host for about 6–10 h. Additionally, infection can be transmitted due to crushing of the tick during removal.

Ticks can attach and feed anywhere on the body but are most commonly found in the scalp, behind the ear, or in the groin, axilla, or perineum [6]. A thorough examination of the skin is imperative on any patient who presents with signs or symptoms in which the differential includes a tick-borne illness. Ticks have been found, after admission to the hospital, by parents, residents in training, nurses, or technicians [7]. When one tick is found, continued search for other ticks is recommended. Because tick paralysis is more common in girls, a very thorough search of what is often very thick, long hair is crucial. A fine-tooth comb can often aid in the search.

Risk factors for tick-borne illnesses include living in endemic areas and outdoor activities such as camping, hiking, gardening, walking dogs, golfing, or simply playing the backyard.

Prevention of tick-borne illness is mainly based on avoiding areas where ticks and their hosts are known to thrive in the late spring, summer, and early fall months. Light-colored clothing that covers the arms and lower legs is required including long-sleeved shirts buttoned at the cuffs and long pants tucked into socks or boots.

Clothing can be sprayed with permethrin (Permanone). Pretreated clothing with permethrin can be purchased and is considered safe for use by adults and children [5]. DEET-containing products (N,N-diethyl-meta-toluamide) can be applied to the skin as protection against tick bites. Both the Environmental Protection Agency (EPA) and the American Academy of Pediatrics (AAP) have concluded that, when used properly, DEET products are safe for both adults and children with the AAP recommending a 10–30% concentration for children older than 2 months old. Picaridin, 5–10% concentration, is also now available in the United States and safe for children [5, 8].

If time is spent outdoors, the body should be thoroughly searched for ticks. High-risk areas include the head, neck, axilla, and scrotum. Any ticks found should be removed as soon as possible with fine-tipped tweezers using steady pressure to gently pull back- and upward to remove the tick from the skin. If tweezers are not available, then fingers with gloves or tissues can be used. Alternative removal methods such as application of isopropyl alcohol, petroleum jelly, or a hot extinguished match are not recommended and are more likely to result in transmission of organisms [5].

Keeping grass mowed and avoiding plants or shrubberies that attract hosts such as deer are important. Fencing to deter deer and walls to deter mice can help keep these hosts away from property [9].

Vaccines are not available and prophylactic antibiotic treatment after known tick exposure is not recommended [5].

Spotted fever group rickettsiosis, ehrlichiosis, and anaplasmosis are all reportable conditions in the United States. It is important that providers check with their local health departments for an accurate list of reportable conditions. A brief summary of Rocky Mountain spotted fever and some of the more serious tick-borne illnesses mentioned in this chapter can be found in Table 16.2.

Rocky Mountain Spotted Fever

Rocky Mountain spotted fever is caused by the organism *Rickettsia rickettsia*, the most common rickettsial infection in the United States [10]. Transmitted by the dog tick *Dermacentor variabilis* (Fig. 16.1), *R. rickettsia* is an intracellular pathogen that infects vascular endothelial cells and, less often, underlying smooth muscle cells of small and medium vessels. This infection causes direct vascular injury, prostaglandin production that may cause increase vascular permeability, and perivascular lymphocytic infiltrate. Clotting factor activation results but rarely disseminated intravascular coagulation (DIC). Infection leads to this systemic vasculitis that is characterized by petechial skin lesions. Untreated RMSF can have potentially fatal consequences.

Although RMSF has been reported in all areas of the contiguous United States, predominance is in the Southern and Eastern regions [11, 12]. According to the CDC, the incidence of RMSF is now reported under a new category called spotted fever group (SFG) rickettsiosis that captures other spotted fever group *Rickettsia* species. The number of SFG cases has been steadily increasing since 2000, peaking in 2012 to 14.2 cases per million persons [1]. Whether this is truly an increase in disease or just improved reporting is controversial. Transmission of *R. rickettsia* has been seen after blood products transfusions [1].

Table 16.2 Tick-borne illnesses clinical and laboratory findings

Disease	Incubation period	Clinical characteristics	Laboratory findings
RMSF *R. Rickettsii*	Symptoms appear 3–12 days after initial tick bite	Diffuse macular or papular rash starting on wrists and ankles (often palms/soles) spreading to arms, legs, trunk, associated with systemic symptoms such as fever, headache, myalgias, and malaise	Thrombocytopenia, increased hepatic transaminase levels, normal or increased white blood cell count with increased immature neutrophils, hyponatremia, increased serum urea nitrogen, creatinine, and bilirubin
Lyme disease	Symptoms appear 7–14 days after initial tick bite but may be as long as 30 days	Erythema migrans, solitary erythematous lesion, at site of tick bite followed weeks to months later by multiple erythema migrans, neurological, or cardiac sequelae, followed months to years later by arthritis	Mild thrombocytopenia, mild leukopenia, increased hepatic transaminase levels
Ehrlichiosis, *E. Chaffeensis*	Symptoms appear 1–2 weeks after tick bite, but shorter periods have been reported	Maculopapular rash, not as common as the RMSF rash and less often on palms and soles; leukopenia and thrombocytopenia	Leukopenia, thrombocytopenia, increased hepatic transaminase levels, hyponatremia, anemia
Babesiosis	Symptoms appear 1–6 weeks after tick bite	Fever, fatigue, weakness	Hemolysis of RBCs
Tick paralysis	Symptoms may not appear for several days after tick bite	Acute symmetric ascending paralysis eventually effecting the upper extremities and respiratory muscles; mental status not affected unless hypoxia from respiratory failure ensues	No laboratory abnormalities define tick paralysis

Classic Clinical Presentation

Although clinical symptoms and signs vary somewhat between the tick-borne illnesses, most cases present with nonspecific features such as fever, nausea, and headache. Because of these nonspecific features early on, practitioners will often attribute the illness to more common viral processes such as acute gastroenteritis or bacterial processes such as streptococcal pharyngitis.

RMSF presents classically in approximately 90% of patients with a macular and then maculopapular rash (small 1–5 mm lesions) 2–4 days after onset of fever [13]

Fig. 16.2 RMSF rash
adult (Image appears with
permission from VisualDx)

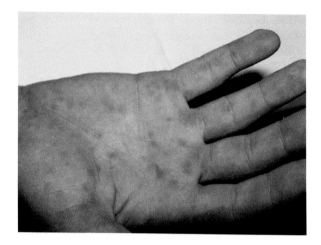

Fig. 16.3 RMSF rash
child (Image appears with
permission from VisualDx)

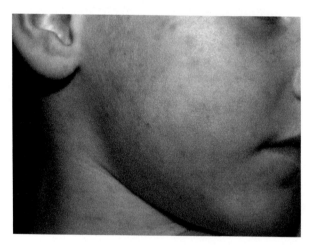

(Fig. 16.2). The rash may soon become petechial or purpuric in about 50% of cases. Classically beginning on the wrists and ankles, and often involving palms and soles, the rash soon spreads to the arms, legs, and trunk. The rash may be transient or localized to one region of the body [5]. The rash is typically not pruritic. Darker skin may make the rash less noticeable. Children develop the rash more often than adults and develop the rash earlier in the course of the illness [1, 11] (Fig. 16.3). The rash may even be absent in up to 10% of cases making the diagnosis more difficult and a fatal outcome more likely [1, 14]. In severe cases, distal areas such as fingers and toes may develop necrosis due pathogen-induced damage to the small vessels.

Atypical Presentation

An atypical presentation would be late onset or absence of rash, significant gastro-intestinal symptoms early in the disease, or lack of headache [1].

Associated Systemic Symptoms

RMSF clinical presentation includes fever, headache, chills, myalgias, and fatigue. Nausea, vomiting, abdominal pain, anorexia, and photophobia have also been noted [1]. Headache is usually more present in adults. Especially in children, abdominal pain may be a prominent complaint, and an erroneous diagnosis of gastroenteritis can occur early on before the rash is present. Pedal edema is especially noticeable in children. The classic triad of RMSF (fever, rash, and headache) is present in only 5% of patients in the first few days but up to 60–70% of patients by the second week [5, 15, 16]. Rash, fever, and a history of a tick bite are equally insensitive [5]. Other less common symptoms include diarrhea, conjunctival suffusion, peripheral edema (more often in children), calf pain, transient hearing loss, hepatomegaly, or splenomegaly [1].

Time Course of Disease (Incubation Period After Exposure to Infectious Agent or Drug Exposure)

Symptoms of RMSF typically present 3–12 days after an infected tick bite. Patients who go on to develop severe disease generally present with symptoms sooner [1].

Common Mimics and Differential Diagnosis

Early RMSF has similar symptoms to many common disorders. Headache and fever may be attributed to viral syndrome, meningitis, or encephalitis. The maculopapular rash may be thought due to drug reaction, viral syndrome, scarlet fever, or Kawasaki disease. Abdominal pain associated with RMSF has been mistaken for appendicitis, cholecystitis, or gastroenteritis [1]. Significant cutaneous necrosis or vasculitis of RMSF may be mistaken for meningococcemia or an idiopathic vasculitis such as Kawasaki disease in children.

Key Physical Exam Findings and Diagnostic Features

The key physical exam finding of RMSF is the maculopapular, and then often vasculitic, rash starting on the distal extremities.

Laboratory tests are generally not revealing with the total leukocyte count usually normal or slightly elevated with increased numbers of immature neutrophils. Mild thrombocytopenia ($<150,000/mm^3$) occurs in about 60% of patients, and half of patients may have mild hyponatremia (<135 mEq/L) or transaminitis. Thrombocytopenia is thought due to increased destruction at the areas of pathogen-induced vascular injury. Other laboratory abnormalities include increases in serum urea nitrogen or creatinine and bilirubin. A prolonged prothrombin or partial thromboplastin time can also be seen. If analyzed, cerebrospinal fluid (CSF) may show a predominance of lymphocyte or monocyte pleocytosis (usually <100 cells/microL) and increased protein concentration (100–200 mg/dL) [1, 11]. Azotemia can be present and is likely due to hypovolemia.

Serology testing using indirect fluorescent antibody (IFA) testing to RMSF *Rickettsia* can be performed. Typically IgG and IgM antibodies do not appear until 7–10 days after the onset of symptoms, and therefore IFA testing cannot be used in the decision to treat in the first few days of the illness.

Management

Treatment for RMSF should be started as soon as possible. In several studies, patients, ultimately diagnosed with RMSF, were shown to seek care early on in the illness when the diagnosis was not as obvious [5]. Mortality due to RMSF has been shown to be linked in delays to antimicrobial treatment [5]. Treatment therefore may need to be started when clinical suspicion of RMSF is high and not wait for definitive diagnosis. Serum antibodies to *Rickettsia* causing RMSF may not be positive for 7–10 days into the illness, and therefore serology testing may be negative when the patients present early in the course of the illness. If the decision is made to test for disease, then antimicrobial therapy should probably be started.

Doxycycline is the drug of choice for the treatment of RMSF for both adults and children. Five- to 7-day duration of therapy is usually curative [16, 17] (Table 16.3). Chloramphenicol had been the treatment of choice because of the perceived risk of permanent teeth staining by doxycycline but has now fallen out of favor and is not available orally in the United States. Chloramphenicol is less effective, does not provide treatment for ehrlichiosis which can be difficult to differentiate from RMSF, and has its own toxicity including aplastic anemia. Concerns over a short course use of doxycycline and its effects on teeth also appear unfounded. The CDC and the American Academy of Pediatrics (AAP) have recommended doxycycline as the treatment of choice for all children with suspected rickettsial disease [1, 5].

Other antibiotics such as beta-lactams, macrolides, aminoglycosides, and sulfonamides are not effective against RMSF. Severe doxycycline allergy such as anaphylaxis or Stevens-Johnson may require the use of an alternative antibiotic, inpatient desensitization, and/or consultation with an infectious disease expert.

The use of doxycycline during pregnancy remains inconclusive as controlled studies regarding teeth staining or teratogenicity have not been reported [1].

More severe presentation or inability to take oral antibiotics should prompt inpatient treatment. Fever should typically subside within 24–48 h after treatment if antibiotics are started in the first 4–5 days of illness.

Complications

Complications include end-stage manifestations such as meningoencephalitis, cerebral edema, acute renal failure, cutaneous necrosis, non-cardiogenic pulmonary edema (acute respiratory distress syndrome, ARDS), arrhythmia, shock, and seizures.

Table 16.3 Antibiotic treatment of tick-borne illnesses

Tick-borne illness	Adults	Children
RMSF, *R. rickettsii*	Doxycycline 100 mg PO or IV BID for 5–7 days	Doxycycline 2 mg/kg PO or IV BID for 5–7 days (for children <45 kg)
Lyme disease	Doxycycline 100 mg PO BID for 10–21 days Amoxicillin 500 mg PO TID for 14–21 days Cefuroxime axetil 500 mg PO BID for 14–21 days	Doxycycline 2 mg/kg PO BID (max dose 100 mg) for 10–21 days Amoxicillin 50 mg/kg PO divided TID (max dose 500 mg) for 14–21 days Cefuroxime 30 mg/kg PO per day divided BID (max dose 500 mg) for 14–21 days
Ehrlichiosis	Doxycycline 100 mg PO BID for 10 days Rifampin 300 mg PO BID for 10 days	Doxycycline 2 mg/kg PO BID (max dose 100 mg) for 10 days Rifampin 10 mg/kg PO BID (max dose 300 mg) for 10 days
Babesiosis, *B. microti*	(1) Atovaquone 750 mg orally every 12 h plus azithromycin 500 mg/d orally on day 1 and then 250 mg/d from day 2 onward for 7–10 days (2) Quinine 650 mg orally every 6–8 h plus clindamycin 600 mg orally every 8 h for 7–10 days#* For severe disease, consider clindamycin 300–600 mg IV every 6–8 h or 600 mg PO every 6–8 h plus quinine 650 mg PO every 6–8 h # Regiment (2) better tolerated *Treatment of choice during pregnancy	(1) Atovaquone 20 mg/kg orally every 12 h (max 750 mg/dose) plus azithromycin 10 mg/kg orally on day 1 (max 500 mg) and then 5 mg/kg (max 250 mg/d) orally from day 2 onward for 7–10 days@ (2) Quinine 8 mg/kg orally every 8 h (max 650 mg/d) plus clindamycin 7–10 mg/kg orally every 6–8 h (max 600 mg/dose) for 7–10 days# For severe disease, consider clindamycin 7–10 mg/kg IV every 6–8 h (max 600 mg/dose) or 7–10 mg/kg PO every 6–8 h (max 600 mg/dose) @ Used safely in kids >5 kg # Regiment (2) better tolerated
Tick paralysis	Removal of the tick Given that tick paralysis is not an infectious process, no specific antibiotic treatment is warranted unless evidence of an infectious process exists	Removal of the tick Given that tick paralysis is not an infectious process, no specific antibiotic treatment is warranted unless evidence of an infectious process exists

A small portion of patients with severe RMSF may suffer long-term sequelae such as peripheral neuropathy, hemiparesis, or deafness [16].

Mortality due to RMSF has significantly decreased as a result of antimicrobial therapy. Prior to antibiotics, mortality generally ranged from 20% to 30% [10]. Recent data from the CDC shows a case fatality rate of less than 1% since 2001 [1]. Mortality is highest in the very young (<4 years old), 3–4%, and the elderly (>60 years old), 4–9% [1, 10]. Other risk factors for complications include male gender, black race, chronic alcohol abuse, and G6PD (glucose-6-phosphate dehydrogenase) deficiency. Treatment for RMSF should ideally begin within 5 days of the start of symptoms; delay in treatment has also been shown to contribute to mortality [10, 13].

Lyme Disease

Lyme disease, caused primarily by the bacterial spirochete *Borrelia burgdorferi*, is endemic to the Northeastern and Upper Midwestern states with some presence in the Pacific Northwest. Illnesses in travelers to endemic areas and false-positive testing can account for reports of Lyme disease in non-endemic areas. The tick vector is *Ixodes ricinus.*

Classic Clinical Presentation

Clinical manifestations of Lyme disease present classically in three stages: early localized, early disseminated, and late disease; some patients may initially present with a later stage symptomatology.

The *early localized stage* presents with an erythematous expanding patch often with central clearing located at the site of the tick bite. The rash, known as erythema migrans (EM), is usually nonpruritic and nontender and may have purpuric, vesicular, or pustular components (Figs. 16.4 and 16.5). In adults, EM lesions are often found in or near the axilla, inguinal region, popliteal fossa, or belt line. In children, the EM lesions are more often found in the head and neck, arms and legs, and back areas [18]. Eighty percent of adult and pediatric patients manifest the rash [19, 20].

If the early localized stage is not treated, the spirochete will then enter the blood stream resulting in the *early disseminated stage*, manifesting as disseminated erythema migrans lesions. Neurological sequelae include lymphocytic meningitis, cranial nerve palsies (especially facial nerve), radiculopathy (Bannwarth syndrome), peripheral neuropathy, or rarely cerebellar ataxia or encephalomyelitis. Lyme disease is one of the few causes of bilateral facial nerve palsies. Lyme meningitis will present similarly to other viral meningitis in addition to erythema migrans, possible

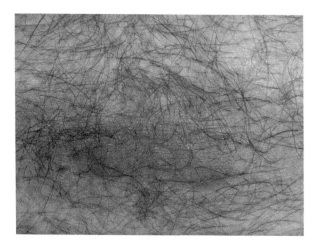

Fig. 16.4 Lyme disease, erythema migrans (Image appears with permission from VisualDx)

Fig. 16.5 Lyme disease, erythema migrans. Image appears with permission from Centers for Disease Control and Prevention (CDC)

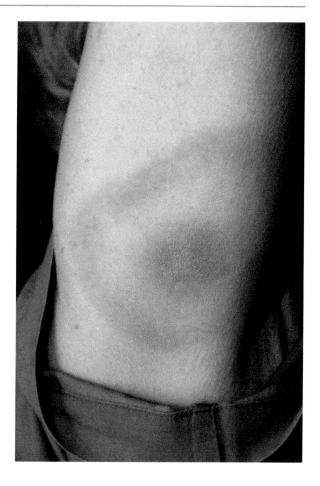

cranial nerve palsy or palsies, papilledema, prolonged duration of symptoms, and minimal polymorphonuclear cells in the CSF. Facial nerve palsy without signs of central nervous system infection (e.g., severe headache, vomiting, nuchal rigidity, or papilledema) does not necessarily require a lumbar puncture.

Cardiac sequelae can include atrioventricular heart block or sometimes myoperi-carditis. Early disseminated stage can occur weeks to months after the tick bite. Ocular findings include conjunctivitis, keratitis, and uveitis.

Late disease stage results in intermittent or persistent arthritis involving usually one or more large joints especially the knees (Fig. 16.6). Rarely, neurological symptoms such as mild encephalopathy ("Lyme encephalopathy") or polyneuropathy may persist. Late disease presents months to a few years after the tick bite and may be the presenting sign of Lyme disease.

Patients with Lyme disease almost always also present with classic signs and symptoms such as erythema migrans, facial nerve palsy, or arthritis of larger joints. If these classic signs or symptoms are not present in the setting of nonspecific consti-tutional signs and symptoms, then Lyme disease is not the likely diagnosis [1, 5, 11].

Fig. 16.6 Lyme disease arthritis (Image appears with permission from Emily Rose MD)

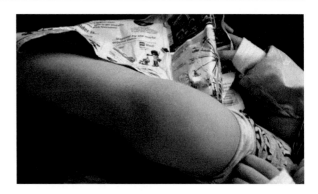

Atypical Presentation

Not all Lyme disease cases manifest all three stages. In some cases, disseminated erythema migrans, arthritis, or neurological symptoms may be the first presentation.

Associated Systemic Symptoms

Constitutional symptoms such as fatigue, headache, myalgias, and arthralgias are seen in close to half of affected patients. Fever may not be as common [21]. Respiratory or gastrointestinal symptoms are not common with Lyme disease.

Time Course of Disease (Incubation Period After Exposure to Infectious Agent or Drug Exposure)

Early localized signs of erythema migrans appears usually within 7–14 days after the tick bite but as long as 30 days. Early disseminated may take weeks to months with late Lyme disease presenting, sometimes, years later.

Common Mimics and Differential Diagnosis

Hypersensitivity to a tick bite can mimic Lyme disease. Hypersensitivity will result in a small lesion, <5 cm, which will defervesce by 24–48 h. Erythema migrans lesion will continue to grow in size.

STARI (southern tick-associated rash illness) has an erythema migrans-like rash, similar to the rash of Lyme disease. Found in the Southeastern and South Central areas of the United States, STARI does not appear to progress to disseminated illness as Lyme disease does if left untreated.

Nummular eczema results in multiple circular lesions, 2–10 cm in diameter, located on the trunk and extremities that are intensely pruritic.

Tinea corporis (ringworm), a dermatophytic infection, manifests as an enlarging pruritic circular or oval erythematous patch or plaque with central clearing and erythematous border.

Erythema multiforme manifests as distinctive target lesions.

Key Physical Exam Findings and Diagnostic Features

The key physical exam finding is the classic rash of erythema migrans.

Laboratory findings include erythrocyte sedimentation rate more than twice normal. Other laboratory abnormalities such as elevated serum creatine phosphokinase, leukocytosis, leukopenia, or anemia are seen much less frequently. Serological testing is not sensitive enough during early localized disease and so is not helpful in making the diagnosis. Blood cultures for *B. burgdorferi* are not commercially available.

Management

Treatment for early Lyme disease (erythema migrans) is the same whether the patient has the initial erythema migrans lesion or multiple from more disseminated disease without evidence of neurological or cardiac involvement. The goal is to reduce the risk of development of late Lyme disease. Amoxicillin, doxycycline, or cefuroxime axetil are considered first-line therapy for patients with Lyme disease (Table 16.3). Doxycycline is often used because of its effectiveness against *Anaplasma phagocytophilum*, a potential coinfecting organism. Although doxycycline's effect on the teeth of young children appears unfounded [5], amoxicillin is a viable alternative.

In the United States, macrolides such as azithromycin or erythromycin are not recommended as first-line therapy for erythema migrans. Macrolides may be used in patients who are intolerant of the first-line therapy antibiotics, but patients should be closely monitored for inadequate response to treatment. First-generation cephalosporins such as cephalexin are not effective against Lyme disease. Early Lyme disease (erythema migrans) may be mistaken for cellulitis. In endemic areas, it's important for providers to consider treatment of "cellulitis" with an antibiotic that also treats erythema migrans, such as amoxicillin-clavulanate or cefuroxime.

Early disseminated Lyme disease presenting with acute neurological findings such as meningitis, facial nerve palsy, and/or motor or sensory neuropathies often requires intravenous antibiotic treatment. Studies are limited but it appears high-dose penicillin is effective, as is ceftriaxone or cefotaxime. Facial nerve palsy even meningitis has been treated successfully in Europe using oral doxycycline. Guidelines from the American Academy of Neurology (2007) and the Infectious Diseases Society of America (2006) both still recommend parenteral therapy. Consultation with an infectious disease specialist is recommended [21].

Up to 15% of patients with early Lyme disease, especially those with multiple skin lesions, may experience a worsening of symptoms during the first 24 h of treatment. What is thought to be a Jarisch-Herxheimer reaction is due to the immune response to antigens released by the treated organisms [21].

From 4% to 28% of Lyme disease patients will also be infected with other organisms transmitted by *Ixodes* ticks. In the United States, these include *A. phagocytophilum* (causes human granulocytic anaplasmosis) and *Babesia microti* (causes babesosis) [22, 23]. Because of this, doxycycline is considered the drug of choice in areas where coinfection is high.

Complications

Coinfection with another tick-borne illness may occur. In the Unites States, other organisms transmitted by the *Ixodes* tick include *Anaplasma phagocytophilum* and *Babesia microti*. Patients with Lyme disease who are persistently febrile after 48 h of antimicrobial treatment warrant a search for a coinfection. Anemia, leukopenia, and/or thrombocytopenia may occur with these other coinfections.

Unlike syphilis, another spirochete disease, current evidence shows that Lyme disease occurring during pregnancy poses no threat for a congenital abnormality or fetal demise [21].

Some patients treated for Lyme disease may experience persistent nonspecific symptoms such as fatigue or musculoskeletal pain. The Infectious Diseases Society of America (IDSA) defines this post-Lyme disease syndrome as requiring a prior history of Lyme disease treated with an accepted regimen and resolution or stabilization of initial symptoms. Later, subjective symptoms such as fatigue, musculoskeletal pain, or cognitive difficulties occur within 6 months of the Lyme disease diagnosis and persist for at least 6 months [24]. Other diagnoses such autoimmune, malignancy, or psychiatric illnesses must be excluded. There is no evidence that these patients have persistent *Borrelia burgdorferi* infections [5, 24]. Prolonged courses of antibiotics to treat these persistent symptoms have not been shown to be helpful. The Infectious Diseases Society of America (IDSA) specifically recommends against treating persistent Lyme disease symptoms with prolonged courses of antibiotics [5, 24].

Ehrlichiosis

The most important ehrlichial disease is human monocytic ehrlichiosis (HME) caused by *Ehrlichia chaffeensis*. Two other *Ehrlichia* species also cause human disease but less frequently – *E. ewingii* and EML agent ehrlichiosis. Human granulocytic anaplasmosis (HGA), previously known as human granulocytic ehrlichiosis, is caused by *Anaplasma phagocytophilum*. In some references, HGA and HME are both considered ehrlichial diseases; in other references the diseases are separated as anaplasmosis and ehrlichiosis. Although these are considered separate diseases, their clinical and laboratory presentations are similar. This section will focus mainly on HME caused by *E. chaffeensis*.

Incidence of ehrlichiosis has been on the rise over time in the United States [1, 25]. In 2012, the annual incidence of ehrlichiosis was 3.2 cases per million persons with wide variation by state [1]. In some states, ehrlichiosis may be more common than RMSF.

E. chaffeensis (causing HME) is most commonly transmitted by the lone star tick (*Amblyomma americanum*). *A. phagocytophilum* (causing HGA) is most commonly transmitted by the *Ixodes* tick species, *I. scapularis* (black-legged tick) in the Eastern United States and *I. pacificus* (Western black-legged tick) in the Western United States [1].

Ehrlichiosis cases have been reported in the Southeastern United States and extending into the Midwest and New England states. Highest reported rates include Arkansas, Delaware, Missouri, Oklahoma, Tennessee, and Virginia.

White-tailed deer appears to be an important host for a number of *Ehrlichia* species. It has been reported that ehrlichiosis can be transmitted via maternal-child transmission, blood transfusion, or direct contact with a slaughtered deer [26].

Ehrlichia are obligate intracellular bacteria that grow in animal and human leukocytes. The organisms multiply in cytoplasmic membrane-bound vacuoles and form clusters of bacteria called morulae. In fatal cases, the greatest burden of bacteria has been found in the spleen, lymph nodes, and bone marrow [1]. The patient's systemic inflammatory response is likely responsible for most of the clinical findings of ehrlichiosis [1].

Classic Clinical Presentation

The clinical presentation of ehrlichiosis is similar to RMSF and can run the spectrum from subclinical to acute to chronic infection.

Compared with RMSF, the rash associated with HME is present less often occurring in only one-third of adults and two-thirds of children. The rash varies ranging from maculopapular or petechial to diffuse erythema (Fig. 16.7). The rash appears a few days later than in RMSF and is less often petechial. The ehrlichial rash is typically on the extremities and trunk less commonly involving the palms and soles. The rash occurs more often in children than in adults [1].

Atypical Presentation

Subclinical infections of ehrlichiosis may go unrecognized.

Fig. 16.7 Ehrlichiosis
(Image appears with
permission from VisualDx)

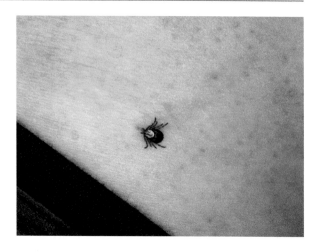

Associated Systemic Symptoms

Most patients with ehrlichiosis are febrile but many may be low grade. Nonspecific symptoms such as headache, myalgias, and malaise may occur in up to two-thirds of patients; cough, vomiting, and arthralgias can occur in up to 50% of patients [26]. Children have a similar presentation to adults. Neurological symptoms such as altered mental status, stiff neck, and clonus can happen but are not common. When CSF is evaluated, lymphocytic pleocytosis and elevated protein levels may be found [27].

Time Course of Disease (Incubation Period After Exposure to Infectious Agent or Drug Exposure)

The incubation period for ehrlichial diseases appears to be 1–2 weeks but shorter time frames have been seen.

Common Mimics and Differential Diagnosis

Ehrlichiosis has often been called "spotless" RMSF but *R. rickettsii* may also result in a spotless infection. The combination of leukopenia and no rash in the setting of tick-borne illness makes ehrlichiosis more likely. The differential diagnoses also include viral infections such as mononucleosis or *West Nile virus*, thrombotic thrombocytopenic purpura, malignancies, or liver disorders such as viral hepatitis or cholangitis.

Key Physical Exam Findings and Diagnostic Features

Laboratory results include leukopenia (<4000/mm^3) occurring in 60% of patients and up to 90% of patients showing thrombocytopenia, elevated transaminases,

Fig. 16.8 Peripheral blood smear of *E. chaffeensis* (ehrlichiosis) morulae (Image appears with permission from Centers for Disease Control and Prevention (CDC))

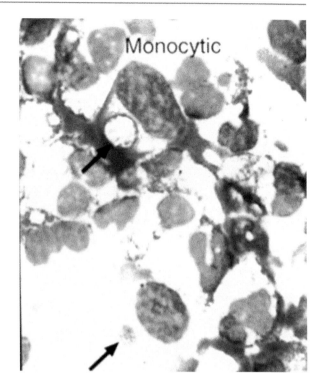

lactate dehydrogenase, and alkaline phosphatase. Anemia and elevated creatinine may also be seen [1, 11, 28]. CSF evaluation may show a lymphocytic pleocytosis with CSF white blood cells typically <250 cells/microL (higher in children) and elevated protein.

In some patients, morulae may be observed in monocytes in peripheral blood or in CSF (Fig. 16.8). Visualization of morulae still requires confirmatory testing. Culture of the *Ehrlichia* bacteria is very difficult. The preferred method is the indirect fluorescent antibody (IFA) test. Antibodies, however, are not detectable for the first 2–3 weeks of the illness.

Management

When ehrlichiosis is the most reasonable diagnosis (history of tick bite or tick exposure during spring or summer months in an endemic area with a fever, leukopenia, and/or thrombocytopenia), then doxycycline is the treatment of choice. As stated in the section on RMSF, doxycycline has not been shown to have the risk of staining permanent teeth like tetracycline and therefore is safe to use in both adults and children (Table 16.3). Currently, no guidelines exist for the treatment of ehrlichiosis in pregnant women, but doxycycline has been used to treat severe ehrlichiosis in pregnant women [10].

Complications

Mortality rate for ehrlichiosis is estimated to 3% with highest rates among children less than 10 years old and older individuals greater than 70 years old [1]. Patients who are immunocompromised or have chronic illnesses are also at higher risk for death [1]. Complications include seizures, coma, and respiratory renal or hepatic failure. A septic or toxic shock-like illness as a sequelae of ehrlichiosis has also been reported [26]. Due to a limited number of cases, it is unclear of the real effects of ehrlichiosis on pregnant women or the fetus. There is no evidence currently that untreated ehrlichiosis results in persistent symptoms.

Babesiosis

Background

Babesiosis is caused by protozoa of the genus *Babesia* and is endemic to geographic areas similar to Lyme disease typically in the Northeast and Midwest parts of the United States.

Most cases of babesiosis in the Northern Hemisphere occur from May to September with predominance in July and August [29]. In 2014, over 1700 cases of babesiosis were reported to the CDC [30].

Babesia are obligate parasites of red blood cells (RBCs) causing a febrile hemolysis and renal failure. Babesiosis (or Babesia infection) was first described in cattle in the days of the Pharaohs but was only found to cause human disease in the 1950s. *B. microti* is the most common species in the Unites States with organisms. Organisms similar to *B. microti* have been found in Europe, Asia, and Australia. *B. divergens* is predominantly found in Europe with organisms similar to *B. divergens* found in the Midwest and West Coast of the Unites States. *B. duncani* has also been found on the West Coast [29].

The tick vector of babesiosis is the *Ixodes scapularis* tick species (also known as the deer tick or black-legged tick) which also transmits Lyme disease.

Classic Clinical Presentation

Babesiosis classic clinical presentation ranges from asymptomatic to severe illness and can be fatal. Twenty-five percent of seropositive adults and 50% of seropositive children are asymptomatic in certain endemic areas [11].

Classic symptoms can range from mild to severe symptoms. Mild symptoms include gradual onset of fever, fatigue, and weakness due to the parasite-mediated hemolysis of RBCs. Severe illness may show signs of severe hemolysis such as jaundice or hemoglobinuria.

Nearly all *B. divergens* found in Europe and *B. divergens*-like organism illnesses found in the Midwest and Washington state appear to cause symptomatic disease, usually severe, in asplenic patients [29].

Patients with babesiosis infections are often coinfected with other tick-borne illnesses. Reports show two-thirds of babesiosis patients also suffer from concurrent Lyme disease and one-third concurrent human granulocytic anaplasmosis [31]. Studies vary but it appears babesiosis patients with coinfections will remain symptomatic for longer duration than patients without a coinfection of another tick-borne illness [29].

Atypical Presentation

Asymptomatic infections can occur and generally self-resolve in immunocompetent patients without treatment.

Associated Systemic Symptoms

Fever and nonspecific symptoms are typically present. Fever can wax and wane ranging from low 38 °C to over 40 °C. Fatigue, weakness, chills, and myalgias are common. Other less common symptoms include sore throat, dry cough, vomiting, and diarrhea.

Time Course of Disease (Incubation Period After Exposure to Infectious Agent or Drug Exposure)

Symptoms typically develop 1–6 weeks after the patient has been bitten by the tick. Symptoms may first appear or recur many months after exposure in patients who are or become immunocompromised. Subclinical cases that became more apparent have been reported when the patient underwent a splenectomy for an unrelated illness or developed a malignancy [9, 29].

Common Mimics and Differential Diagnosis

Differential diagnosis of babesiosis includes malaria which also presents with fever, anemia, and associated symptoms such as headache, fatigue, and myalgias. Malaria should be considered in a patient who has traveled to or lived in an endemic area. Diagnosis is made by visualizing parasites on peripheral smear or the use of a rapid diagnostic test for malaria. Other tick-borne illnesses transmitted by the *B. microti* tick vector can have similar presentations to babesiosis. These include human granulocytic anaplasmosis (*A. phagocytophilum*) and *B. miyamotoi* (*B. miyamotoi*) diseases. Diagnosis again would be made via microscopy, polymerase chain reaction, or serology. Rickettsial infections such as Rocky Mountain spotted fever can present with similar nonspecific symptoms, but also a petechial or purpuric rash may develop. Viral hepatitis infections will typically show a significantly elevated transaminitis and positive viral serologies.

Key Physical Exam Findings and Diagnostic Features

Hepatosplenomegaly may be present. Lymphadenopathy is not present. Lab results classically show anemia and thrombocytopenia. Hemolysis results in increased reticulocyte count, increased bilirubin, decreased haptoglobin, and increased lactate dehydrogenase. White blood cell counts (WBCs) can range from decreased to increased. Liver function tests are typically increased [9, 11, 28, 29].

Definitive diagnosis of babesiosis is made by manual microscopy of thin blood smears using Wright or Giemsa staining. Early on in the disease, microscopy results may be negative as red blood cells with parasites are few. Repeat microscopy is recommended if concern for babesiosis is still high. Expertise by lab technicians is typically required. Automated cell readers can often miss the parasitemia and are generally not recommended to be used [29].

Polymerase chain reaction (PCR) assay can be used to detect low levels of parasitemia in cases such as early disease or convalescent phase. Serology testing using indirect immunofluorescent antibody test may be positive when microscopy and PCR are both negative. This may occur in cases of asymptomatic carriers or patients who cleared the infection with or without antibiotics [29].

In one review, severe babesiosis was associated with a parasitemia >4%, alkaline phosphatase >125 units/L, and WBC >5 × 10(9)/L. Risk factors for severe illness include asplenism (or decreased function of the spleen), HIV/AIDS with low CD4 cell count, and immunosuppression due to other causes such as cancer treatment.

Parasite serum levels (or parasitemia) range from 1% to 20% with mild cases having levels less than 4% [29].

Management

Asymptomatic patients generally do not require any treatment. Mild symptomatic cases of babesiosis usually self-resolve or respond to a short course 7–10 days of antibiotics. Treatment should be reserved for symptomatic patients with babesial parasites on blood smear or babesial DNA detected by PCR. Treatment is also recommended for asymptomatic patients with babesial parasites on blood smear or babesial DNA detected by PCR for greater than 3 months [29].

Antimicrobial recommendations for *B. microti* infections include two options: (1) atovaquone plus azithromycin or (2) quinine plus clindamycin (Table 16.3). The second regiment is generally better tolerated. Intravenous quinine and clindamycin are recommended for those patients who cannot tolerate oral medications. Higher oral dosages and/or prolonged treatment course up to 6 weeks may be needed in immunocompromised patients [29, 32]. The Centers for Disease Control recommends quinine plus clindamycin for the treatment of babesiosis in pregnant patients. Atovaquone has been used safely in kids >5 kg [33].

Treatment for other babesiosis infections such as *B. divergens* or *B. duncani* also includes the use of quinine/quinidine plus clindamycin [29].

Adverse effects of the atovaquone plus azithromycin treatment include diarrhea and rash. Quinine plus clindamycin can result in diarrhea and symptoms of cinchonism (tinnitus, decreased hearing, and vertigo). QT prolongation can be seen with quinine and quinidine and less often, azithromycin [29].

Patients with evidence of severe babesiosis require hospitalization. The 2006 Infectious Diseases Society of America (IDSA) guidelines recommend oral quinine plus intravenous clindamycin for cases of severe disease [32]. Due to quinine toxicity, some have recommended a three-drug regimen (atovaquone plus azithromycin plus clindamycin), but this regimen has not been clinically studied [29]. Intravenous quinidine, if required, can result in ventricular arrhythmias, hypotension, hypoglycemia, and QT prolongation or torsades de pointe on cardiac monitoring.

Red blood cell (RBC) exchange transfusion can be useful for clearing the body of infected RBCs, removing inflammatory mediators and toxic results of RBC lysis. RBC exchange transfusion should be considered for patients with evidence of severe disease such as severe anemia (hemoglobin <10 g/dL) with high counts of parasitemia ($\geq$10%). Exchange transfusion is also recommended for those patients with high parasitemia and risk for severe complications such pulmonary, renal, or hepatic. It can be also considered in those with severe disease even if parasitemia is not high (<10%). RBC transfusion can be considered in moderately ill patient cases with milder parasitemia but hemoglobin $\leq$10 mg/dL [29].

Infections caused by *B. divergens* are usually severe and therefore RBC exchange transfusion is recommended. For all severe cases, consultation with experts in hematology is recommended.

Complications

Although babesiosis resolves without sequelae in most patients, infections can be life threatening especially in asplenic or other immunocompromised states [9, 11, 28]. Serious complications include splenic infarct, acute respiratory distress syndrome, disseminated intravascular coagulation, congestive heart failure, and liver or renal failure. In one study, 5% of patients infected with *B. microti* died [9]. Severe disease is more likely in older patients or those with splenectomies, malignancies, or other immunocompromised conditions. Nausea and vomiting with hyperbilirubinemia appear to be predictive of severe disease [9, 34]. Babesiosis has been known to be recurrent or relapsing [29].

Tick Paralysis

Tick paralysis occurs worldwide with a predominance of cases in the Pacific Northwest of the United States and Southwest Canada [7]. Australia has also reported cases of tick paralysis. As stated earlier, tick paralysis is caused by a neurotoxin that is produced in the tick's salivary gland. While fully engorged and still attached to the host, the tick transmits the toxin to the host (Fig. 16.9). The true incidence of tick paralysis in the United States remains unclear as reporting is not mandatory, and many cases are likely attributed to other causes of flaccid paralysis such as Guillain-Barré syndrome.

Although tick bites are very common, tick paralysis is extremely rare. Even when reporting was mandatory, the Department of Health in the state of Washington only reported 33 cases from 1946 to 1996 [6]. Most cases of tick paralysis are in children with a predominance of cases in females. This may be due to long hair in young girls that allows the ticks' camouflage [7].

Classic Clinical Presentation

Tick paralysis in North America presents as an acute symmetric ascending paralysis, beginning in the lower extremities, evolving over hours to days. Deep tendon reflexes are usually diminished or absent. Pain is typically rare. If the tick is not removed, the paralysis will continue on to the upper extremities and then cranial nerves. Respiratory muscles will eventually weaken and the patient will be at risk for respiratory failure and death. Patients will remain alert and only become altered as respiratory failure with hypoxia and hypercarbia ensues [7].

Laboratory studies are typically normal in tick paralysis with CSF showing classically normal WBCs and protein. MRI imaging of the brain will be normal.

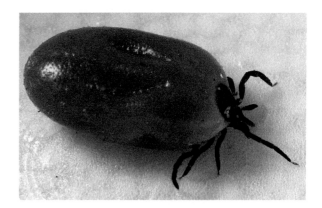

Fig. 16.9 Tick engorged with blood (Image appears with permission from Centers for Disease Control and Prevention (CDC))

Atypical Presentation

Scattered cases of focal weakness have been reported with almost all of them occurring in Australia. A tick or group of ticks is usually found near the site of weakness such as unilateral facial or upper extremity weakness. Pupillary dilation has been seen in the Australian version of tick paralysis. Flaccid paralysis with pupillary dilation in North America should suggest botulism or possibly diphtheria [7].

Associated Systemic Symptoms

Prodromic symptoms can occur that include paresthesias, myalgias, irritability, and fatigue. Patients are typically afebrile. These symptoms are followed often within hours by the flaccid paralysis.

Time Course of Disease (Incubation Period After Exposure to Infectious Agent or Drug Exposure)

Ticks associated with tick paralysis only begin to secret toxin once they have become engorged with blood. Symptoms and signs of tick paralysis may not present for several days after a patient is first bitten as it takes time for the tick to become finally engorged and start to secrete the toxin. Once the tick has been removed from the patient's body, North American cases (*Dermacentor* spp.) will typically see remission of symptoms. Australian cases (*Ixodes* sp.) will typically still see progression of symptoms for an additional 24–48 h.

Common Mimics and Differential Diagnosis

Guillain-Barré syndrome (GBS) is typically the most common cause of a flaccid paralysis. Just as with tick paralysis, GBS will present rarely with fever or pain. Unlike tick paralysis, sensory findings are frequently seen as a prodrome in GBS. The ascending paralysis associated with GBS is usually slower onset than with tick paralysis. Both tick paralysis and GBS can involve the cranial nerves with GBS most often involving cranial nerve VII but also III, IV, and VI. Pupils are rarely dilated in GBS. And CSF will show elevated protein in GBS. MRI imaging is usually normal. Miller-Fischer variant of GBS typically presents with ophthalmoplegia, ataxia, and areflexia without muscular weakness.

Transverse myelitis may also present with flaccid paralysis and may present with fever depending upon the cause. Pain and sensory complaints are common. Dilated pupils are absent. CSF evaluation in transverse myelitis will show an elevated WBC and often protein. MRI imaging is typically abnormal showing variable areas of enhancement indicating inflammation.

Spinal cord compression can also present with flaccid paralysis. Fever is usually absent except in some cases of epidural abscesses. Pain and sensory complaints are also common. Pupil dilation is absent. CSF results will be variable depending upon the cause. MRI imaging will be abnormal. Spinal cord ischemia or infarction should also be considered with many similar findings.

Botulism can also be mistaken for tick paralysis. Botulism also presents without fever, pain, or sensory complaints. Dilated pupils are present. CSF evaluation will be normal. And MRI imaging will also be normal.

Poliomyelitis was once a common cause of acute paralysis but is now only seen in Afghanistan, Pakistan, and Nigeria. A viral encephalomyelitis can also present with a flaccid paralysis but, unlike tick paralysis, will present with fever and often altered mental status or pain. Sensory complaints are not common and dilated pupils are absent. CSF evaluation in a patient with encephalomyelitis will be abnormal with elevated WBC and protein. MRI imaging will also be abnormal. Other enteroviruses, *West Nile* and *Powassan virus*, have all both been identified as causes of encephalomyelitis [7, 35, 36].

Key Physical Exam Findings and Diagnostic Features

Key physical exam findings include a painless symmetric ascending flaccid paralysis without fever or sensory findings. CSF evaluation is normal. Finding an engorged tick on the patient's body with improvement of the symptoms (24–48 h later in Australian cases) after removal is diagnostic. If evaluated, electrophysiologic tests in patients with tick paralysis show a diffuse reduction in the compound muscle action potentials. GBS will show similar results. North American tick paralysis cases may show reduced sensory and motor nerve conduction studies, but Australian cases will typically be normal [7].

Management

Any patient diagnosed with an ascending flaccid paralysis is at risk for respiratory complications and therefore requires cardiac and pulmonary monitoring. A thorough search for and then removal of the tick is imperative and is the definitive treatment. Symptoms can progress even after tick removal. North American cases generally improve faster than Australian cases. Once the tick (or ticks) are found and removed, symptoms generally begin to improve rapidly and are usually completely resolved by 24 h. Australian cases can continue to progress for some time. Until symptoms have resolved, supportive care is typically all that is required.

Complications

If an ascending paralysis is unrecognized, the patient is at risk for respiratory failure, hypoxia, and death. Even though tick paralysis is potentially fatal, today in the era of critical care, death is rare [6].

Bottom Line: Clinical Pearls

1. For many tick-borne illnesses, decision to treat should be based on clinical symptoms rather than waiting for confirmatory testing.
2. Early empiric antimicrobial treatment can prevent severe disease and death.
3. Doxycycline is the treatment of choice for rickettsial infections in both adults and children.
4. Coinfections by two or more tick-borne illnesses are not uncommon.
5. Providers should be aware of the reportable diseases in their area.

References

1. Biggs HM, Behravesh CB, Bradley KK, et al. Centers for Disease Control and Prevention (CDC). Diagnosis and management of tickborne rickettsial diseases: rocky mountain spotted fever and other spotted fever group rickettsioses, ehrlichioses, and anaplasmosis – United States. MMWR. 2016;65(2):1–44.
2. Marshall GS, Stout GG, Jacobs RF, et al. Antibodies reactive to *Rickettsia rickettsii* among children living in the southeast and south central regions of the United States. Arch Pediatr Adolesc Med. 2003;157:443–8.
3. Openshaw JJ, Swerdlow DL, Krebs JW, et al. Rocky Mountain spotted fever in the United States, 2000-2007: interpreting contemporary increases in incidence. Am J Trop Med Hyg. 2010;83:174–82.
4. Dahlgren FS, Mandel EJ, Krebs JW, et al. Increasing incidence of Ehrlichia chaffeensis and Anaplasma phagocytophilum in the United States, 2000-2007. Am J Trop Med Hyg. 2011;85:124–31.
5. Buckingham SC. Tick-borne diseases of the USA: ten things clinicians should know. J Infect. 2015;71:S88–96.
6. Dworkin MS, Shoemaker PC, Anderson DE. Tick paralysis: 33 human cases in Washington State, 1946-1996. Clin Infect Dis. 1999;29(6):1435–9.
7. Edlow JA, McGillicuddy DC. Tick paralysis. Infect Dis Clin N Am. 2008;22:397–413.
8. American Academy of Pediatrics 2017 Summer Safety Tips. https://www.aap.org/en-us/about-the-aap/aap-press-room/news-features-and-safety-tips/pages/summer-safety-tips.aspx.
9. Vannier E, Krause PJ. Human babesiosis. N Engl J Med. 2012;366:2397–407.
10. Sexton DJ, McClain MT. Clinical manifestations and diagnosis of Rocky Mountain spotted fever. UpToDate May 18, 2016.
11. Mukkada S, Buckingham S. Recognition of and prompt treatment for tick-borne infections in children. Infect Dis Clin N Am. 2015;29:539–55.
12. Woods CR. Rocky Mountain spotted fever in children. Pediatr Clin N Am. 2013;60:455–70.
13. Helmick CG, Bernard KW, D'Angelo LJ. Rocky Mountain spotted fever: clinical, laboratory, and epidemiological features of 262 cases. J Infect Dis. 1984;150:480.
14. Sexton DJ, Corey GR. Rocky Mountain "spotless" and "almost spotless" fever: a wolf in sheep's clothing. Clin Infect Dis. 1992;15:439–48.
15. Buckingham SC, Marshall GS, Schutze GE, et al. Clinical and laboratory features of Rocky Mountain spotted fever in children. J Pediatr. 2007;150:180–4.
16. Chen LF, Sexton DJ. What's new in Rocky Mountain spotted fever? Infect Dis Clin N Am. 2008;22:415–43.
17. Pickering LK, Baker CJ, Kimberlin DW, Long SS, editors. Rocky Mountain spotted fever In Red book: 2012 report of the committee on infectious diseases. 29th ed. Elk Grove Village: American Academy of Pediatrics; 2012. p. 623–625.

18. Feder HM Jr. Lyme disease in children. Infect Dis Clin N Am. 2008;22:315–26.
19. Steere AC, Sikand VK. The presenting manifestations of Lyme disease and outcomes of treatment. N Engl J Med. 2003;348:2472–24.
20. Shapiro E. Lyme disease: clinical manifestations in children. UpToDate June 26, 2016.
21. Hu L. Treatment of Lyme disease. UpToDate June 19, 2017
22. Swanson SJ, Neitzel D, Reed KD, Belongia EA. Coinfections acquired from ixodes ticks. Clin Microbiol Rev. 2006;19:708.
23. Steere AC, McHugh G, Suarez C, et al. Prospective study of coinfection in patients with erythema migrans. Clin Infect Dis. 2003;36:1078.
24. Wormser GP, Dattwyler RJ, Shapiro ED, et al. The clinical assessment, treatment, and prevention of Lyme disease, human granulocytic anaplasmosis, and babesiosis: clinical practice guidelines by the Infectious Diseases Society of America. Clin Infect Dis. 2006;43(9):1089–134.
25. Nichols Heitman K, Dahlgren FS, Drexler NA, et al. Increasing incidence of ehrlichiosis in the United States: a summary of national surveillance of Ehrlichia chaffeensis and Ehrlichia ewingii infections in the United States, 2008-2012. Am J Trop Med Hyg. 2016;94:52.
26. Sexton DJ, McClain MT. Human ehrlichiosis and anaplasmosis. UpToDate Aug 15, 2016.
27. Ratnasamy N, Everett ED, Roland WE, et al. Central nervous system manifestations of human ehrlichiosis. Clin Infect Dis. 1996;23:314.
28. Buckingham SC. Tick-borne diseases in children: epidemiology, clinical manifestations and optimal treatment strategies. Paediatr Drugs. 2005;7:163–76.
29. Gelfand JA, Vannier EG. Clinical manifestations, diagnosis, treatment and prevention of babesiosis. UpToDate Mar, 2017.
30. CDC Babesiosis. Surveillance for Babesiosis – United States 2014, Annual Summary reported Feb 29, 2016. https://www.cdc.gov/parasites/babesiosis/resources/babesiosis_surveillance_summary_2016.pdf.
31. Diuk-Wasser MA, Vannier E, Krause PJ. Coinfection by Ixodes tick-borne pathogens: ecological, epidemiological and clinical consequences. Trends Parasitol. 2016;32:30–42.
32. Sanchez E, Vannier E, Wormser GP, et al. Treatment and prevention of Lyme disease, human granulocytic anaplasmosis, and babesiosis: a review. JAMA. 2016;315:1767–77.
33. CDC Babesiosis. Treatment DPDx Laboratory identification of parasitic diseases of public health concern. Updated Nov 29, 2013. https://www.cdc.gov/dpdx/babesiosis/tx.html.
34. Mareedu N, Schotthoefer A, et al. Risk factors for severe infection, hospitalization, and prolonged antimicrobial therapy in patients with babesiosis. Am J Trop Med Hyg. 2017;97(4):1218–25.
35. Jeha LE, Sila CA, Lederman RJ, Prayson RA, Isada CM, Gordon SM. West Nile virus infection: a new acute paralytic illness. Neurology. Jul 8 2003;61(1):55–9.
36. Jackson AC. Leg weakness associated with Powassan virus infection–Ontario. Can Dis Wkly Rep. Jun 17 1989;15(24):123–4.

Henoch-Schönlein Purpura

Julie Furmick and Dale Woolridge

Background

Henoch-Schönlein purpura (HSP) is the most common vasculitis seen in children with an incidence of 10–20 per 100,000 [1, 2]. It is a systemic, immune-mediated small vessel vasculitis that most commonly affects the vessels supplying the skin, GI tract, kidney, and joints. It was named after both Henoch and his student Schönlein, who identified the association of joint pain, purpura with microscopic hematuria, in 1837 [3, 4]. The mean age of those affected is 6 years, and 90% of presentations occur before the age of 10 years. Caucasian children are most commonly affected, with 85% of cases occurring in white children with a male predominance 2:1 [2, 4]. Pathogenesis is driven by IgA deposits within the walls of small vessels, particularly those within the skin, small bowel, and renal glomeruli. This is a clinical diagnosis but a skin biopsy can be done to confirm diagnosis. Leukocytoclastic vasculitis (LCV) is seen with demonstration of immune complexes deposited within the wall of small-sized arteries [5].

Classic Clinical Presentation

Patients with HSP present with a palpable purpuric rash, pinpoint petechiae, and coalescent ecchymosis that usually concentrate to the lower extremities and buttocks; the propensity of the rash to aggregate in this pattern simply represents that these are pressure-dependent areas [2]. The rash may present in different locations depending on the age of the patient, and infants may have lesions on the face and

J. Furmick
Department of Pediatrics, University of Arizona, Tucson, AZ, USA
e-mail: jfurmick@peds.arizona.edu

D. Woolridge (✉)
Department of Emergency Medicine, University of Arizona, Tucson, AZ, USA
e-mail: dale@aemrc.arizona.edu

Fig. 17.1 Urticarial phenotype of Henoch-Schönlein purpura (HSP)

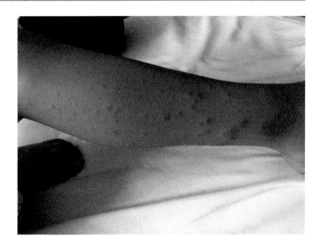

back. The second most common symptom is arthritis which usually affects large joints such as the knees and ankles. Painful joints may inhibit walking and associated lower extremity edema is common. Up to 75% of patients will have vague abdominal pain and vomiting, and roughly half of all patients diagnosed with HSP will have varying degrees of renal manifestations from mild proteinuria to severe, progressive glomerulonephritis [3].

The rash of HSP can vary significantly. Figures 17.1, 17.2, and 17.3 demonstrate this variability. Figure 17.4 demonstrates the pedal edema that is often seen in HSP. Figure 17.5 demonstrates the limited distribution of the rash on the upper extremities as compared to the lower extremities. Figure 17.6 demonstrates a slightly different appearance of HSP with a mild purpuric rash on the posterior aspect of the lower extremities, faint ecchymosis noted on the left heel, and mild edema of the feet bilaterally. Both of these patients represent a classical presentation of HSP.

The European League Against Rheumatism and Pediatric Rheumatology International Trials Organization published the diagnostic criteria in 2010 including palpable purpura as a mandatory criterion, plus one of the following findings: diffuse abdominal pain, leukocytoclastic vasculitis (LCV) with predominant IgA deposits on skin biopsy, acute arthritis or arthralgias in any joint, and renal involvement as evidenced by proteinuria and/or hematuria. The sensitivity and specificity of these classification criteria are 100% and 87%, respectively [5].

Atypical Presentation

The order of presentation of symptoms in HSP helps significantly in making the diagnosis. The typical presentation starts with the classic purpuric rash followed by one or more of the following symptoms: arthralgias, abdominal pain, and/or nephritis. The diagnosis becomes difficult when the symptoms present out of order or prior to rash presentation. Also there are a large variety of symptoms seen in this disease process; Table 17.1 reviews these various symptoms as well as the frequency at which they appear.

Fig. 17.2 Common purpuric type rash with Henoch-Schönlein purpura (HSP)

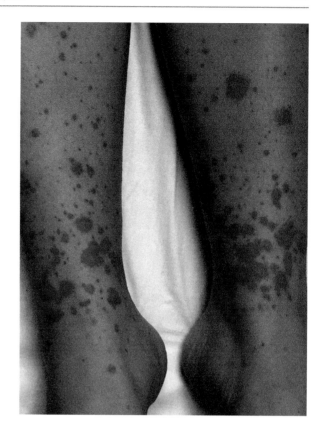

Fig. 17.3 Pinpoint petechiae often seen with Henoch-Schönlein purpura (HSP)

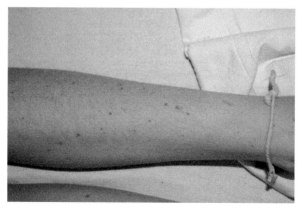

Joint pain can be a presenting sign in up to 25% of patients, preceding the rash by up to 1 week [6]. Gastrointestinal complaints occur in up to 65% of patients with HSP, with the most common complaints being dull, periumbilical pain. Notably, however, 15% of the time abdominal pain can be the presenting symptom preceding the rash [3]. Stools may be hemoccult positive in 30% of patients [7]. Abdominal US usually shows abdominal wall thickness, edema, and even mild ascites. Severe

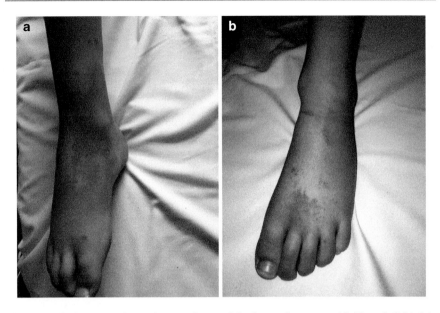

Fig. 17.4 Coalescent ecchymosis as well as pedal edema often seen with Henoch-Schönlein purpura

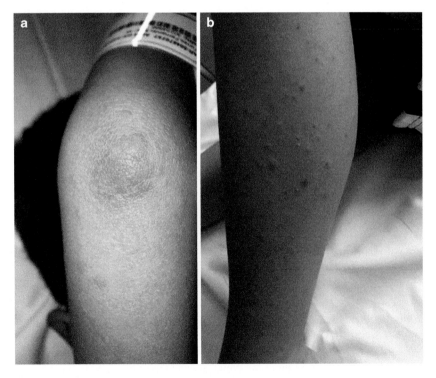

Fig. 17.5 Demonstrates the variability in the presentation of Henoch-Schönlein purpura. Above is a patient with palpable, pinpoint lesions on the upper extremities

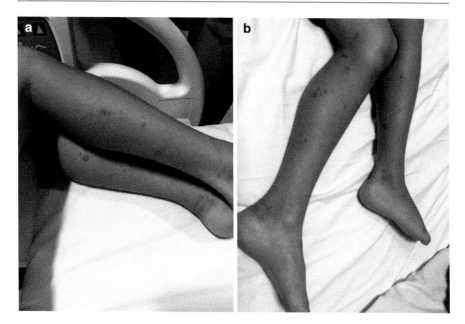

Fig. 17.6 Pictured are the lower extremities of the same patient in Fig. 17.5. This demonstrates the propensity of the rash to effect dependent areas such as the lower extremities

Table 17.1 Illustrates common clinical presentation of Henoch-Schönlein purpura (HSP) [2, 3]

Clinical diagnosis of HSP	Signs and symptoms
Rash (purpuric, pinpoint petechiae, coalescent ecchymosis)	+
Arthritis (usually large joints: knees/ankles)	+
Abdominal pain ± nausea/vomiting	+
Renal manifestations	±
Extremity edema	±
Scrotal pain/edema	±

bowel wall edema may lead to intussusception which most commonly is ileoileal. Small bowel intussusception is diagnosed by ultrasound and the treatment is surgical. Enema neither makes the diagnosis nor is the treatment for ileoileal intussusception. Undiagnosed and untreated intussusception may progress to bowel wall necrosis and perforation. Pleural effusions, carditis, and respiratory failure may rarely occur and are treated with steroid administration [8]. Between 2% and 8% of patients can have neurological involvement, ranging in severity as demonstrated in Table 17.1. One case report espoused status epilepticus as the presenting symptom [9]. Isolated scrotal pain and/or penile swelling may also be an atypical presentation of HSP [10].

Nephritis may rarely be the initial manifestation prior to the onset of the rash. A limited subset of patients can present with severe nephritic or nephrotic syndrome, but most of the time these symptoms are delayed weeks to months after the appearance of the rash. Follow-up is important because renal complications such as hypertension, hematuria, proteinuria, or acute renal failure have been reported up to 10 years after initial presentation [2].

Another well-described atypical presentation is bullous HSP. Lesions present as vesicles and bullae rather than palpable purpura. Figures 17.7, 17.8, 17.9, 17.10, and 17.11

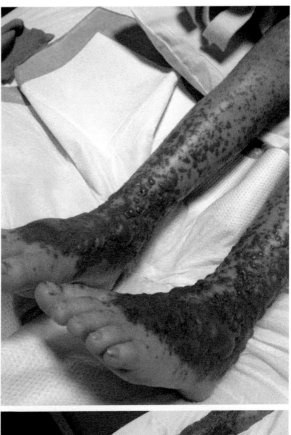

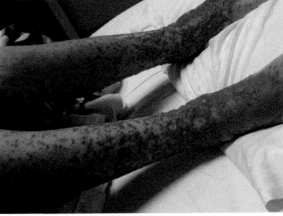

Fig. 17.7, 17.8, 17.9, 17.10, and 17.11 Patient with bullous Henoch-Schönlein purpura on day 1 of presentation

Fig. 17.7, 17.8, 17.9, 17.10, and 17.11 (continued)

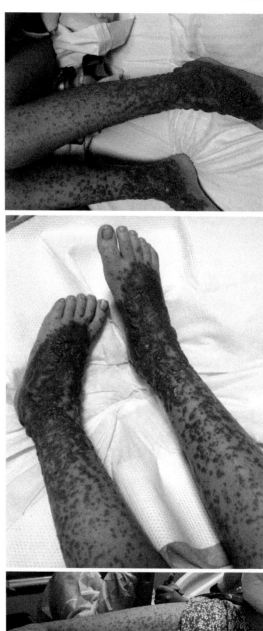

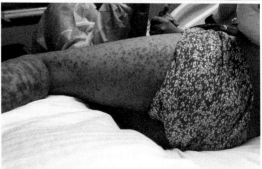

demonstrates bullous HSP on day 1 of presentation. Figure 17.12 is also on day 1 of presentation but demonstrates the dependent nature of the disease process; the rash becomes progressively more severe distally. The onset of the bullous rash is rarely the presenting feature of this disease process and has rarely been described in the literature. Though not supported by robust evidence, most patients report symptomatic improvement with steroid treatment. Figures 17.13 and 17.14 represent our patient after 4 days of oral prednisone at 1 mg/kg.

Fig. 17.12 The upper extremities of patient with bullous Henoch-Schönlein purpura on day 1 of presentation; demonstrates the dependent nature of this rash as lower extremities are much more severely affected

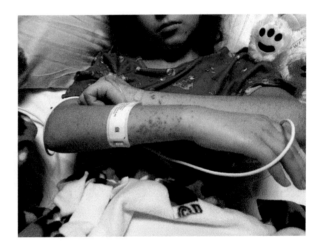

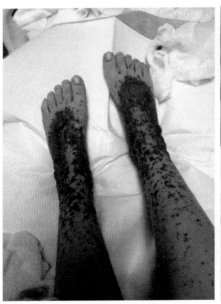
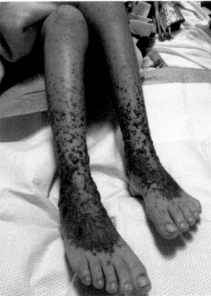

Fig. 17.13 and 17.14 After day 4 of treatment with steroids

Associated Systemic Symptoms (Table 17.2)

Table 17.2 Illustrates variety of symptoms seen with Henoch-Schönlein purpura (HSP) [1, 6, 9, 11, 14, 15, 21]

System	Symptom/location	Incidence	Note
General	Non-pitting edema noted on scalp, face, trunk, extremities	50% of patients	Does not correlate to the degree of proteinuria or serum albumin
Skin	Palpable purpuric rash	100% of patients	Not always presenting symptom
MSK	Migratory arthritis knees, ankles	80% of patients	May be presenting symptom in 15–25% of patients
Gastrointestinal	Colicky abdominal pain, vomiting	75% of patients	Abdominal symptoms can proceed rash by 2 weeks in 10–20% of patients
	GI bleed	30% of patients	
	Occult GI bleed	20% of patients	
	Gross GI bleed	10% of patients	
	Intussusception	0.7–13.6 of patients	Ileoileal (51%) Ileocolic (39%) Jejuno-jejunal (7%)
	Other GI complications (including ischemia, necrosis, and perforation)	Rare complication, incidence not cited in literature	Perforation, usually ileal, may appear in patients on steroids usually in the 2nd week of treatment [14]
Renal	Ranges in severity:	30–50% of patients	97% of renal manifestation are present by 6 months
	Microscopic hematuria	40%	
	Gross hematuria	10%	
	Proteinuria	25%	
	Nephrotic syndrome	5%	
	ESRD	1%	
Central nervous system	Headache, behavioral changes, encephalopathy, seizures, ataxia, neuropathy	Incidence not well established, less than 2–8%	
Genital	Testicular involvement (pain, swelling, tenderness)	10–20% of patients	Can mimic testicular torsion
Pulmonary involvement	Ranges from pneumonia to alveolar hemorrhage	8% of patients	More common in adults
Recurrence of symptoms	Milder and shorter than primary insult, usually occurring within 12 months of acute phase of disease	33% of patients	Pre-existing renal disease usually does not progress

Time Course of Disease

Most patients present in fall to winter, often following an upper respiratory infection. Though there have been multiple drugs, pathogens, and environmental exposures linked to this disease process, the exact cause remains unknown. Positive beta-hemolytic strep throat cultures have been reported in 10–30% of patients, and antistrepolysin titers are elevated in 20–50% of patients presenting with HSP. However, 12–20% of asymptomatic children are colonized with *S. pyogenes* making a direct correlation unlikely [12, 13].

The majority of patients present first with a rash followed by joint pain, pedal edema, abdominal pain, nausea, vomiting, and infrequently with hematuria. However, presentation varies; abdominal or joint pain can precede the rash as seen in Table 17.1, which might make diagnosis difficult if rash is not evident. The rash can also change from throughout the disease process. Figure 17.15 represents day 1 of disease and Fig. 17.16 represents day 3 demonstrating the progression of the rash to a more coalescent ecchymosis appearance.

The diagnosis of HSP is clinical; all labs are usually normal including the urinalysis if there is no renal involvement. Urinalysis is the most commonly abnormal

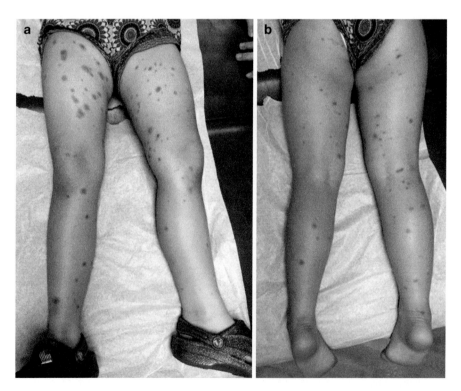

Fig. 17.15 Demonstrates classic palpable purpuric rash Henoch-Schönlein purpura (HSP), picture taken on day 1 on presentation

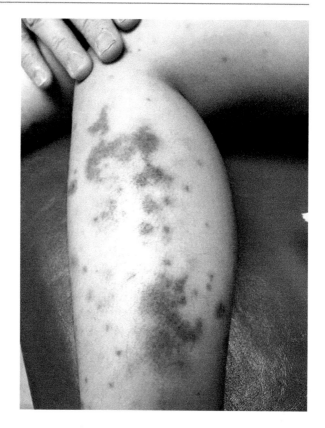

Fig. 17.16 This is the same patient pictured in Fig. 17.15 on day 3 of presentation. This demonstrates the progression of the rash from palpable purpuric rash to coalescent ecchymosis.

laboratory finding which may be significant for hematuria or proteinuria depending on renal involvement. HSP is typically a self-limited process, lesions typically last 3–10 days, and there is a complete resolution of symptoms by 6 weeks in the majority of patients [2]. However, roughly 1/3 of patients will relapse within 1 year of presentation. Relapse is usually less severe.

Nephritis, if present, is the only symptom that has the potential to progress to a chronic disease process. Hematuria is common and usually self-resolves; however when accompanied by nephrotic-range proteinuria, 20% will go on to develop chronic kidney disease.

Common Mimics and Differential Diagnosis

Diagnosing HSP is challenging when the classic rash is not the presenting symptom. When joint pain presents several weeks before the rash, rheumatologic diseases such as systemic lupus erythematosus (SLE) or juvenile idiopathic arthritis (JIA) may be considered first. Additionally infectious concerns such as septic joint versus transient synovitis may confound the clinical picture. Similarly, if nephritic/nephrotic syndrome is the presenting symptom, a wide range of differential diagnoses from urinary tract infection (UTI), systemic infection, drug, or toxin to primary renal pathology could be considered the inciting event.

In atypical HSP, labs may help to rule out other diagnoses. Laboratory evaluation often includes CBC, sedimentation rate, ANA, double-stranded DNA, antineutrophil cytoplasmic antibody, and complement levels. These studies will all be normal in HSP but can be used to differentiate between other rheumatologic processes. IgA can be elevated in about 50% of patients. A skin biopsy may be performed to confirm the diagnosis and will demonstrate granulocytic infiltration of the small vessels with IgA deposits within the vessel walls.

Imaging may be indicated in those patients with severe abdominal pain in order to exclude alternative diagnoses or rare complications of HSP including intussusception and bowel wall necrosis/perforation.

Key Physical Exam Findings

The classic key physical exam findings include a palpable purpuric rash about 2–10 cm in diameter, pinpoint petechiae, and coalescent ecchymosis, as seen in Fig. 17.2. In some rare cases, these lesions can present like vesicles and bullae rather than, or in addition to, the rash described above. Dermatologic findings present in areas of dependence, so the rash is usually in the lower extremities, but in young infants the rash may be found throughout the body. Patients typically have pitting edema in the areas affected by the rash. On physical exam, patients may have an antalgic gait or refusal to bear weight from lower extremity joint pain. Patients often have abdominal distention and pain from involvement of the vessels within the small bowel and dark, tea-colored, frothy urine if there is renal involvement.

Diagnosis and Management

The initial workup for HSP depends on the severity of symptoms. Figure 17.17 outlines a diagnostic algorithm for HSP. Urinalysis should be obtained on first evaluation and then weekly during active stages of disease and monthly thereafter for 6 months after diagnosis. Labs are not required but may help rule out other diagnoses if the diagnosis is not clear on presentation [1]. If patient remains asymptomatic during this time period, renal disease is unlikely to occur. If patient develops hypertension, proteinuria, or hematuria during this screening process, referral to pediatric nephrology is warranted. An abdominal US may be indicated depending on the degree of abdominal symptoms. Skin biopsy is the most diagnostic for LCV and is the most reliable tool for diagnosis HSP [5].

Acetaminophen and NSAIDs are used for joint pain, fever, or muscle aches, but caution should be used with NSAIDs and renal involvement. Ranitidine may be effective in some patients with mild GI symptoms [16]. The role of steroids in the treatment of HSP is somewhat controversial. Steroids may decrease discomfort but

Fig. 17.17 Algorithm for diagnosing and treating renal complications of Henoch-Schönlein purpura [1]

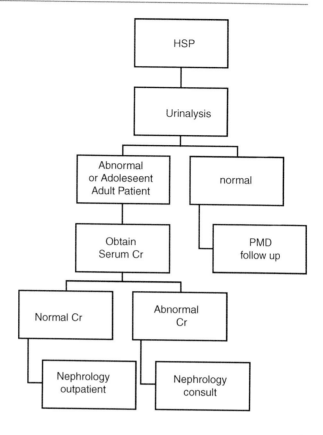

does not impact the disease course of HSP or decrease sequelae. There are two randomized, double-blind, placebo-controlled trials with different results, one demonstrating a decrease in intensity and duration of joint pain and abdominal pain and milder renal manifestations in 171 patients [17]. The second study showed no significant difference in disease processes between steroid and placebo groups among 40 patients [18]. In 2013, another randomized, double-blind, placebo-controlled trial was completed in which 352 children were randomized and demonstrated that early treatment with steroids does not reduce the prevalence of proteinuria 1 year after disease onset in HSP [19].

There was another study showed that 44% of patients treated with steroids improved within the first 24 h compared to spontaneous improvement of only 14% within the first 24 h of those not treated. However, when compared at day 3, improvement was the same in both groups [20]. Therefore, the role of steroids is unclear, and the natural history of this disease is spontaneous improvement. Those with severe renal manifestations may warrant immunosuppression or cell cycle inhibitors. Other treatment options include intravenous immunoglobulin (IVIG), plasmapheresis, or transplantation if end-stage renal failure (ESRD) is reached [2].

Complications

There are several rare complications of HSP delineated in Table 17.1 that affect less than 1% of the patient population. These include intussusception, bowel wall necrosis, and perforation as well as neurological involvement including seizures, encephalopathy, and ataxia.

The most common complication is HSP nephritis. This usually occurs weeks to months after initial presentation and is mild and demonstrates limited microscopic hematuria without significant proteinuria. Overall, these patients have an excellent prognosis with less than 1% progressing to ESRD. Prognosis is more guarded in those patients who present with nephrotic range proteinuria; as many as 5% of these patients progress to ESRD. The severity of symptoms tends to be milder in those under the age of 2 years and more severe in adults [6].

Bottom Line

HSP is the most common vasculitis affecting children. It is a clinical diagnosis characterized by non-thrombocytic purpuric rash, joint and abdominal pain, and some degree of nephritis in about 50% of patients. Urine should be obtained in all patients to assess for renal involvement. A creatinine should be obtained in patients with abnormal urinalysis and in all adolescents/adults. Most patients fully recover within 4–6 weeks and the prognosis of HSP, including HSP nephritis, is excellent. Spontaneous and complete resolution of nephritis typically occurs in those who present with mild renal symptoms (hematuria and proteinuria); however, those who present with nephrotic syndrome have about a 5% chance of developing chronic renal disease. Follow-up is essential as renal involvement usually presents 4–6 weeks after initial disease presentation.

Clinical Pearls
- HSP is the most common vasculitis that affects children.
- Symptoms include:
  - Non-thrombocytic purpuric rash.
  - Joint and abdominal pain.
  - Fifty percent of patients have some degree of nephritis.
- Urinalysis (UA) should be obtained on first evaluation, if negative follow-up should be arranged for weekly urinalyses during active disease, then monthly thereafter for the next 6 months.
- Treatment is largely symptomatic support.

References

1. Marcdante KJ, Kliegman RM. Nelson essentials of pediatrics. Philadelphia: Elsevier/Saunders; 2015.
2. Reid-Adam J. Henoch-Schönlein Purpura. Pediatr Rev. 2014;35(10):447–9.
3. Sharieff GQ, Francis K, Kuppermann N. Atypical presentation of Henoch-Schoenlein purpura in two children. Am J Emerg Med. 1997;15(4):375–7. https://doi.org/10.1016/s0735-6757(97)90130-3.
4. Maguiness S, Balma-Mena A, Pope E, Weinstein M. Bullous Henoch-Schönlein purpura in children: a report of 6 cases and review of the literature. Clin Pediatr. 2010;49(11):1033–7. https://doi.org/10.1177/0009922810374977.
5. Yang Y-H, Yu H-H, Chiang B-L. The diagnosis and classification of Henoch–Schönlein purpura: An updated review. Autoimmun Rev. 2014;13(4-5):355–8. https://doi.org/10.1016/j.autrev.2014.01.031.
6. Saulsbury FT. Clinical update: Henoch-Schönlein purpura. Lancet. 2007;369(9566):976–8. https://doi.org/10.1016/s0140-6736(07)60474-7.
7. Chang WL, Yang YH, Lin YT, Chiang BL. Gastrointestinal manifestations in Henoch-Schönlein purpura: a review of 261 patients. Acta Paediatr. 2004;93(11):1427.
8. Mrusek S, Krüger M, Greiner P, Kleinschmidt M, Brandis M, Ehl S. Henoch-Schönlein purpura. Lancet. 2004;363(9415):1116. https://doi.org/10.1016/s0140-6736(04)15895.
9. Mannenbach MS, Reed AM, Moir C. Atypical presentation of Henoch-Schönlein Purpura. Pediatr Emerg Care. 2009;25(8):513–5. https://doi.org/10.1097/pec.0b013e3181b0a46f.
10. Tewary KK, Khodaghalian B, Narchi H. Acute penile pain and swelling in a 4-year-old child with Henoch-Schonlein purpura. Case Rep. 2015;2015(apr09 1) https://doi.org/10.1136/bcr-2013-202341.
11. Pacheva IH, Ivanov IS, Stefanova K, et al. Central nervous system involvement in Henoch-Schonlein purpura in children and adolescents. Case Rep Pediatr. 2017;2017:1–6. https://doi.org/10.1155/2017/5483543.
12. Ferretti, JJ, Stevens, DL, Fischetti, VA; Streptococcus pyogenes: Basic Biology to Clinical Manifestations, 2016; University of Oklahoma Press. Oklahoma City: University of Oklahoma Health Sciences Center.
13. Shaikh N, Leonard E, Martin JM. Prevalence of streptococcal pharyngitis and streptococcal carriage in children: a meta-analysis. Pediatrics. 2010;126(3):e557–64.
14. Schwartz RH, Wientzen RL, Pedreira F, Feroli EJ, Mella GW, Guandolo VL. Penicillin V for group A streptococcal pharyngotonsillitis. A randomized trial of seven vs ten days' therapy. JAMA. 1981;246(16):1790–5.
15. Ebert EC. Gastrointestinal Manifestations of Henoch-Schonlein Purpura. Dig Dis Sci. 2008;53(8):2011–9. https://doi.org/10.1007/s10620-007-0147-0.
16. Wu C-S, Tung S-Y. Henoch-Schönlein Purpura Complicated by Upper Gastrointestinal Bleeding with an Unusual Endoscopic Picture. J Clin Gastroenterol. 1994;19(2):128–31. https://doi.org/10.1097/00004836-199409000-00011.
17. Narin N, Akçoral A, Aslin MI, Elmastas H. Ranitidine administration in Henoch-Schönlein vasculitis. Pediatr Int. 1995;37(1):37–9. https://doi.org/10.1111/j.1442-200x.1995.tb03682.x.
18. Ronkainen J, Koskimies O, Ala-Houhala M, et al. Early prednisone therapy in Henoch-Schönlein purpura: a randomized, double-blind, placebo-controlled trial. J Pediatr. 2006;149(2):241–7. https://doi.org/10.1016/j.jpeds.2006.03.024.
19. Huber A. A randomised, placebo controlled trial of prednisone in early Henoch-Schonlein Purpura. http://isrctnorg. 2012. https://doi.org/10.1186/isrctn85109383.
20. Dudley J, Smith G, Llewelyn-Edwards A, et al. Randomised, double-blind, placebo-controlled trial to determine whether steroids reduce the incidence and severity of nephropathy in Henoch-Schonlein Purpura (HSP). Arch Dis Child. 2013;98(10):756–63. https://doi.org/10.1136/archdischild-2013-303642.
21. Tizard EJ, Hamilton-Ayres MJJ. Henoch Schonlein purpura. Arch Dis Child Educ Pract. 2008;93(1):1–8. https://doi.org/10.1136/adc.2004.066035.

Necrotizing Infections

18

Tiffany M. Abramson and Stuart Swadron

Background

Necrotizing fasciitis (NF) is a rare soft tissue infection that results in high morbidity and mortality. It is characterized by necrosis of the superficial fascia and subcutaneous tissue, allowing for rapid spread of bacteria along tissue planes, early sepsis, and organ failure. Prompt recognition and emergent surgical debridement are crucial to avoid the loss of life or limb associated with NF [1].

Necrotizing fasciitis has a global prevalence of 0.4 cases per 100,000 per year [1, 2] and is even less common in the pediatric population. While it is often associated with trauma, many cases do not have an identifiable portal of entry for the pathogens. It most commonly affects the limbs, abdominal wall, and perineum.

Classic Clinical Presentation

In addition to the swelling, pain, and erythema that are characteristics of most soft tissue infections, findings concerning for NF include tenderness beyond the area of erythema, tense edema, indistinct margins, and bronzing of the skin. The patient's pain is frequently out of proportion to what might be expected from the physical examination, however, occasionally the patient may exhibit an inappropriate indifference or a subtle alteration of mental status. Drainage from the wound is often described as having the consistency of "dishwater" fluid. As the infection progresses, the infected area may become anesthetic due to the destruction of the cutaneous nerves. Later, other skin findings may develop including bullae, crepitus, and

T. M. Abramson (✉) · S. Swadron
LAC+USC Medical Center- Department of Emergency Medicine, Keck School of Medicine, Los Angeles, CA, USA
e-mail: Tiffany.Abramson@med.usc.edu

necrosis. Lastly, rapid progression of the infection is typically seen despite antibiotic treatment [1–5] (Table 18.1) (Figs. 18.1, 18.2, 18.3, and 18.4).

Necrotizing fasciitis is more common in males. Risk factors for NF include diabetes, cirrhosis, obesity, steroid use, alcohol abuse, and immunocompromised states. However, it may occur in young, healthy, immunocompetent individuals as well [6]. While adults more commonly have a polymicrobial infection affecting the extremities, pediatric infections tend to affect the trunk primarily and are often caused by a single pathogen [7].

Necrotizing fasciitis is sometimes classified into four subtypes based on the pathogen involved; however, this classification is less relevant in the acute care setting where specific bacteriologic diagnosis must wait until after emergent surgical intervention [2] (Table 18.2).

Table 18.1 Key Physical Exam Findings

Exam findings
Pain out of proportion to examination findings
Pain and induration beyond margins of erythema
Tense edema
Violaceous skin discoloration
Crepitus
Bullae
Skin necrosis
Cutaneous anesthesia
Dishwater discharge from wound
Systemic toxicity
Progression of infection despite antibiotics
Fever
Tachycardia
Hypotension

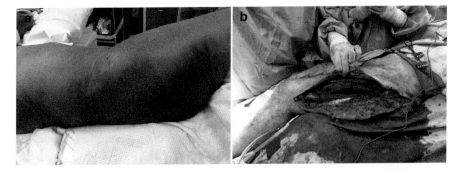

Fig. 18.1 (**a**) Subtle skin findings in a case of necrotizing fasciitis demonstrating bronzing of the skin with indistinct margins. (**b**) Surgical debridement of the same case demonstrating extensive necrosis along the fascial plane despite only exhibiting subtle skin findings. (Photo Credit: Demetrios Demetriades, MD PHD)

Fig. 18.2 Necrotizing
fasciitis of the groin and
perineum with extensive
skin findings
demonstrating erythema,
edema, bullae, and
necrosis. (Photo Credit:
Saman Kashani, MD and
Talib Omer, MD)

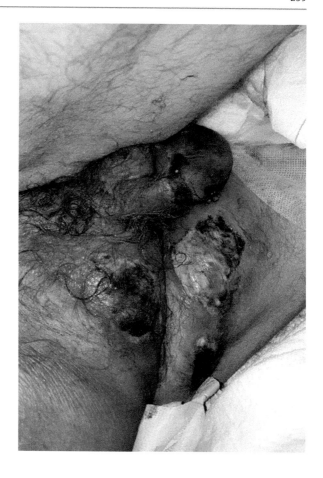

Fig. 18.3 Necrotizing
fasciitis involving the thigh
demonstrating rapidly
expanding erythema,
extensive bullae formation,
and "dishwater" drainage
from the affected area.
(Photo Credit: Emily Rose,
MD)

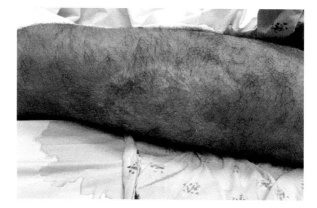

Fig 18.4 Necrotizing fasciitis of the arm demonstrating extensive external findings including bullae, necrosis, "dishwater" drainage, and erythema. (Photo Credit: Garrett Sterling, MD)

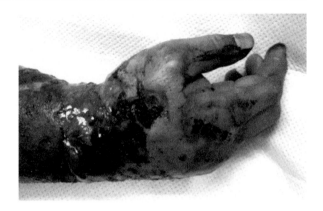

Table 18.2 Classification of Necrotizing Fasciitis

	Pathogen	Clinical pearl
Type I	Polymicrobial	Immunodeficient hosts, diabetes mellitus. Most common, more indolent
Type II	Monomicrobial (*Streptococcus pyogenes*)	Associated with wounds, postsurgical, IV drug use. More aggressive
Type III	Gram-negative (*Clostridium, Vibrio*)	Seafood ingestion, water contamination. Highest mortality
Type IV	Fungal (Candida, Zygomycetes)	Trauma associated, immunocompromised and immunocompetent. Aggressive with rapid spread

Cirrhotic patients are at a higher risk of NF in general, and, specifically, they are more susceptible to *Vibrio vulnificus* than the general population [4]. They may contract an infection with Vibrio species either by eating shellfish or through direct contact with salt water. They initially present with gastrointestinal symptoms and non-bloody diarrhea and then later develop skin lesions. In addition to the typical broad-spectrum antibiotic coverage and early surgical consult that is used in the treatment of all cases of NF, doxycycline is added for specific antibiotic coverage of the *Vibrio* species found in saltwater and seafood. *Intravenous drug users* are also at unique risk of NF; black tar heroin is specifically associated with NF caused by clostridial species.

Atypical Presentation

Necrotizing fasciitis is a challenging, "high-stakes" diagnosis. Some cases will present initially with minimal findings on examination but with telltale pain out of proportion to those findings. Typical examination findings such as bullae, crepitus, or fever may be absent. In some cases, examination findings will be obvious but the patient will demonstrate an inappropriate indifference to impressive physical findings. Finally, concerning laboratory abnormalities or a change in the patient's vital signs are often the prompt for the clinician to consider NF [1].

Associated Systemic Symptoms

Patients with NF may initially appear well but quickly develop systemic symptoms. They are often febrile and/or tachycardic out of proportion to their fever. Without prompt resuscitation and surgical debridement, patients progress quickly to severe sepsis and septic shock with multiple organ system failure [1, 4].

Time Course of Disease

Necrotizing fasciitis typically has a very rapid course. It starts with an inoculation of the superficial fascia through hematogenous spread or a skin wound, rapidly tracks along the fascial planes, and causes systemic illness. However, in cases caused by methicillin-resistant staphylococcal aureus (MRSA), there may be a much slower progression of disease [3].

Common Mimics and Differential Diagnosis

In an early presentation, it may be difficult to distinguish NF from a simple cellulitis or abscess. For this reason, NF should at least be considered as part of the differential diagnosis whenever evaluating a soft tissue infection. Of note, NF is one of many infections that falls under the larger category of necrotizing soft tissue infections (NSTI). This broader category includes gas gangrene, myositis, invasive streptococcal cellulitis, Fournier's gangrene, and necrotizing fasciitis. While the final diagnosis may vary, the initial presentation of all NSTIs are similar. Moreover, all NSTIs are managed with aggressive resuscitation and emergent surgical intervention.

Management

Diagnosis

Diagnosis of NF is based on history and physical examination. While it is primarily a clinical diagnosis, imaging and laboratory testing may be helpful early in the disease course or in equivocal cases. This workup should not delay surgical consultation when there is more than a minimal concern for NF [1, 2, 4].

Plain X-rays may reveal a characteristic gas pattern along fascial planes. While not sensitive, this sign is specific and can lead to a rapid disposition to the operating room. Computed tomography (CT) is more sensitive than plain X-rays at identifying gas in the fascial planes as well as other signs of NF. Magnetic resonance

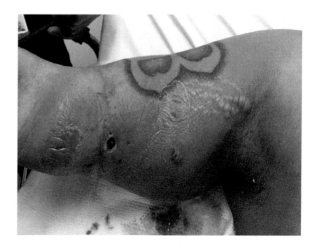

Fig. 18.5 A case of NF demonstrating erythema, edema, bullae, and dishwater drainage from an opening in the affected area. (Photo Credit: Tiffany M. Abramson, MD)

(MR) is extremely sensitive for NF but the time required to perform MR makes it difficult to justify if NF is suspected [8]. Point-of-care ultrasound (POCUS) can be used to identify fascial and subcutaneous tissue thickening, abnormal fluid collections along the fascia, and subcutaneous air consistent with NF. Ultrasound is inexpensive and noninvasive and can be performed concurrently with resuscitation in critically ill patients [9]. No imaging modality should delay surgical treatment (Fig. 18.5).

Laboratory testing is not diagnostic but can be suggestive of NF. Laboratory abnormalities associated with NF include marked leukocytosis, hyponatremia, hyperglycemia, anemia, elevated creatinine, and markedly elevated C-reactive protein (CRP). The LRINEC (Laboratory Risk Indicator for Necrotizing Fasciitis) is a diagnostic scoring system that uses these values to evaluate the severity of soft tissue infection. While laboratory findings may be suggestive of NF, their absence does not exclude NF [10, 11]. Ultimately, the diagnosis can only be confirmed or excluded by surgical debridement.

Treatment

Necrotizing fasciitis is a surgical emergency. The focus should be on getting the patient to the operating room as soon as possible with fluid resuscitation and antibiotics started once the diagnosis is considered. The definitive treatment is surgical and no testing or other intervention should delay surgical debridement. Typically, patients require multiple return visits for further debridement as the infection often progresses despite the initiation of treatment and initial debridement.

Patients with NF require aggressive fluid resuscitation and broad-spectrum antibiotics including empiric MRSA coverage. Clindamycin is sometimes recommended as the first or "anchor" antibiotic, as it is thought to be a suppressor of the toxin associated with Group A streptococcal NF. The addition of intravenous

Table 18.3 Treatment of Necrotizing Fasciitis

Definitive therapy	Adjunctive therapy	Therapy for refractory cases
Surgical debridement	Broad-spectrum antibiotics: 1. Carbapenem or beta-lactam-beta-lactamase inhibitor (i.e., meropenem, piperacillin-tazobactam), *plus* 2. MRSA coverage (i.e. vancomycin, linezolid), *plus* 3. Clindamycin (antitoxin effects)	IVIG
	IV fluid resuscitation	Hyperbaric oxygen
	Vasopressor agents	

immunoglobulin therapy (IVIG) has been shown to inhibit streptococcal and staphylococcal virulence factors and may also play a role in management [1, 2, 6, 12] (Table 18.3).

Complications

Worse outcomes are associated with truncal involvement, significant comorbidities, and, most importantly, delay in surgical management. A delay of more than 12 h between presentation and surgical intervention is associated with increased mortality [2]. Without treatment, NF has a mortality of 100% [1]. Even with aggressive resuscitation, broad-spectrum antibiotics, and surgical debridement, there is still a 17–30% mortality rate which rises to 12–45% if the trunk is involved [1, 2, 4]. Furthermore, there is a high degree of morbidity as these patients often have a prolonged hospital course, amputations, and extensive soft tissue loss.

> **Bottom Line: Necrotizing Soft Tissue Infection Clinical Pearls**
> * Early recognition is critical.
> * Necrotizing fasciitis has a high mortality rate, 17–30% with treatment, 100% without treatment [1, 2, 4].
> * Exam findings include bullae, crepitus, tense edema, bronzing of skin, violaceous erythema, rapid progression, and pain beyond the area of induration [1–6].
> * Systemic findings may develop, but vital sign abnormalities and fever may be late findings.
> * A telltale sign is pain out of proportion to physical examination findings [1, 4, 5].
> * Necrotizing fasciitis is associated with multiple laboratory abnormalities including hyponatremia, hyperglycemia, leukocytosis, anemia, elevated creatinine, and elevated CRP, but their absence does not preclude the diagnosis [10, 11].

- Staphylococcal, streptococcal, and polymicrobial infections are common [4].
- Initial management is emergent surgical consultation along with aggressive fluid resuscitation and broad-spectrum antibiotics with MRSA coverage [2, 6].
- Definitive management is surgical debridement in the operating room [1].

References

1. Misiakos EP, Bagias G, et al. Early diagnosis and surgical treatment for necrotizing fasciitis: A multicenter study. Front Surg. 2017;4:5.
2. Liebling M, Marzi I. Necrotizing fasciitis: treatment concepts and clinical results. Eur J Trauma Emerg Surg. 2018;44(2):279–90.
3. Miller LG, et al. Necrotizing fasciitis caused by community-associated methicillin-resistant staphylococcus aureus in Los Angeles. N Engl J Med. 2005;352(14):1445.
4. Goh T, Goh LH, et al. Early diagnosis of necrotizing fasciitis. Br J Surg. 2014;101(1):e119–25.
5. Edlich RF, et al. Modern concepts of the diagnosis and treatment of necrotizing fasciitis. J Emerg Med. 2010;39(2):261.
6. Smeets L, et al. Necrotizing fasciitis: diagnosis and treatment. Rev Med Liege. 2006;61(4):240.
7. Bingol-Kologlu M, Yildiz RV, et al. Necrotizing Fasciitis in children: diagnostic and therapeutic aspects. J Pediatr Surg. 2007;42(11):1892–7.
8. Simpfendorfer CS. Radiologic approach to musculoskeletal infections. Infect Dis Clin North Am. 2017;31(2):299–324.
9. Wronski M, et al. Necrotizing fasciitis: early sonographic diagnosis. J Clin Ultrasound. 2011;39(4):236–9.
10. Wong CH, et al. The LRINEC (laboratory risk indicator for necrotizing fasciitis) score: a tool for distinguishing necrotizing fasciitis from other soft tissue infections. Crit Care Med. 2004;32(7):1535.
11. Bechar J, Sepehripur S, et al. Laboratory risk indicator for necrotizing fasciitis (LRINEC) score for the assessment of early necrotizing fasciitis: a systematic review of the literature. Ann R Coll Surg Engl. 2017;99(5):341–6.
12. Madsen MB, Hjortrup PB, et al. Immunoglobulin G for patients with necrotizing soft tissue infection (INSTINCT): a randomized, blinded, placebo-controlled trial. Intensive Care Med. 2017;43(11):1585–93.

Erythroderma

19

Katrina Harper-Kirksey

Background

Erythroderma is a severe and potentially life-threatening dermatitis described as an intense and widespread erythema typically involving greater than 90% of the body surface area, with a variable degree of exfoliative skin scaling (see Figs. 19.1 and 19.2) [1, 2]. It is a manifestation of a wide range of cutaneous and systemic diseases including infection, malignancy, and drug hypersensitivity reactions [3].

There are numerous systemic and cutaneous diseases known to be associated with erythroderma (Tables 19.1 and 19.3). The most common trigger of erythroderma is an exacerbation of an underlying dermatitis, most commonly psoriasis (Fig. 19.3) (23%), atopic dermatitis, and contact dermatitis [4–7]. Drug reaction is another important cause of erythroderma, implicated in 20% of cases, with at least 135 drugs suspected as potential causative agents [5–8, 10]. A common malignancy associated with erythroderma is cutaneous T-cell lymphoma (CTCL) [3, 7, 9]. Idiopathic erythroderma, where no cause can be elucidated despite thorough serial investigations, occurs in approximately 30% of cases. "Red man's syndrome" associated with rapid vancomycin infusion is considered to be an example of idiopathic erythroderma [3–5, 8, 10, 11].

Because erythroderma is often associated with scaling and extensive erythema, it is often difficult to discern the typical features characteristic of the preexisting, underlying condition. For this reason, diagnosis and management strategies can be challenging [1, 2].

Erythroderma is thought to be mediated by a complicated process of inflammatory cell interactions, resulting in a dramatic turnover of epidermal cells [12]. It is a rare condition, with an incidence rate of approximately 1 per 100,000 adults [13].

K. Harper-Kirksey, MD
Department of Emergency Medicine, Department of Anesthesia Critical Care, NYU Langone Medical Centers, New York, NY, USA
e-mail: Katrina.Harper-Kirksey@nyumc.org

© Springer International Publishing AG, part of Springer Nature 2018
E. Rose (ed.), *Life-Threatening Rashes*, https://doi.org/10.1007/978-3-319-75623-3_19

Fig. 19.1 Widespread erythema and areas of sparing in a patient with unclear etiology of erythroderma. (Used with permission from Rothe et al. [3])

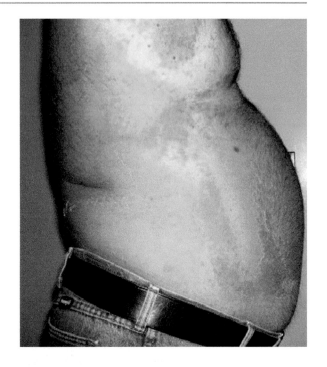

Fig. 19.2 Diffuse erythema and scaling of a 14-year-old girl with erythroderma of unknown etiology. (Source (open access): https://www.ncbi.nlm.nih.gov/pmc/articles/PMC2800861/)

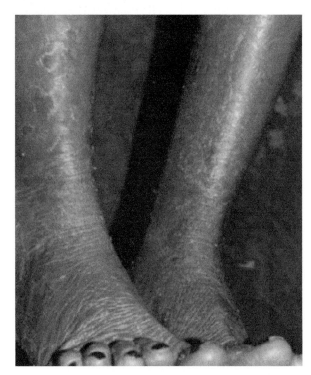

Table 19.1 Common causes of erythroderma (remembered by mnemonic IDSCALP) [54]

I	*Idiopathic – 30%*
	Infections (HIV, HSV, dermatophytosis, scabies)
D	*Drug allergy – 20%*
S	*Seborrheic dermatitis – 2%*
	Sarcoidosis
C	*Contact dermatitis – 3%*
	Connective tissue diseases
A	*Atopic dermatitis – 10%*
	Autoimmune (systemic lupus/dermatomyositis/bullous pemphigoid/pemphigus foliaceus/lichen planus/graft vs host disease)
L	*Lymphoma and leukemia – 14%* (including Sezary syndrome)
P	*Psoriasis – 23%* (including reactive arthritis/pityriasis rubra pilaris)

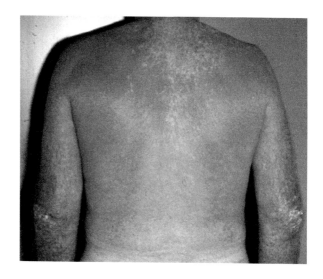

Fig. 19.3 Patient with erythrodermic psoriasis and classic plaques on elbows. (Used with permission from Rothe et al. [3])

Erythroderma is rare in children and occurs at an average age of 42–61 years [14]. When age of onset is less than 40 years, the condition is typically a result of atopic dermatitis, seborrheic dermatitis, staphylococcal scalded skin syndrome, or a hereditary ichthyosis [14, 15]. It is more common in males and has no racial predilection [3–7, 9, 16].

Classic Clinical Presentation

The typical presentation of erythroderma is characterized by erythematous patches which progressively increase in size and coalesce to cover most of the body's surface, with occasional islands of sparing [17]. Scaling can occur as large sheets or small flakes and generally erupt 2–6 days after the onset of erythema. Pruritus is common and is most severe in patients with atopic dermatitis and Sezary syndrome

Fig. 19.4 Patient with
Sezary and skin fissuring.
(Used with permission
from Rothe et al. [3])

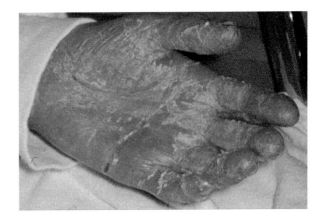

Fig. 19.5 Diffuse alopecia
in a patient with chronic
idiopathic erythroderma.
(Used with permission
from Rothe et al. [3])

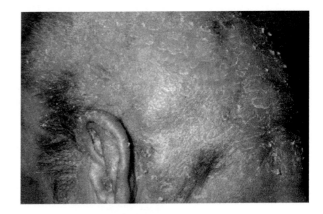

(a leukemic variant of cutaneous T-cell lymphoma where atypical lymphocytes known as Sezary cells are found in peripheral blood; see Fig. 19.4) [50]. The skin may feel leathery secondary to excessive scratching and there may be eyelid and periorbital involvement [18].

Especially in chronic conditions, patches of hypopigmentation can be observed, and hair and nails may shed [19]. Nails may also become ridged, thickened, and brittle [9, 17, 20, 21]. Individuals with long-standing erythroderma may present with cachexia, vitiligo, diffuse alopecia (see Fig. 19.5), and thickened palms and soles (Table 19.2) [18, 22].

Atypical Presentation

Table 19.2 Classic features of erythroderma

Skin	Widespread erythema Variable degree/character of scaling (2–6 days after erythema) Pruritus (can lead to lichenification)
Eyes	Eyelid swelling may lead to ectropion (eyelid eversion), blepharitis, epiphora (excessive tearing), ectropion (eyelid eversion)
Palms/soles	May develop yellowish, diffuse keratoderma
Nails	Dull, ridged, thickened May develop onycholysis and shed (onychomadesis)
Lymph nodes	Generalized lymphadenopathy which may be reactive or suggestive of lymphoma
Hair	Telogen effluvium (scaling of the scalp) leading to varying degrees of hair loss

Table 19.3 Uncommon causes of erythroderma

Stevens-Johnson syndrome
Toxic epidermal necrolysis
Toxic shock syndrome
Stasis dermatitis (venous eczema)
Seborrheic dermatitis
Staphylococcal scalded skin syndrome
Blistering diseases including pemphigus and bullous pemphigoid
Sezary syndrome
Rare congenital ichthyotic conditions

Associated Systemic Symptoms

Systemic symptoms related to erythroderma itself or to the primary disease can be observed. Many of these features can lead to serious sequelae and are discussed further in the complications section. Patients often are unwell appearing and report chills, fever, fatigue, and malaise. Lymphadenopathy and (rarely) splenomegaly can be observed. Hepatomegaly is seen in 1/3 of cases and is most common in drug-induced erythroderma [7, 22]. Significant protein loss exceeding 9 g/ m^2 body surface per day as a consequence of skin exfoliation can lead to hypoalbuminemia, edema, and muscle wasting [12]. As a result, patients may experience loss in temperature regulation and up to 50% of patients develop pretibial and pedal edema [2, 3].

When erythroderma occurs secondary to drug reaction, eosinophilia can be observed along with systemic symptoms characteristic of DRESS (drug reaction and systemic symptoms; see Chap. 20) [2].

Time Course of Disease

Erythroderma may develop rapidly over hours to days or more gradually over weeks to month (see Table 19.4) [22]. Patients may initially present as medically stable or with life-threatening complications [3].

The duration of erythroderma is highly variable and is determined by the underlying cause. Erythroderma as a result of primary skin disease is typically a gradual course with a median duration of 10 months but can go on to last years [7].

The disease evolves more rapidly when it is a result of drug hypersensitivity reaction, lymphoma, or leukemia. In the setting of systemic disease, symptoms may persist from weeks to years – dependent on the course of the underlying disorder. Conversely, in the case of drug-induced erythroderma, resolution of disease can occur in as little as 2–6 weeks after discontinuation of the offending agent [3]. Patients with DRESS, however, may take longer to recover – over weeks to months with possible relapse (*see* Chap. 20).

Common Mimics and Differential Diagnosis

The diagnosis of erythroderma is difficult given it is usually a manifestation of an underlying diagnosis or exacerbation of primary disorder (Table 19.5). Additionally, the characteristic physical findings of erythroderma generally obscure underlying disease features.

Key Physical Exam Findings and Diagnosis Features

As the list of causative factors of erythroderma continues to expand, it becomes more difficult to pinpoint the precipitating diagnosis [22]. Because of this, a thorough history of presenting illness is of utmost importance in diagnosing erythroderma [23]. Patients must be asked about all medications, preexisting medical conditions, allergies, and previous diagnoses of rash and skin disorders [7, 22].

Table 19.4 Typical course of disease according to etiology [22]

	Onset	Features	Duration
Primary cutaneous	Slower/indolent	Erythematous patches of increasing size with variable islands of sparing Subsequent scaling	Variable
Drug-induced	Abrupt	Morbilliform or urticarial followed by erythematous patches which increase in size	Comparatively quick resolution
Systemic	Gradual	Initially characteristic of disease before patches form and coalesce	Variable
Idiopathic			Unpredictable

Table 19.5 Common mimics of erythroderma, often implicated as precipitating factors

Acanthosis nigricans
Allergic contact dermatitis
Bullous pemphigoid
Contact dermatitis
Cutaneous T-cell lymphoma
Familial benign pemphigus (Hailey-Hailey disease)
Graft-versus-host disease
Lichen planus
Malignancy
Pediatric atopic dermatitis
Pemphigus foliaceus
Pityriasis rubra pilaris
Plaque psoriasis
Reactive arthritis
Rapid vancomycin infusion
Sarcoidosis
Seborrheic dermatitis
Stasis dermatitis

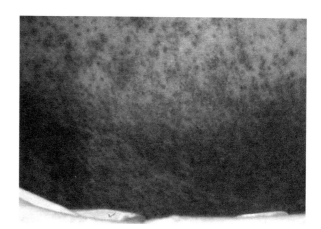

Fig. 19.6 Elderly patient with near erythroderma. Microscopy confirmed scabies infestation. (Used with permission from Rothe et al. [3])

Physical examination is crucial in attempts to detect an underlying etiology as well as to evaluate for systemic involvement and potential complications (i.e., organomegaly, lymphadenopathy, peripheral edema, infection, heart failure, and potential respiratory compromise) [7, 18, 24].

Following a detailed history and physical, a skin biopsy, laboratory studies, imaging, and histology may useful adjuncts to derive a definitive diagnosis and exclude clinical mimics (see Fig. 19.6). These ancillary studies are often nonspecific, although with repeat testing the diagnosis may become apparent over time (Table 19.6) [11, 15, 16].

Table 19.6 Diagnostic features of underlying disorders

Skin exam features [3, 18, 26]	Blisters and crusting: secondary infection, autoimmune blistering disorders (bullous pemphigoid, pemphigus foliaceus Large scales: psoriasis Fine scales: atopic dermatitis/dermatophyte infection Burn-like scale: seborrheic dermatitis Islands of sparing/yellow tinge to the skin/hyperkeratosis of the palms and soles: pityriasis rubra pilaris (PRP)
Laboratory testing	Leukocytosis, increased ESR, anemia, hypoalbuminemia, and hyperglobulinemia are frequent findings in all causes Eosinophilia in patients with DRESS Increased IgE may be noted in atopic dermatitis Consider peripheral blood smears and bone marrow examination if leukemia is considered
Skin biopsy	Consider if cause unknown although tend to be nonspecific Repeated biopsies may be necessary Skin scrapings may show hyphae or mites
Imaging [22]	If cause is unknown, imaging may be performed as a survey for occult malignancy Chest radiograph can identify infections, inflammatory disorders such as sarcoidosis with hilar lymphadenopathy, and congestive heart failure
Cultures/PCR	Evaluation for suprainfection, fungal infections, herpes simplex virus, and varicella zoster virus
Histological [27–30]	In all comers, hyperkeratosis, acanthosis, spongiosis, and perivascular inflammatory infiltrate are frequent findings in general May otherwise be nonspecific
Immunofluorescence [22, 31]	Of benefit in autoimmune blistering disease or connective tissue disease (i.e., immunoglobulins at the dermal-epidermal junction)

Management

Erythroderma is a dermatologic emergency which requires a dermatology consultation and hospital admission for severe cases to avoid potentially catastrophic complications. The principle management consists of discontinuation of all offending medications, maintaining skin moisture and integrity (through aggressive wound care), adequate hydration and nutrition, electrolyte repletion, and antibiotics for secondary infection (Table 19.7). Erythroderma as an isolated process will persist until the underlying condition is addressed, and the primary etiology may impact disease course and management options. Therefore, once the underlying diagnosis is established, targeted therapy should be administered promptly (Table 19.8).

If a cause can be identified, then specific treatment should be initiated. Notably, systemic steroid should be avoided in psoriasis and staphylococcal scalded skin syndrome.

Table 19.7 Initial management

Systemic symptoms [3]	Replacement of fluid and electrolytes Monitoring hemodynamic status Monitoring and regulation of body temperature Nutritional support Treatment of skin inflammation and pruritus Discontinuation of all offending/unnecessary medications Diuretics for refractory edema
Skin inflammation and pruritus [3, 22, 32]	Topical corticosteroids and oral antihistamines Oatmeal baths or warm wet compresses (no more than a quarter of the body at a time) Bland emollients or petrolatum for patient comfort
Infections	Blood cultures Broad-spectrum antibiotic coverage (to include MRSA) Antiviral medications where appropriate

Table 19.8 Targeted treatment modalities

Atopic dermatitis [22, 33–36]	Avoiding allergens Topical and systemic steroids In refractory cases: cyclosporine, methotrexate, azathioprine, mycophenolate mofetil, and/or interferon
Psoriasis [37–40, 51–53]	Topical steroids Phototherapy Methotrexate Retinoids (i.e., acitretin) Cyclosporine In refractory cases: tumor necrosis factor (TNF) inhibitors, interleukin (IL) inhibitors, phosphodiesterase type 4 [PDE-4] inhibitors (i.e., infliximab, adalimumab, etanercept, ustekinumab, secukinumab) *this therapy can cause mycosis fungoides to progress
Mycosis fungoides [41–45]	Topical corticosteroids Topical chemotherapy Topical retinoids May consider phototherapy and radiotherapy In refractory cases: interferon, oral retinoids, histone deacetylase inhibitors, monoclonal antibodies, photopheresis, and chemotherapy Rarely stem cell transplantation considered
Cutaneous T-cell lymphoma [25]	Methotrexate Potent topical steroids Chemotherapy UV light
Sezary syndrome [46]	Extracorporeal photochemotherapy Systemic retinoids Interferon
Pityriasis rubra pilaris (PRP) [22, 47]	Systemic retinoids as first line Topical steroids as adjunct to palms, soles, face, skin folds, and extremities May consider *methotrexate*, TNF-alpha inhibitors, *cyclosporine*, and azathioprine
Drug induced [2, 7, 35]	Discontinue causative agents Short-course oral steroids or pulse intravenous IV steroid therapy
Idiopathic erythroderma [1, 5, 9, 11]	Low to mid-potency topical corticosteroids Oral antihistamines In refractory cases: systemic corticosteroids

Complications

While the physiologic demands of erythroderma are tolerated by many patients, those at the extremes of age and patients with multiple comorbidities may suffer life-threatening consequences (see Table 19.9). The shunting of blood through the skin due to peripheral vasodilation can result in high-output heart failure [3]. These patients can present with tachycardia and pulmonary edema. Increased skin perfusion also results in temperature dysregulation and fluid and electrolyte imbalance. Exfoliation and protein loss result in edema and leave patient's susceptible to secondary infections [12]. Acute respiratory distress syndrome (ARDS) is also a common complication.

End-organ damage may develop such as hepatitis, myocarditis, and/or interstitial nephritis [2].

Mortality rates range between 4 and 64% depending on the patient population [7, 22].

> **Bottom Line: Erythroderma Clinical Pearls**
> In the majority of cases, erythroderma results from an underlying condition and cannot itself be prevented [22]. Individuals who develop erythroderma as a result of drug hypersensitivity should be instructed to avoid the offending agent in the future. Erythroderma as a result of underlying inflammatory skin condition will usually abate with treatment but may recur at any time. Idiopathic erythroderma is characterized by a more unpredictable course. Overall, prognosis of erythroderma is dependent on the underlying cause and is generally favorable if the underlying disease can be effectively treated [48–50].

Table 19.9 Physiologic derangements

Protein loss
Edema
Hypoalbuminemia
Fluid loss
Temperature dysregulation
Electrolyte and metabolic disturbances
High output cardiac failure
Sepsis from superinfection

References

1. Khaled A, Sellami A, Fazaa B, Kharfi M, Zeglaoui F, Kamoun MR. Acquired erythroderma in adults: a clinical and prognostic study. J Eur Acad Dermatol Venereol. 2010;24:781–8.
2. Usatine RP, Smith MA, Chumley HS, Mayeaux EJ Jr. Erythroderma. In: Usatine RP, Smith MA, Chumley HS, Mayeaux Jr EJ, editors. The color atlas of family medicine. 2nd ed. New York: McGraw-Hill; 2013.

3. Rothe MJ, Bernstein ML, Grant-Kels JM. Life-threatening erythroderma: diagnosing and treating the "red man". Clin Dermatol. 2005;23:206–17.
4. Pal S, Haroon TS. Erythroderma: a clinico-etiologic study of 90 cases. Int J Dermatol. 1998;37:104.
5. Akhyani M, Ghodsi ZS, Toosi S, Dabbaghian H. Erythroderma: a clinical study of 97 cases. BMC Dermatol. 2005;5:5.
6. Rym BM, Mourad M, Bechir Z, et al. Erythroderma in adults: a report of 80 cases. Int J Dermatol. 2005;44:731.
7. Grant-Kels JM, Fedeles F, Rothe MJ. Exfoliative dermatitis. In: Goldsmith LA, Katz SI, Gilchrest BA, Paller AS, Leffell DJ, Wolff K, editors. Fitzpatrick's dermatology in general medicine. 8th ed. New York: McGraw Hill Medical; 2012.
8. Sheen YS, Chu CY, Wang SH, Tsai TF. Dapsone hypersensitivity syndrome in non-leprosy patients: a retrospective study of its incidence in a tertiary referral center in Taiwan. J Dermatol Treat. 2009;20:340.
9. Li J, Zheng HY. Erythroderma: a clinical and prognostic study. Dermatology. 2012;225:154–62.
10. Sigurdsson V, Toonstra J, van Vloten WA. Idiopathic erythroderma: a follow-up study of 28 patients. Dermatology. 1997;194:98.
11. Thestrup-Pedersen K, Halkier-Sørensen L, Søgaard H, Zachariae H. The red man syndrome. Exfoliative dermatitis of unknown etiology: a description and follow-up of 38 patients. J Am Acad Dermatol. 1988;18:1307.
12. Kanthraj GR, Srinivas CR, Devi PU, et al. Quantitative estimation and recommendations for supplementation of protein lost through scaling in exfoliative dermatitis. Int J Dermatol. 1999;38:91.
13. Sigurdsson V, Steegmans PH, van Vloten WA. The incidence of erythroderma: a survey among all dermatologists in the Netherlands. J Am Acad Dermatol. 2001;45:675.
14. Sarkar R, Garg VK. Erythroderma in children. Indian J Dermatol Venereol Leprol. 2010;76:341. Sarkar R, Basu S, Sharma RC. Neonatal and infantile erythrodermas. Arch Dermatol. 2001;137:822
15. Fraitag S, Bodemer C. Neonatal erythroderma. Curr Opin Pediatr. 2010;22(4):438–44.
16. Sigurdsson V, Toonstra J, Hezemans-Boer M, van Vloten WA. Erythroderma. A clinical and follow-up study of 102 patients, with special emphasis on survival. J Am Acad Dermatol. 1996;35:53.
17. Sehgal VN, Srivastava G, Sardana K. Erythroderma/exfoliative dermatitis: a synopsis. Int J Dermatol. 2004;43:39–47.
18. Sterry W, Steinhoff M. Erythroderma. In: Bolognia JL, Jorizzo JL, Schaffer JV, eds. Dermatology.3rd ed. Philadelphia: Elsevier Saunders; 2012:171–181.
19. Bi MY, Curry JL, Christiano AM, et al. The spectrum of hair loss in patients with mycosis fungoides and Sézary syndrome. J Am Acad Dermatol. 2011;64:53.
20. Klein A, Landthaler M, Karrer S. Pityriasis rubra pilaris: a review of diagnosis and treatment. Am J Clin Dermatol. 2010;11:157.
21. Rosenbach M, Hsu S, Korman NJ, Lebwohl MG, Young M, Bebo BF Jr, et al. Treatment of erythrodermic psoriasis: from the medical board of the National Psoriasis Foundation. J Am Acad Dermatol. 2010;62(4):655–62.
22. Mistry N, Gupta A, Alva A, Sibbald G. A review of the diagnosis and Management of Erythroderma (generalized red skin). In: Advances in skin and wound care: Woltkers Kluwer Health; 2015. p. 228–36. www.woundcarejournal.com.
23. Yuan XY, Guo JY, Dang YP, Qiao L, Liu W. Erythroderma: a clinical-etiological study of 82 cases. Eur J Dermatol. 2010;20(3):373–7.
24. Lancrajan C, Bumbacea R, Giurcaneanu C. Erythrodermic atopic dermatitis with late onset casepresentation. J Med Life. 2010;3:80–3.
25. Botella-Estrada R, Sanmartin O, Oliver V, Febrer I, Aliaga A. Erythroderma. A clinicopathological study of 56 cases. Arch Dermatol. 1994;130:1503–7.
26. Griffiths WA. Pityriasis rubra pilaris. Clin Exp Dermatol. 1980;5:105. PMID7398119

27. Megna M, Sidikov AA, Zaslavsky DV, Chuprov IN, Timoshchuk EA, Egorova U, et al. The role of histological presentation in erythroderma. Int J Dermatol. 2017;56(4):400–4.
28. Ram-Wolff C, Martin-Garcia N, Bensussan A, Bagot M, Ortonne N. Histopathologic diagnosis of lymphomatous versus inflammatory erythroderma: a morphologic and phenotypic study on 47 skin biopsies. Am J Dermatopathol. 2010;32(8):755–63.
29. Zip C, Murray S, Walsh NM. The specificity of histopathology in erythroderma. J Cutan Pathol. 1993;20:393.
30. Vasconcellos C, Domingues PP, Aoki V, et al. Erythroderma: analysis of 247 cases. Rev Saude Publica. 1995;29:177.
31. Armstrong AW, Bagel J, Van Voorhees AS, Robertson AD, Yamauchi PS. Combining biologic therapies with other systemic treatments in psoriasis: evidence-based, best-practice recommendations from the medical Board of the National Psoriasis Foundation. JAMA Dermatol. 2015;151(4):432–8.
32. Bruno TF, Grewal P. Erythroderma: a dermatologic emergency. CJEM. 2009;11(3):244–6.
33. Guttman-Yassky E, Dhingra N, Leung DY. New era of biologic therapeutics in atopic dermatitis. Expert Opin Biol Ther. 2013;13(4):549–61.
34. Shimizu H. Shimizu's textbook of dermatology. 1st ed. Tokyo: Hokkaido University Press/ Nakayama Shoten; 2007. p. 122–5.
35. Katsarou A, Armenaka M. Atopic dermatitis in older patients: particular points. J Eur Acad Dermatol Venereol. 2011;25(1):12–8.
36. Gelbard CM, Hebert AA. New and emerging trends in the treatment of atopic dermatitis. Patient Prefer Adherence. 2008;2:387–92.
37. Strober BE. Successful treatment of psoriasis and psoriatic arthritis with etanercept and methotrexate in a patient newly unresponsive to infliximab. Arch Dermatol. 2004;140:366.
38. Barland C, Kerdel FA. Addition of low-dose methotrexate to infliximab in the treatment of a patient with severe, recalcitrant pustular psoriasis. Arch Dermatol. 2003;139:949–50.
39. Ladizinski B, Lee KC, Wilmer E, Alavi A, Mistry N, Sibbald RG. A review of the clinical variants and the management of psoriasis. Adv Skin Wound Care. 2013;26:271–84.
40. Zattra E, Belloni Fortina A, Peserico A. Alaibac M. Erythroderma in the era of biological therapies. Eur J Dermatol. 2012;22(2):167–71.
41. Rupoli S, Canafoglia L, Goteri G, Leoni P, Brandozzi G, Federici I, et al. Results of a prospective phase II trial with oral low dose bexarotene plus photochemotherapy (PUVA) in refractory and/or relapsed patients with mycosis fungoides. Eur J Dermatol. 2016;26(1):13–20.
42. Sokolowska-Wojdylo M, Florek A, Zaucha JM, Chmielowska E, Giza A, Knopinska-Posluszny W, et al. Polish lymphoma research group experience with bexarotene in the treatment of cutaneous T-cell lymphoma. Am J Ther. 2016;23(3):e749–56.
43. Chung CG, Poligone B. Cutaneous T cell lymphoma: an update on pathogenesis and systemic therapy. Curr Hematol Malig Rep. 2015;10(4):468–76.
44. Galper SL, Smith BD, Wilson LD. Diagnosis and management of mycosis fungoides. Oncology (Williston Park). 2010;24(6):491–501.
45. Wilcox RA. Cutaneous T-cell lymphoma: 2016 update on diagnosis, risk-stratification, and management. Am J Hematol. 2016;91(1):151–65.
46. Al Hothali GI. Review of the treatment of mycosis fungoides and Sézary syndrome: a stage-based approach. Int J Health Sci (Qassim). 2013;7(2):220–39.
47. Leger M, Newlove T, Robinson M, Patel R, Meehan S, Ramachandran S. Pityriasis rubra pilaris. Dermatol Online J. 2012;18(12):14.
48. Boyd AS, Menter A. Erythrodermic psoriasis. Precipitating factors, course, and prognosis in 50 patients. J Am Acad Dermatol. 1989;21:985.
49. Kubica AW, Davis MD, Weaver AL, et al. Sézary syndrome: a study of 176 patients at Mayo Clinic. J Am Acad Dermatol. 2012;67:1189.
50. Kim YH, Bishop K, Varghese A, Hoppe RT. Prognostic factors in erythrodermic mycosis fungoides and the Sezary syndrome. Arch Dermatol. 1995;131:1003.

51. Wang J, Wang YM, Ahn HY. Biological products for the treatment of psoriasis: therapeutic targets, pharmacodynamics and disease-drug-drug interaction implications. AAPS J. 2014;16(5):938–47.
52. Cather JC, Crowley JJ. Use of biologic agents in combination with other therapies for the treatment of psoriasis. Am J Clin Dermatol. 2014;15(6):467–78.
53. Zattra E, Belloni Fortina A, Peserico A. Alaibac M. Erythroderma in the era of biological therapies. Eur J Dermatol. 2012;22(2):167–71.
54. Umar, S, Kelly P. Erythroderma (Generalized Exfoliative Dermatitis) clinical presentation. Medscape. (updated June 4 2018). Retrieved 2018 from https://emedicine.medscape.com/article/1106906-overview.

DRESS Syndrome: Drug Reaction with Eosinophilia and Systemic Symptoms/Drug-Induced Hypersensitivity Syndrome (DHS)

20

Matthieu P. DeClerck and Brittney K. DeClerck

Background

Drug reaction with eosinophilia and systemic symptoms (DRESS) syndrome, also known as drug-induced hypersensitivity syndrome (DHS), is a rare but potentially lethal adverse drug reaction that classically manifests as a morbilliform rash with associated fever, lymphadenopathy, hematologic abnormalities, and multi-organ manifestations. While anticonvulsants and sulfonamides are the most common offending agents, many other drugs can cause DRESS syndrome. Systemic involvement can manifest with hematologic, hepatic, renal, pulmonary, cardiac, neurologic, gastrointestinal, and endocrine abnormalities [1].

The list of potential offending medications is long (see Table 20.1), but the most common culprits include carbamazepine, phenytoin, phenobarbital, lamotrigine, allopurinol, dapsone, and sulfasalazine [1]. DRESS syndrome is relatively rare, with an incidence of 1/5000 to 1/10,000 prescriptions of each of the causal agents [2–5]. Most cases affect adults without gender predilection, but rare cases have been reported in children [1]. DRESS syndrome carries a 10% mortality risk, usually due to hepatic failure [1].

The pathophysiology of DRESS syndrome remains incompletely understood but involves reactivation of herpesviruses (HHV-6, HHV-7, Epstein-Barr virus [EBV], and cytomegalovirus [CMV]), against which the body mounts a strong immune response [2, 6, 7]. The offending medications may not only affect epigenetic control mechanisms, thereby promoting viral reactivation, but also induce an antiviral T-cell response by interacting with the major histocompatibility complex receptors in

M. P. DeClerck (✉)
Keck School of Medicine, LAC+USC Medical Center, Los Angeles, CA, USA
e-mail: mdeclerc@usc.edu

B. K. DeClerck
Keck School of Medicine, Los Angeles, CA, USA
e-mail: brittney.declerck@med.usc.edu

© Springer International Publishing AG, part of Springer Nature 2018
E. Rose (ed.), *Life-Threatening Rashes*, https://doi.org/10.1007/978-3-319-75623-3_20

Table 20.1 Common drugs associated with DRESS

Drug category	Drug name
Anticonvulsant	Carbamazepine, lamotrigine, phenobarbital, phenytoin, valproic acid, zonisamide
Antimicrobial	Ampicillin, cefotaxime, dapsone, ethambutol, isoniazid, linezolid, metronidazole, minocycline, pyrazinamide, quinine, rifampin, sulfasalazine, streptomycin, trimethoprim-sulfamethoxazole, vancomycin
Antiviral	Abacavir, nevirapine, zalcitabine
Antidepressant	Bupropion, fluoxetine
Antihypertensive	Amlodipine, captopril
Biologic	Efalizumab, imatinib
NSAID	Celecoxib, ibuprofen
Miscellaneous	Allopurinol, epoetin alfa, mexiletine, ranitidine

individuals with genetic susceptibility [2]. Two theories currently exist regarding the pathophysiology of DRESS syndrome:

1. Patients with predisposing genetic mutations lack the ability to metabolize certain medications leading to the accumulation of active drug metabolites that then trigger an autoimmune response and/or induce the reactivation of herpesviral infections [1].
2. The reactivation of herpesviruses (mainly HHV-6, but also CMV, EBV, and HHV-7) is triggered by an allergic immune response to a drug with the subsequent activation of T-cell populations (particularly cytotoxic CD8$^+$ lymphocytes) that cause direct tissue damage [1].

In both hypotheses, drug-related reactivation of herpesviral infections directly influences the immune attack on the patient's skin and affected organs leading to the clinical manifestations of DRESS syndrome. Clinical features of DRESS, such as fever, edema, lymphadenopathy, hematologic expansion, and hepatitis, are consistent with those seen in a typical herpesvirus infection and support the hypothesis of a viral infection as a trigger of the syndrome.

Classic Clinical Presentation

The common initial symptoms of DRESS syndrome are fever, malaise, lymphadenopathy, and a skin eruption. A telling feature of DRESS syndrome is the delay of the onset of symptoms in relation to exposure to the offending medication. These symptoms typically occur 2–6 weeks following the initiation of the offending agent, which is prolonged in contrast to other types of drug eruptions [1, 2]. Medications taken for more than 3 months or initiated less than 2 weeks before the onset of DRESS syndrome are unlikely to be the culprit.

A diffuse morbilliform rash with associated pruritus is the most common cutaneous finding [1]. Occasionally the rash can generalize and progress to erythroderma (>90% involvement). The rash typically begins on the face with characteristic associated facial edema that appears similar to angioedema (Fig. 20.1). The rash then progresses

Fig. 20.1 DRESS patient with morbilliform rash and facial edema

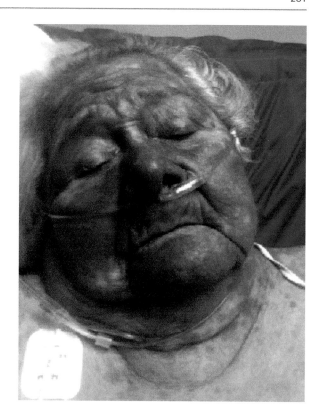

Fig. 20.2 DRESS patient with morbilliform rash progressing from the face to trunk and upper extremities

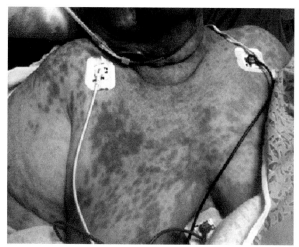

to the upper trunk and arms (Fig. 20.2) and can also involve the lower extremities (Fig. 20.3). The rash often involves more than 50% of body surface area (BSA) [1]. Other possible cutaneous manifestations include vesicles, bullae, targetoid plaques, purpura, pustules, scaling, and mucosal inflammation with erosions [1] (Fig. 20.4).

Fig. 20.3 DRESS patient
with morbilliform rash that
progressed from the face
and trunk to lower
extremities

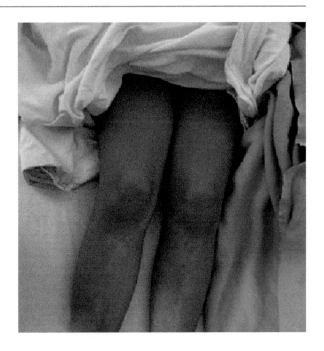

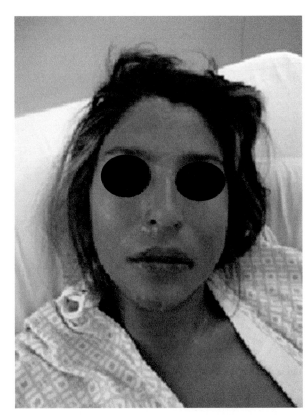

Fig. 20.4 DRESS patient
with facial eruption and
edema as well as oral and
ocular mucosal
inflammation and erosion

Atypical Presentation

There are rare cases of DRESS syndrome that exist without "D" (causative drug relation), "R" (rash), "E" (eosinophilia), or "SS" systemic symptoms [9]. In one review of 216 cases over a 15-year period in France, they found a morbilliform eruption in only 70% of cases and eosinophilia in only 50% of cases [10].

Associated Systemic Symptoms

Hematologic and lymphatic involvement are common. Hematologic abnormalities occur in 30–90% of cases and diffuse lymphadenopathy occurs in 30–60% of cases [6, 8, 9]. Hematologic abnormalities include lymphocytosis, eosinophilia, and atypical lymphocytes (mononucleosis-like). Thrombocytopenia and anemia may also be present as part of a hemophagocytic syndrome. Lymphadenopathy is commonly present at cervical lymph nodes but can be found elsewhere and is typically found at multiple sites.

Associated systemic symptoms other than fever, malaise, and rash are directly related to the organ system involved (Table 20.2). Systemic involvement of at least one visceral organ occurs in approximately 90% of patients. The liver is the most common organ affected with 60–80% of cases showing liver impairment. Renal involvement occurs in 10–30% of cases and lung involvement occurs in 5–25% of cases [11–13]. Hepatic necrosis with fulminant liver failure is the most common cause of mortality in DRESS syndrome. Other organ systems that may be involved include the heart, gastrointestinal tract, pancreas, thyroid, neurologic system (brain and peripheral nerves), muscles, and eyes [9]. Clinical symptoms, laboratory abnormalities, and imaging studies will reflect specific organ involvement (Table 20.2). While multiple drugs can cause DRESS syndrome, some specific drugs have a predilection for specific organ dysfunction (Table 20.2) [16].

Key Physical Exam Findings and Diagnostic Features

A thorough history and physical examination should be performed. DRESS syndrome should be suspected in patients who have received a high-risk medication initiated within the past 2–6 weeks who present with a constellation of the following signs and symptoms [2]:

- Morbilliform skin eruption that may progress to confluent and infiltrated erythema or exfoliative dermatitis.
- Facial edema.
- Fever (38–40°C).
- Enlarged cervical lymph nodes and/or generalized lymphadenopathy
- Systemic manifestations with organ involvement (hepatitis, nephritis, pneumonitis, carditis).
- Histopathology of the skin biopsy can help exclude other entities but is most commonly non-specific.

Table 20.2 Systemic manifestations, related drugs, and clinical findings

Systemic manifestation	Common offending drug	Clinical findings
Cutaneous (majority of cases)	Any	Erythematous morbilliform rash Facial edema Generalized erythroderma Pustular eruption Targetoid lesions Mucositis
Hematologic (30–90% of cases)	Any	Leukocytosis with eosinophilia (>700/microL) Atypical lymphocytosis Thrombocytopenia Anemia
Lymphatic (75% of cases)	Any	Cervical or generalized lymphadenopathy
Hepatic (60–80% of cases)	Phenytoin, minocycline, dapsone	Hepatosplenomegaly Hepatitis with elevated liver enzymes Hepatic necrosis with liver failure Hepatic coagulopathy
Renal (10–30% of cases)	Allopurinol, carbamazepine, dapsone	Renal insufficiency Elevated BUN and creatinine Impaired creatinine clearance Urine eosinophils Interstitial nephritis Renal failure
Pulmonary (5–25% of cases)	Minocycline	Acute interstitial pneumonitis Lymphocytic interstitial pneumonia Pleuritis Acute respiratory distress syndrome Atypical chest X-ray or chest CT scan
Cardiac	Ampicillin, minocycline	Myocarditis Cardiomegaly and pleural effusion on CXR ST and TW changes on EKG Systolic dysfunction with decreased EF, wall thickening, and pericardial effusion on echo Elevation of cardiac enzymes (BNP, CK, and troponin)
Gastrointestinal	Any	Gastroenteritis with dehydration Ulcerations/mucosal erosions with GI bleeding Colitis Pancreatitis
Endocrine	Any	Thyroiditis (autoimmune/Graves' thyroiditis) Sick euthyroid syndrome
Neurologic	Any	Meningitis Encephalitis Polyneuritis Brain lesions on MRI
Others	Any	Myositis with rhabdomyolysis Uveitis

Since DRESS syndrome cannot be diagnosed solely on the clinical signs and symptoms, a thorough initial evaluation for DRESS syndrome to exclude other causes would include CBC, BMP, LFTs, urinalysis, 24-h urine protein and urinary eosinophil count, CPK, LDH, ferritin, triglycerides, calcium, PTH, TSH, PT/PTT, lipase, serum protein electrophoresis, CRP, quantitative PCR (HHV-6, HHV-7, EBV, and CMV), blood culture, viral hepatitis serologies, and ANA.

Laboratory studies in DRESS syndrome:

- CBC: eosinophilia, lymphocytosis, atypical lymphocytes
- Liver function tests: ALT > 2× upper limit, Alk Phos >1.5× upper limit)
- Creatinine and urinalysis (moderately increased creatinine, proteinuria, urinary sedimentation rate, eosinophilia)

Imaging/diagnostic studies in DRESS syndrome:

- CXR/CT chest: interstitial pneumonitis and/or pleural effusion
- Echocardiogram and electrocardiogram: pericarditis and/or myocarditis
- Brain MRI: brain lesions
- Skin biopsy: non-specific but can help to exclude other causes

Diagnosis

There is no reliable standard for the diagnosis of DRESS syndrome. Diagnostic criteria are based on clinical and laboratory findings. There are three known scoring systems that may be helpful in making the diagnosis of DRESS syndrome. The most commonly used in the United States and Europe is known as RegiSCAR [11]. The following table (Table 20.3) presents a scoring system for classifying DRESS cases as definite, probable, or no case based on the 201 cases reviewed in the RegiSCAR's multinational registry [11, 18].

Common Mimics and Differential Diagnosis

DRESS has several similarities to other drug-induced rashes and life-threatening rashes that should remain in the differential diagnosis for DRESS. Table 20.4 outlines a few of the features that distinguish DRESS from these similar rashes (Table 20.4).

Management

The cornerstone of treatment of DRESS syndrome is prompt diagnosis, discontinuation of the offending medication, aggressive supportive therapy, and high-dose steroids [8, 16]. Topical corticosteroids can be used for symptomatic relief, but

Table 20.3 Scoring system for classifying DRESS

Clinical feature		Present		Absent
Fever ≥ 38.5°C (101.3°F)		0		−1
Enlarged lymph nodes (>1 cm size, at least 2 sites)		1		0
Eosinophilia: ≥700 or ≥10% (leucopenia)	≥1500 or ≥20%	1	2	0
Atypical lymphocytes		1		0
Rash ≥50% of body surface area		1		0
Rash suggestive (≥2 of facial edema, purpura, infiltration, desquamation)		1		0
Skin biopsy suggesting alternative diagnosis		−1		0
Organ involvement: one	Two or more	1	2	0
Disease duration >15 days		0		−2
Investigation for alternative cause (blood cultures, ANA, serology for hepatitis viruses, mycoplasma, chlamydia) ≥3 done and negative		1		0

Total score < 2, excluded; 2–3, possible; 4–5, probable; ≥6, definite

Table 20.4 Differential diagnosis

Rash	Clinical presentation
Non-specific drug eruption (morbilliform)	Skin eruption may appear similarly Lacking characteristic facial edema, lymphadenopathy, and systemic findings Onset <2 weeks
Stevens-Johnson syndrome (SJS)	Necrosis of the skin Mucosal involvement No facial edema, lymphadenopathy Systemic findings less common/severe Onset 3–30 days
Toxic epidermal necrolysis (TEN)	Necrosis of the skin +/− mucosal involvement No facial edema, lymphadenopathy Systemic findings less common/severe Onset 3–30 days
Acute generalized exanthematous pustulosis (AGEP)	Superficial pustules starting in skin folds Acute onset (<2 days) after drug exposure Fever and facial edema may be present No lymphadenopathy, systemic findings
Cutaneous lymphoma (MF)	Insidious onset Skin biopsy and T-cell clonality can help differentiate as DRESS can show a pseudo-lymphomatous pattern in the skin and lymph nodes histologically Rash morphology usually different

high-dose systemic steroid therapy is generally required, especially when there is systemic organ involvement [16]. Current clinical recommendations are to start systemic steroids at a dose equivalent to at least 1 mg/kg/day of prednisone with increased dosing based on lack of clinical response or when there is significant organ involvement [8]. Steroids should be continued at that dose until adequate clinical response is obtained. Steroids then need to be tapered slowly, over 3–9 months, in order to prevent relapse [2, 16]. In particularly severe cases or in those unresponsive to oral steroids, high-dose IV methylprednisolone may be required for several days with transition to oral prednisone [16].

No prospective randomized trials are available upon which to base the management of DRESS syndrome. Antiviral agents, such as ganciclovir, foscarnet, or cidofovir, may be indicated if active viral replication is detected. However, there is no current data to support such and the potential toxicities of these agents limit their use [2, 17]. Patients with DRESS syndrome should be managed in an ICU or burn unit for appropriate care and infection control. In addition, appropriate specialists should be consulted based on the affected organ systems.

Disease Progression

Most cases of DRESS syndrome will resolve over the course of 2–9 weeks depending on the severity of the initial disease and institution of appropriate treatment [9]. Without proper treatment, symptoms may be persistent and approximately 20% of cases relapse [14]. Relapse usually occurs due to early termination of steroid therapy, reintroduction to the original offending medication, or reactivation of the involved herpesvirus [14, 15]. Those that develop severe organ involvement can progress to fulminant liver failure requiring liver transplantation, renal insufficiency requiring hemodialysis, or other long-term sequelae based on the affected organ system. Death occurs in 10% of cases, usually secondary to hepatic failure.

Prognosis

The severity of DRESS syndrome and associated complications are related to the organ involvement (Table 20.2) [2]. Most patients with DRESS recover completely in the weeks to months after drug withdrawal and appropriate therapy. Occasionally patients will have a prolonged course with flares despite discontinuation of the offending medication [2, 16]. Patients developing liver failure or multi-organ involvement are at risk for chronic complications or death [2]. Careful continued clinical monitoring is crucial as organ involvement may be delayed, and flares may occur, particularly when the glucocorticoid dose is tapered too fast or other drugs are introduced [2].

Complications

End-organ dysfunction can occur almost at any site, and multi-organ failure can lead to shock and disseminated intravascular coagulation. Liver failure is the most common cause of death, but renal and cardiac involvement can become severe and are often more difficult to control with steroids than the hepatic involvement.

Endocrinopathies, such as thyroiditis, more often occur late and require continued clinical observation for several months. Other complications include dehydration and electrolyte imbalances, secondary bacterial or fungal infections, and sepsis related to the breakdown of the skin barrier.

Bottom Line: DRESS Clinical Pearls
- Consider the diagnosis of DRESS syndrome in a patient with rash, facial edema, lymphadenopathy, eosinophilia, and systemic symptoms/organ involvement.
- Delayed onset of rash after drug exposure. Occurs at 2–6 weeks after drug initiation (longer than most other drug eruptions).
- Promptly discontinue the offending drug.
- Obtain labs to evaluate for systemic organ involvement and appropriate imaging studies as indicated.
- Admit to the intensive care or unit burn unit (if severe erosions) with prompt dermatology consultation.
- Treatment includes high-dose steroid therapy of ≥ prednisone 1 mg/kg/day, perhaps IV methylprednisolone 1 g/day for several days in severe cases.
- Prolonged steroid taper is required to prevent relapse (3–9 months).
- Closely monitor patients' clinical symptoms and labs after resolution for relapse or late complications (i.e., endocrinopathies).

References

1. Husain Z, Reddy BY, Schwartz RA. Dress syndrome: Part I. Clinical perspectives. J Am Acad Dermatol. 2013;68:693.
2. Descamps V, Ranger-Rogez S. Dress syndrome. Joint Bone Spine. 2014;81:15–21.
3. Fiszenson-Albala F, Auzerie V, Mahe E, et al. A 6-month prospective survey of cutaneous drug reactions in a hospital setting. Br J Dermatol. 2003;149:1018–22.
4. Tennis P, Sterns RS. Risk of serious cutaneous disorders after initiation of use of phenytoin, carbamazepine, or sodium valproate: a record linkage study. Neurology. 1997;49:542.
5. Guberman AH, Besag FM, Brodie MJ, et al. Lamotrigine-associated rash: risk/benefit consideration in adults and children. Epilepsia. 1999;40:985.
6. Shiohara T, et al. Drug-induced hypersensitivity syndrome (DIHS). A reaction induced by a complex interplay among herpesviruses and antiviral and antidrug immune responses. Allergol Int. 2006;55:1–8.
7. Picard D, et al. Drug reaction with eosinophilia and systemic symptoms (DRESS): a multiorgan antiviral T cell response. Sci Transl Med. 2010;2(46):46ra62.
8. Tas S, et al. Management of drug rash with eosinophilia and systemic symptoms (DRESS syndrome): an update. Dermatology. 2003;206:353–6.
9. Cacoub P, Mussett P, Descamps V, et al. The DRESS syndrome: a literature review. Am J Med. 2011;124:588.
10. Peyriere H, et al. Variability in the clinical pattern of cutaneous side-effects of drugs with systemic symptoms: dose a DRESS syndrome really exist? Br J Dermatol. 2006;155:422–8.

11. Kardaun SH, Sekula P, Valeyrie-Allanore L, et al. Drug reaction with eosinophilia and systemic symptoms (DRESS): an original multisystem adverse drug reaction. Results from the prospective RegiSCAR study. Br J Dermatol. 2013;169:1071.
12. Lee T, Lee YS, Yoon SY, et al. Characteristics of liver injury in drug-induced systemic hypersensitivity reactions. J Am Acad Dermatol. 2013;69:407.
13. Lin IC, Yang HC, Strong C, et al. Liver injury in patients with DRESS: a clinical study of 72 cases. J Am Acad Dermatol. 2015;72:984.
14. Tetart F, Picard D, Janela B, et al. Prolonged evolution of drug reaction with eosinophilia and systemic symptoms: clinical, virologic, and biologic features. JAMA Dermatol. 2014;150:206.
15. Tohyama M, Hashimoto K, Yasukawa M, et al. Association of human herpesvirus 6 reactivation with the flaring and severity of drug-induced hypersensitivity syndrome. Br J Dermatol. 2007;157:934.
16. Husain Z, Reddy BY, Schwartz RA. Dress Syndrome: Part II. Management and therapeutics. J Am Acad Dermatol. 2013;68:702.
17. Moling O, et al. Treatment of DIHS/DRESS syndrome with combined N-acetylcysteine, prednisone and valganciclovir--a hypothesis. Med Sci Monit. 2012;18:cs57–63.
18. Kardaun SH, Sidoroff A, Valeryrie-Allanore L, et al. Variability in the clinical pattern of cutaneous side-effects of drugs with systemic symptoms: does a DRESS syndrome really exist? Br J Dermatol. 2007;156:609.

Ebola Virus

21

Emily Rose

Background

The Ebola virus (EV) is one of the most virulent and deadly pathogens of humans. It is endemic in certain regions of Africa and sporadic outbreaks have been recognized since 1976 [1]. The West Africa epidemic, the largest recorded outbreak, began in December 2013 and lasted until 2016 and had an approximately 40% fatality rate [2, 3]. Prior outbreaks were fatal in approximately 80–90% of cases [4]. The first recognized outbreaks of Ebola virus were in Zaire and Sudan in 1976.

Ebola is present in bodily fluids and infection is spread by direct contact with bodily fluids from an infected animal or human (see Table 21.1). Outbreaks typically start with human contact with an infected animal and then spread from human to human. The earlier Ebola outbreaks have occurred in Central Africa, in areas of relatively low population density in regions where the residents rarely traveled from home. In contrast, the 2014–2016 Ebola outbreak in West Africa was the historically largest and most fatal outbreak as it occurred in both a populous area with communal migration. The West African epidemic began with a 2-year-old child in late 2013 in Guinea. It then spread to Liberia, Sierra Leone, Nigeria, Senegal, and Mali. Likely an underestimate of total cases, there were 28,603 Ebola cases and 11,301 known EV deaths [5]. There were 881 healthcare workers infected with Ebola, 60% of whom died. Though this epidemic has been contained, there is potential for continued transmission and potential for another epidemic. Providers must be vigilant and consider the possibility of this diagnosis, particularly in patients with a recent travel history. The natural reservoir of the virus remains unknown, but bats are suspected to play a role [1]. There is no evidence that the virus has been transmitted by mosquitoes [5, 6].

E. Rose
Division of Emergency Medicine, Keck School of Medicine of the University of Southern California, Los Angeles County + USC Medical Center, Los Angeles, CA, USA
e-mail: emilyros@usc.edu

© Springer International Publishing AG, part of Springer Nature 2018
E. Rose (ed.), *Life-Threatening Rashes*, https://doi.org/10.1007/978-3-319-75623-3_21

Table 21.1 Infectious body fluids in Ebola+

Blood[a]
Feces[a]
Vomit[a]
Urine
Semen
Saliva
Aqueous humor
Vaginal fluid
Breast milk
Tears
Sweat

+Ebola virus can be present in fluids long after it is no longer detected in the serum
+The virus remains on surfaces/objects for hours (days if within bodily fluid) and is inactivated by cooking
[a]Most infectious bodily fluids

Classic Clinical Presentation

Ebola infection typically presents with an abrupt onset of fever and chills with typical viral prodrome symptoms such as fatigue, headache, and decreased appetite. See Table 21.2 for classic symptoms. Fevers are typically 39–40 °C early in disease and wide swings in temperature may occur including hypothermia [7]. Similar to typhoid fever, there is a pulse-temperature dissociation (relative bradycardia) [4, 6–8]. Vomiting and diarrhea are common and were severe and the predominant symptoms associated with the 2014–2016 epidemic. The gastrointestinal symptoms typically occur within the first few days of illness with profuse watery diarrhea; patients not uncommonly lose up to 10 L per day [9–11]. The severe fluid loss and dehydration not uncommonly leads to hypotension and progresses to hypovolemic shock and severe lethargy [9].

Ebola and Marburg viruses previously were classified as hemorrhagic fever viruses due to the description of both internal and external hemorrhage in patients. However, only a small percentage (approximately 5% in one report) [2] develop clinically significant hemorrhage, and this typically occurs late in severe disease when the patient is in severe shock so this classification was removed. However, some degree of bleeding occurs in most patients and presents as petechiae, ecchymosis, oozing from venipuncture sites, and mucosal bleeding. Profuse hemorrhage is common in the terminal phase of the illness and in pregnant patients. Spontaneous miscarriage is common in pregnant women [12]. Hiccups are commonly described in Ebola victims, the pathophysiology of which is not entirely clear and they are most frequently described in fatal cases. Paralytic ileus and inability to tolerate oral hydration frequently occur. Oral ulcers, thrush, and dysphagia are also common complaints [9, 13–15].

Most deaths occur between days 7 and 12 of illness. Terminal infections may have multiple severe manifestations typically in the second week of illness. Shock

Table 21.2 Common Ebola infection symptoms	Fever
	Headache
	Myalgias
	Vomiting
	Diarrhea
	Conjunctival injection
	Red discoloration of soft palate
	Petechiae
	Ecchymosis
	Oozing from venipuncture sites
	Mucosal bleeding
	Erythematous maculopapular rash (may desquamate)

with resultant multi-organ system failure may occur. Patients may develop meningoencephalitis with altered mental status and seizures [16–18]. Nearly all patients that are alive day 13 of illness survive [9].

Atypical Presentation

Mild and asymptomatic cases of Ebola can occur [1, 19, 20]. In one cohort, as many as 71% of seropositive individuals did not have the Ebola disease [21]. In another group, 46% of asymptomatic close contacts with Ebola victims were seropositive [22]. It is estimated overall that approximately 27% of Ebola infections are asymptomatic [23].

Ocular symptoms may occur during the acute infection or during convalescence. As many as 18% of patients in one report developed uveitis in either the acute phase or during recovery [24]. Symptoms included blurry vision, photophobia, and blindness.

Chest pain and shortness of breath have also been described but are not predominant symptoms.

Pregnant women may be infected and shedding virus without fever or other classic presenting symptoms [12]. Fetal mortality is high when Ebola infects pregnant women. Often, fetal death may occur even when the mother fully recovers from infection [25].

Disease Time Course

Fairly abrupt onset of symptoms typically occurs 6–12 days after exposure (the current documented range from exposure to symptoms is 2–21 days) [5, 26]. See Table 21.3 for common symptom progression. There is currently no evidence that asymptomatic people are infectious, but asymptomatic pregnant women have been shown to have significant viral titers and presumed ability to infect others even when asymptomatic. However, exposure to infected tissue or fluids may potentially transmit disease or cause delayed symptoms (see section "Complications" below).

Table 21.3 Clinical timeline of Ebola infection

Day	Clinical features
0–3	*Prodromal symptoms*: fever, malaise, myalgias
3–10	*Fever and gastrointestinal symptoms*: nausea, vomiting, diarrhea, abdominal pain
	Also, headache, conjunctival injection, arthralgias, asthenia, rash
7–12	*Recovery*: symptom resolution
	Shock: altered level of consciousness, hemodynamic compromise, multi-organ system failure
≥10	*Complications*: gastrointestinal hemorrhage, secondary infections, meningoencephalitis
	Convalescence: persistent arthralgias, myalgias, fatigue, uveitis, blindness, hearing loss, persistent neurocognitive deficits

Adapted from Chertow et al. [9]

Outcome is typically apparent at the second week of illness. Fatal cases are typically initially severe and/or rapidly progress to multi-organ failure within the second week of infection. Survivors typically improve in the second week of illness. High viral load during presentation may correlate with a worse outcome or prolonged recovery [9].

Delayed symptoms may frequently occur (see section "Complications" below). Infected virus may be recovered from patient tissue long after symptoms have resolved and serum titers are negative. The ramifications of the viral presence remain unclear.

Pathophysiology

The route of infection may correlate with disease course and final outcome. Contact exposures have longer incubation period and lower mortality rate compared to cases of accidental injection with infected blood [1].

The Ebola virus invades many cell types and is also present in extracellular fluid (see Fig. 21.1). It both invades and inhibits immune response [2]. The rapid viral replication and dissemination occurs particularly in severe and/or fatal infections. Lymphoid depletion and necrosis are seen on autopsy in the spleen, thymus, and lymph nodes in fatal cases [1]. See Fig. 21.1. It appears that EV is cleared fairly rapidly from most bodily fluids but may persist for weeks-months in immunologically privileged sites such as aqueous humor and semen [24]. This may also contribute to the high fetal mortality rate when pregnant women are infected with EV. Higher viral loads appear to correlate with the development of uveitis and other ocular symptoms but do not seem to correlate with the development of arthralgias [24].

Common Mimics and Differential Diagnosis

Ebola frequently occurs concomitantly with malaria, as well as with many other viral infections. Coinfections may obscure the clinical picture and complicate diagnostic ability. See Table 21.4 for differential diagnosis.

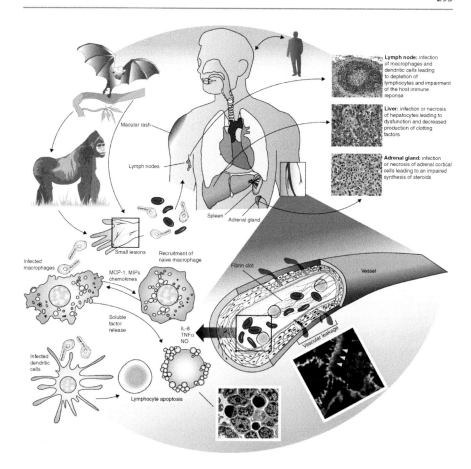

Fig. 21.1 Model of Ebola virus pathogenesis. (Used with permission from Feldmann and Geisbert [1])

Table 21.4 Differential diagnosis of Ebola

Malaria
Acute gastroenteritis
Marburg virus
Lassa fever
Typhoid fever
Meningococcus
Influenza
Measles
Traveler's diarrhea
Yellow fever
Bacterial sepsis
Leptospirosis
Dengue
Streptococcal pharyngitis

Key Physical Exam Findings and Diagnostic Features

The diagnosis of Ebola is suspected in the clinical setting of recent travel/exposure to endemic areas in a patient with fever and viral-type symptoms described above in Clinical Features. Specific physical exam features and diagnostic laboratory findings are discussed below.

Mucocutaneous Features A diffuse, erythematous nonpruritic maculopapular rash that may develop later in the first week of illness (days 5–7). The rash typically involves the face, neck, trunk, and arms and may desquamate [1, 27, 28]. In earlier outbreaks, a rash was described in 25–52% of patients [7]. Patients frequently have conjunctival injection and dark-red discoloration of the soft palate. Petechiae, ecchymosis, oozing from venipuncture sites, and/or mucosal bleeding may occur. See Fig. 21.2 for hemorrhagic manifestations seen in nonhuman primates.

Diagnosis Definitive diagnosis is made by viral antigens or RNA in the blood or other body fluids. Reverse transcription-polymerase chain reaction (RT-PCR) is the standard method of diagnosing Ebola virus. The virus is present in many bodily fluids, but the highest viral load is in the serum and a blood specimen is preferred. A negative RT-PCR collected >72 h after symptom onset rules out Ebola virus disease [9, 29]. However, there is great genetic diversity and potential for viral mutation so the assay accuracy must be vigilantly monitored to ensure virus detection.

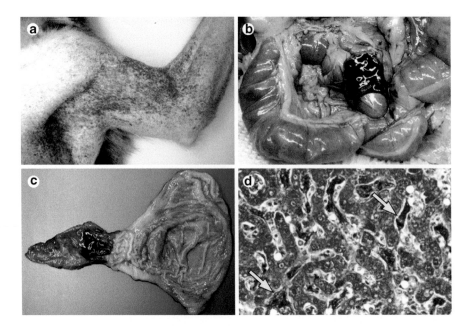

Fig. 21.2 (**a**) Petachiae on the arm an axillary region of a Cynomolgus monkey infected with Sudan Ebola virus. (**b**). Hemorrhage in the ileum of the monkey. (**c**). Hemorrhagic gastroduodenal lesion (**d**). Fibrin thrombi (arrows) in the sinusoids of a rhesus monkey infected with Zaire Ebola virus [1])

Table 21.5 Laboratory abnormalities associated with Ebola infection

Decreased	Increased
Lymphocytes (initially, atypical lymphocytes increase during disease course)	AST
Leukocytes	ALT
Platelets	BUN/Cr (worse with dehydration and shock)
	PT/INR (with shock)

Table 21.6 Personal protective equipment (PPE) required in the care of Ebola patients

Minimum requirements
Disposable/single-use fluid resistant gown to mid-calf or coveralls
Disposable/single-use full face shield
Disposable/single-use face mask
Disposable/single-use two pairs of gloves with at least outer layer of extended cuffs
Surgical scrubs should be worn and no personal items should be worn under PPE
Please see CDC website for specific details (https://www.cdc.gov/vhf/ebola/healthcare-us/ppe/guidance-clinically-stable-puis.html)

Additional Laboratory Findings There are some abnormalities that occur as a result of Ebola infection. And some abnormalities occur because of severe systemic involvement and shock. Leukopenia often initially occurs and then neutrophil counts become elevated with predominance of atypical lymphocytes as the disease progresses [1, 7]. Thrombocytopenia is common, typically 50–100,000 with a nadir around day 8 of illness. Serum transaminases levels are often elevated and may correlate with viral load. DIC may occur in severe illness with abnormal PT/PTT and elevated fibrin degradation products. See Table 21.5.

Management

There is no clinical proven antiviral agent to treat Ebola infection though several experimental agents are available. The mainstay of treatment is targeted supportive care. The hypovolemia and metabolic abnormalities associated with severe gastrointestinal fluid loss should be corrected. Antiemetics and antidiarrheal agents are particularly important in resource limited settings to prevent life-threatening dehydration and shock. Coinfections must be diagnosed and treated. Acute kidney injury must be recognized and renal replacement therapy administered when indicated. Respiratory support including intubation is often required in severe cases [30].

Meticulous use of personal protective wear should be utilized by all healthcare professionals (see Table 21.6) and quarantine strategies enforced to prevent further viral dissemination (see Table 21.7).

Table 21.7 Risk of Ebola transmission

High risk: Percutaneous or mucous membrane exposure to blood or body fluids without PPE. Transmission risk is higher with high viral titers (e.g., patient in later stages of illness or in contact with a corpse)
Moderate risk: Contact within 3 ft. of an infected person for a prolonged period without PPE
Low risk: Exposure to an asymptomatic person

Complications

Acute infections have many secondary infections and severe complications. Patients may develop acute kidney injury secondary to severe fluid loss, but renal abnormalities may develop in the absence of gastrointestinal symptoms. Electrolyte disturbances may occur with severe GI symptoms. Bacterial sepsis may complicate acute infection. Multiorgan failure, shock, and DIC are common in fatal cases [31].

Ebola survivors may have a prolonged convalescent period and delayed complications. Patients may have persistent weakness, fatigue, and chronic headaches for years after initial infection [31]. Arthralgias are common and secondary to desposition of antigen-antibody complexes [32]. Hearing loss, uveitis, and loss of visual acuity may also occur [31, 33]. Uveitis has been reported 14 weeks after initial diagnosis with confirmed Ebola virus in the aqueous fluid [34]. Another patient developed meningitis 9 months after her serum was negative for Ebola, and the active Ebola virus was discovered in the CSF [18].

Asymptomatic patients who no longer test positive for Ebola virus in the serum may also continue to transmit the viral infection via other bodily fluids. One male Ebola survivor sexually transmitted the virus 199 days after initial symptom onset [35]. In response, the World Health Organization (WHO) recommended that "all male survivors be offered semen testing 3 months after disease onset and every month thereafter until two consecutive specimens collected at least one week apart were negative." [36] In a group of 228 male Ebola survivors, 24 (11%) produced at least one semen sample that tested positive for the Ebola virus RNA [36].

Skin sloughing and hair loss may occur secondary to virus-induced necrosis of skin.

> **Bottom Line: Ebola Clinical Pearls**
> - Ebola is extremely contagious and spread via contact with bodily fluids.
> - Asymptomatic patients are unlikely to be infectious but may harbor the virus in "sanctuary sites."
> - Incubation period is 2–21 days (typically 6–12 days).
> - Early symptoms include fever, fatigue, headache, vomiting, and diarrhea; (faint) rash may occur day 5–7 of illness.
> - Faget's sign (sphygmothermic dissociation): fever with relative bradycardia may be a clinical clue of the diagnosis.

- Petechiae, ecchymosis, oozing from venipuncture sites, and mucosal bleeding may occur. Clinically significant hemorrhage may occur in the terminal phase of the disease.
- Treatment includes strict quarantine (standard, contact, and droplet precautions) supportive care and possible experimental medication.
- Fatality rate is 40–70%.
- Sporadic cases may occur at any time, even when there is not any known outbreak.
- Healthcare providers are at high risk for infection, particularly if personal protective equipment is not utilized.

References

1. Feldmann H, Geisbert TW. Ebola haemorrhagic fever. Lancet. 2011;377(9768):849–62.
2. Baseler L, Chertow DS, Johnson KM, Feldmann H, Morens DM. The pathogenesis of Ebola virus disease. Annu Rev Pathol. 2017;12:387–418.
3. Aylward B, Barboza P, Bawo L, et al. Ebola virus disease in West Africa – the first 9 months of the epidemic and forward projections. N Engl J Med. 2014;371(16):1481–95.
4. Bray M, Murphy FA. Filovirus research: knowledge expands to meet a growing threat. J Infect Dis. 2007;196(Suppl 2):S438–43.
5. World Health Organization, Factsheet on Ebola. http://www.who.int/mediacentre/factsheets/fs103/en/. Accessed 8/5/2017.
6. Centers for Disease Control and Prevention. https://www.cdc.gov/vhf/ebola/index.html. Accessed 8/5/2017.
7. Kortepeter MG, Bausch DG, Bray M. Basic clinical and laboratory features of filoviral hemorrhagic fever. J Infect Dis. 2011;204(Suppl 3):S810–6.
8. Bwaka MA, Bonnet MJ, Calain P, et al. Ebola hemorrhagic fever in Kikwit, Democratic Republic of the Congo: clinical observations in 103 patients. J Infect Dis. 1999;179(Suppl 1):S1–7.
9. Chertow DS, Kleine C, Edwards JK, Scaini R, Giuliani R, Sprecher A. Ebola virus disease in West Africa – clinical manifestations and management. N Engl J Med. 2014;371(22):2054–7.
10. Bah EI, Lamah MC, Fletcher T, et al. Clinical presentation of patients with Ebola virus disease in Conakry, Guinea. N Engl J Med. 2015;372(1):40–7.
11. Hunt L, Gupta-Wright A, Simms V, et al. Clinical presentation, biochemical, and haematological parameters and their association with outcome in patients with Ebola virus disease: an observational cohort study. Lancet Infect Dis. 2015;15(11):1292–9.
12. Akerlund E, Prescott J, Tampellini L. Shedding of Ebola virus in an asymptomatic pregnant woman. N Engl J Med. 2015;372(25):2467–9.
13. Dietz PM, Jambai A, Paweska JT, Yoti Z, Ksiazek TG. Epidemiology and risk factors for Ebola virus disease in Sierra Leone-23 May 2014 to 31 January 2015. Clin Infect Dis. 2015;61(11):1648–54.
14. Schieffelin JS, Shaffer JG, Goba A, et al. Clinical illness and outcomes in patients with Ebola in Sierra Leone. N Engl J Med. 2014;371(22):2092–100.
15. West TE, von Saint Andre-von Arnim A. Clinical presentation and management of severe Ebola virus disease. Ann Am Thorac Soc. 2014;11(9):1341–50.
16. Kreuels B, Wichmann D, Emmerich P, et al. A case of severe Ebola virus infection complicated by gram-negative septicemia. N Engl J Med. 2014;371(25):2394–401.

17. de Greslan T, Billhot M, Rousseau C, et al. Ebola virus-related encephalitis. Clin Infect Dis. 2016;63(8):1076–8.
18. Jacobs M, Rodger A, Bell DJ, et al. Late Ebola virus relapse causing meningoencephalitis: a case report. Lancet. 2016;388(10043):498–503.
19. Ebola virus disease update – West Africa. http://www.who.int/csr/don/2014_08_20_ebola/en/. Accessed 8/5/2017.
20. Heymann DL, Chen L, Takemi K, et al. Global health security: the wider lessons from the west African Ebola virus disease epidemic. Lancet. 2015;385(9980):1884–901.
21. Heffernan RT, Pambo B, Hatchett RJ, Leman PA, Swanepoel R, Ryder RW. Low seroprevalence of IgG antibodies to Ebola virus in an epidemic zone: Ogooue-Ivindo region, Northeastern Gabon, 1997. J Infect Dis. 2005;191(6):964–8.
22. Leroy EM, Baize S, Volchkov VE, et al. Human asymptomatic Ebola infection and strong inflammatory response. Lancet. 2000;355(9222):2210–5.
23. Dean NE, Halloran ME, Yang Y, Longini IM. Transmissibility and pathogenicity of Ebola virus: a systematic review and meta-analysis of household secondary attack rate and asymptomatic infection. Clin Infect Dis. 2016;62(10):1277–86.
24. Mattia JG, Vandy MJ, Chang JC, et al. Early clinical sequelae of Ebola virus disease in Sierra Leone: a cross-sectional study. Lancet Infect Dis. 2016;16(3):331–8.
25. Baggi FM, Taybi A, Kurth A, et al. Management of pregnant women infected with Ebola virus in a treatment centre in Guinea, June 2014. Euro Surveill. 2014;19(49):20983.
26. Center for Disease Control and Prevention. https://www.cdc.gov/vhf/ebola/index.html. Accessed 8/5/2017.
27. Parra JM, Salmeron OJ, Velasco M. The first case of Ebola virus disease acquired outside Africa. N Engl J Med. 2014;371(25):2439–40.
28. Lyon GM, Mehta AK, Varkey JB, et al. Clinical care of two patients with Ebola virus disease in the United States. N Engl J Med. 2014;371(25):2402–9.
29. Centers for Disease Control and Infection. https://www.cdc.gov/vhf/ebola/transmission/human-transmission.html. Accessed 8/30/2017.
30. Uyeki TM, Mehta AK, Davey RT Jr, et al. Clinical Management of Ebola Virus Disease in the United States and Europe. N Engl J Med. 2016;374(7):636–46.
31. Clark DV, Kibuuka H, Millard M, et al. Long-term sequelae after Ebola virus disease in Bundibugyo, Uganda: a retrospective cohort study. Lancet Infect Dis. 2015;15(8):905–12.
32. Rowe AK, Bertolli J, Khan AS, et al. Clinical, virologic, and immunologic follow-up of convalescent Ebola hemorrhagic fever patients and their household contacts, Kikwit, Democratic Republic of the Congo. Commission de Lutte contre les Epidemies a Kikwit. J Infect Dis. 1999;179(Suppl 1):S28–35.
33. Kibadi K, Mupapa K, Kuvula K, et al. Late ophthalmologic manifestations in survivors of the 1995 Ebola virus epidemic in Kikwit, Democratic Republic of the Congo. J Infect Dis. 1999;179(Suppl 1):S13–4.
34. Varkey JB, Shantha JG, Crozier I, et al. Persistence of Ebola virus in ocular fluid during convalescence. N Engl J Med. 2015;372(25):2423–7.
35. Mate SE, Kugelman JR, Nyenswah TG, et al. Molecular evidence of sexual transmission of Ebola virus. N Engl J Med. 2015;373(25):2448–54.
36. Purpura LJ, Soka M, Baller A, et al. Implementation of a National Semen Testing and counseling program for male Ebola survivors – Liberia, 2015-2016. MMWR Morb Mortal Wkly Rep. 2016;65(36):963–6.

Potential Bioterrorism Agents with Mucocutaneous Findings (Anthrax, Plague, Tularemia, Smallpox)

22

Mariana Martinez and Emily Rose

General Introduction

The four biochemical agents discussed in this chapter are just a few of the bacteria, viruses, and chemicals which have been weaponized by human societies throughout history. While some of these diseases remain naturally endemic in certain parts of the world, none of them occur frequently, but all have the potential to be rapidly fatal, especially if not recognized early in their clinical course. These characteristics along with their ease of dissemination into a susceptible population make them excellent potential agents for biological terrorism. Recognition of the cutaneous manifestations of each of these infections is key to their diagnosis and, despite their rarity, should be a part of every emergency provider's clinical knowledge base.

Anthrax

Background

The gram-positive, spore-forming *Bacillus anthracis* is capable of causing multiple forms of disease in humans. While primarily a disease of livestock in parts of Asia, Africa, and the Middle East, this bacterium is able to cause respiratory, gastrointestinal, and cutaneous disease in humans when exposed to its spores.

M. Martinez
Department of Emergency Medicine, Los Angeles County + University of Southern California Medical Center, Los Angeles, CA, USA

E. Rose (✉)
Department of Emergency Medicine, Keck School of Medicine of the University of Southern California, Los Angeles County + USC Medical Center, Los Angeles, CA, USA
e-mail: emilyros@usc.edu

There is no known human-to-human transmission. Livestock vaccination programs have made the disease fairly rare in Western countries, but the disease still is endemic in unvaccinated livestock worldwide [1]. Anthrax came to national attention in the United States following the September 11, 2001, terrorist attacks when there were 22 cases of either inhalational or cutaneous anthrax resulting from intentional exposures leading to 5 deaths [2, 3]. Anthrax's resilient spores can easily be transported and aerosolized which facilitates potential utilization as a bioterrorism agent [4].

Classic Clinical Presentation

Anthrax derives its name from the Greek term *anthrakites* meaning "coal-like" which refers to the classic black eschar seen with cutaneous presentations [1]. Cutaneous anthrax is caused by introduction of the spore into a break of skin, most commonly through exposure to infected animal products such as hides. After introduction, patients develop a painless but frequently pruritic papule that becomes vesicular and edematous prior to crusting over into an eschar (Fig. 22.1). The vast majority of lesions (>90%) occur on the face, neck, arms, and hands (areas of most commonly exposed skin) [5].

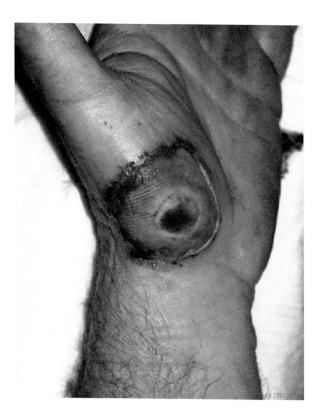

Fig. 22.1 Bullous and necrotic lesion of cutaneous anthrax. (Used with permission from Cinquetti et al. [6])

Fig. 22.2 Forearm wound with necrotic eschar and surrounding erythema and edema. (Used with permission from Cinquetti et al. [6])

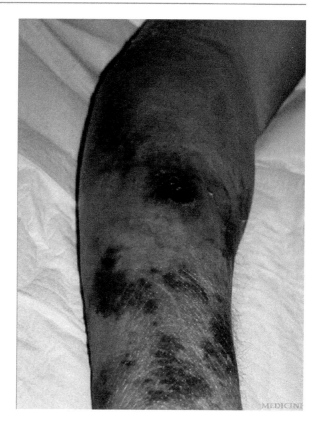

Atypical Presentation

Less commonly patients will present with a primary lesion that is more vesicular containing cloudy fluid; however, a true pustule is unlikely to be a manifestation of cutaneous anthrax [7]. Local edema may occur as well as regional lymphadenopathy and/or lymphangitis (Figs. 22.1 and 22.2). More recently a new form of anthrax infection has been identified in intravenous (IV) drug users due to use of contaminated drugs or needles; lesions are similar to other ones seen in "skin-poppers" but can progress very quickly and require surgical debridement [8].

Associated Systemic Symptoms

Cutaneous anthrax often has associated low-grade fevers and malaise during vesicular phase [9]. Patients also may have lymphangitis and painful lymphadenopathy (Fig. 22.3) [4]. Those with cutaneous disease are also potentially at risk for inhalational or GI disease if they inhaled or ingested spores during their initial exposure and thus should be questioned about and examined for respiratory and GI symptoms that might indicate secondary exposure [10].

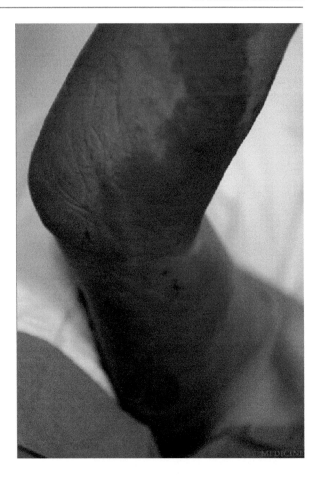

Fig. 22.3 Cutaneous anthrax with associated lymphangitis, bulla, and serous drainage. (Used with permission from Cinquetti et al. [6])

Inhalational anthrax is characterized by sudden onset of fever/malaise with rapidly progressive respiratory decompensation and shock. CXR usually demonstrates pleural effusions and/or mediastinal widening due to hemorrhage and edema of mediastinal lymph nodes [4].

Time Course of Disease

Please see Fig. 22.4 for a summary of the disease time course in cutaneous anthrax.

Common Mimics and Differential Diagnosis

Please see Table 22.1 for differential diagnosis of cutaneous anthrax. The initial painless papule is similar to that of an insect bite and thus has a wide differential [7]. The following eschar has a more characteristic appearance and thus more limited differential. Most of the other diagnoses are also rare, and thus diagnosis is going to be largely guided by history and risk factors for possible exposures.

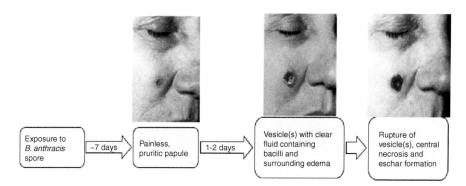

Fig. 22.4 Cutaneous anthrax time course. (Images courtesy of the Center of Disease Control and Prevention Public Health Image Library (ID #1802, 1804, 1807))

Table 22.1 Differential diagnosis of cutaneous anthrax

Disease	Differentiating factors
Brown recluse spider bite	Painful lesion, bite occurrence geographically within spider habitation
Staph furuncle	Painful, erythematous
Ecthyma	No edema or systemic manifestations, surrounding erythema
Ecthyma gangrenosum	Neutropenic patient
Orf	No gelatinous edema, has scab formation but not large eschar
Cutaneous tularemia	Painful ulcer, not always with eschar

Key Physical Exam Findings and Diagnostic Features

Presentation of the classic eschar along with possible exposure to animal hides or other possible source of spore should raise clinical suspicion. Gram stain and culture should be performed on samples from wound or vesicles which should demonstrate gram-positive bacilli. It is important to notify the microbiology lab processing the samples of the possible diagnosis to protect lab workers and to ensure that the results are not disregarded as a contaminant. Punch biopsies can be done for sent out lab testing if gram stain is negative or patient already on antibiotics.

Management

Standard precautions are sufficient for potential cutaneous anthrax cases as there have been no documented cases of person-to-person transmission of anthrax. Contact precautions should be used for draining lesions, and dressings should be disposed of with hazardous waste [9]. State and local public health officials should be notified of any suspected cases. Blood cultures should be done prior to initiation of antibiotics if possible [4].

For simple cutaneous anthrax in adults without signs of systemic involvement the CDC recommends treatment for 60 days with *ciprofloxacin 500 mg BID* or *doxycycline*

100 mg BID. A three-dose vaccine course should also be administered simultaneously. This treatment regimen is similar to that for postexposure prophylaxis as those with cutaneous anthrax are presumed to have pulmonary exposure to spores. Multiple other antibiotic regimens are available in case of shortages or contraindications to these medications. If patient has any sign of systemic involvement or has primary lesions on the head or neck, IV antibiotics with multidrug regimens are preferred along with admission. For inhalational, GI or systemic infections multidrug intravenous regimens are recommended. Shorter courses of treatment may be appropriate for naturally occurring cases rather than those secondary to bioterrorism [11]. *B. anthracis* is not susceptible to many cephalosporins, and thus the antibiotics most commonly used to treat skin flora will be ineffective [9]. Topical therapies are not useful.

Complications

Cutaneous infections when managed with appropriate antibiotics are usually self-limited. With antibiotic treatment lesions will still progress to eschars yet lesions will be sterile. Left untreated, endospores will be carried to regional lymph nodes to macrophages where they become vegetative bacteria. These bacteria then spread throughout the bloodstream leading to massive septicemia [12]. The bacteria carry endotoxins which trigger a chain of cellular events leading to massive edema, shock, and eventually death [4].

> **Bottom Line: Anthrax Clinical Pearls**
> - Cutaneous anthrax is generally nonlethal, but recognition of the characteristic lesion may be the key to diagnosis in more serious respiratory or other forms of the disease.
> - Ensure notification of public health departments in possible cases and exposures to ensure proper testing and treatment.

Plague

Background

Yersinia pestis, the causative agent of plague or the "black death," is widely considered one of the serious agents available for use as a biological weapon [13]. It has previously been used as a biological weapon including by the Japanese army on China during World War II [14]. The gram-negative coccobacillus persists as an endemic disease across the world including in the western United States [15]. It is a zoonotic disease with fleas serving as the main vectors to mammalian hosts such as wild rodents and rats. Transmission to humans is possible via the bite of a carrier flea (*Xenopsylla cheopis*) or handling of infected animal and their bodily fluids.

Intentional dissemination of plague as bioterrorism would likely occur via release of aerosolized *Y. pestis* leading to an outbreak of pneumonic plague. Naturally occurring epidemics are usually preceded by a large death of rats. Currently the United States averages about seven cases per year primarily in New Mexico, Arizona, Colorado, and California [13, 16]. Plague exists in three main clinical forms: bubonic, septicemic, and pneumonic. This chapter will focus on the bubonic form since it is the most common and also the one with the most cutaneous findings.

Classic Clinical Presentation

Bubonic plague manifests with sudden onset of fever and generalized malaise with associated onset of a "bubo" or large, swollen, painful, lymph node in the groin, axilla, or neck. Location of lymphadenopathy is usually dependent on area of original flea bite or exposure. Buboes range in size from 1 to 10 cm with overlying erythema, warmth, and sometimes edema but no fluctuance [17]. Untreated, bubonic plague will progress to disseminated infection/sepsis in about half of cases.

Atypical Presentation

Bubonic plague: Buboes rarely can be fluctuant and suppurate. Skin lesions at the site of inoculation are typically minor but may be pustular and necrotic or develop ulceration or eschar (see Fig. 22.5).

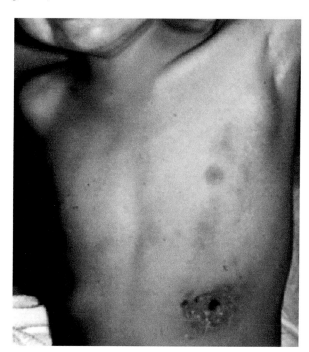

Fig. 22.5 Patient with bubonic plague demonstrating a left axillary bubo and unusual plague ulcer and eschar at the site of the infective flea bite. (Used with permission from Citation: Kasper et al. [18])

Septicemic plague presents as a severe febrile illness with nonspecific associated symptoms such as myalgias, nausea, vomiting, and diarrhea.

Pneumonic plague may develop by primary inhalation of aerosolized particles or via hematogenous spread of the bacteria. Patients typically present with the sudden onset of dyspnea, chest pain, and hemoptysis.

Associated Systemic Symptoms

Patients may have sudden onset of fever, chills, and weakness in the 24 h prior to onset of bubo [13].

Time Course of Disease

Please see Fig. 22.6 for the classic disease time course of bubonic plague.

Common Mimics and Differential Diagnosis

The characteristic "buboes" of plague may be mistaken for cutaneous abscess; however, buboes are usually nonfluctuant and should not be opened via I&D due to risk of aerosolization. Also in the differential is any condition that can cause regional lymphadenitis (malignancy, tuberculosis, tularemia, cat scratch fever, chancroid).

Key Physical Exam Findings and Diagnostic Features

Diagnosis of bubonic plague is primarily a clinical one based on possible exposure to infected animal (or human) in endemic area along with appearance of characteristic buboes (Figs. 22.5, 22.6, and 22.7) and systemic symptoms. Lymph node aspirate and blood cultures should be collected but may not be useful in the acute setting due to the time it may take for them to offer results. *Yersinia* grows well on culture media and culture samples may be obtained from serum, sputum, aspiration of buboes, or cerebrospinal fluid as clinically indicated.

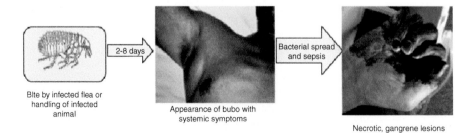

Fig. 22.6 Time course of Bubonic plague. (Images courtesy of the Center of Disease Control and Prevention Public Health Image Library and Christina Nelson MD, MPH (ID #2045 and 16,551))

Fig. 22.7 Cervical and submandibular buboes in a patient with bubonic plague. (From http://www.who.int/csr/disease/plague/en/)

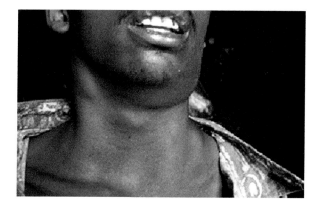

Management

There is no person-to-person spread of bubonic plague; however, those who develop septicemia and secondary pneumonic plague can spread the disease by respiratory droplet. Those with suspected pneumonic plague should remain in droplet precautions for at least 48 h; others can remain with standard precautions [14]. Lymph node aspiration should be done for gram stain and culture, but full incision and drainage should not due to risk of aerosolization [17]. Blood cultures should also be drawn prior to initiation of antibiotics. Laboratory personnel must be notified prior to sending samples as they must be handed with special precautions [19]. The traditional treatment for plague is streptomycin; however, this medication is infrequently used and often unavailable. Gentamicin is an effective alternative treatment and may be used in children and pregnant women. Tetracycline and doxycycline are FDA approved for plague prophylaxis and may be used to treat acute infection in patients who cannot tolerate aminoglycosides [13]. Fluoroquinolones have limited human data but have successfully treated plague in animal studies.

Complications

Plague responds well to early treatment if recognized and antibiotic therapy initiated early. Untreated, *Y. pestis* invades the bloodstream and spreads leading to septicemic plague and potentially secondary pneumonic plague, both of which can be rapidly fatal. Treatment is most successful when initiated on the first day of illness. Complications from septicemic plague include shock, DIC, and meningitis [13]. Large, ecchymotic, and gangrenous lesions that occur with late septicemic plague are the reasons why it has been commonly called the "black death." Untreated bubonic plague has a mortality rate of 50–60% [17].

> **Bottom Line: Plague Clinical Pearls**
> - Bubonic plague is in the differential of the toxic patient with regional lymphadenopathy.
> - Buboes should not be incised and drained as this may aerosolize the bacteria and potentially cause infection.
> - Consider the plague in an ill patient with pneumonia and hemoptysis.

Tularemia

Background

Tularemia, caused by the bacteria *Francisella tularensis*, is very infectious and requires very few organisms to cause disease. It exists as primarily as a disease of rural environments throughout Europe and North America. In the United States, it is most prevalent in the south-central states such as Missouri and Arkansas [20]. Ticks, flies, and mosquitos act as vectors with small mammals such as rabbits being the usual hosts. Similar to plague, humans can become infected either by bites from carrier insects or handling infected animals. However, due to great infectivity of the bacteria, humans can also become infected via contact with infected water, soil, or aerosolized organisms. There have been no documented cases of human-to-human transmission. Depending on the mode of exposure, tularemia is able to cause pulmonary, oropharyngeal, ocular, or cutaneous disease. The cutaneous or ulceroglandular form is the most commonly encountered form. Similar to the other agents discussed in this chapter, tularemia would most likely be aerosolized in a bioterrorism event. Most patients in this setting would present with pneumonic tularemia or typhoidal tularemia (fever, myalgias, sore throat, abdominal pain, and diarrhea). However, any form of tularemia may occur, particularly if food and water supplies are contaminated. Direct inoculation of mucosal and skin surfaces may occur and result in oculoglandular, pharyngeal, ulceroglandular, or glandular tularemia [21].

Classic Clinical Presentation

Ulceroglandular tularemia usually presents with a local papule which becomes pustular then ulcerates within a few days and may have a central eschar. The ulcer is generally tender. Usually single lesions range in size from 0.4 to 3 cm with "heaped-up" edges (see Fig. 22.8) [17]. Patients are frequently febrile and may also have enlarged, tender regional lymph nodes after appearance of papule (see Fig. 22.9). These lymph nodes can become fluctuant and drain. Both lesions can remain for months even with antibiotic therapy.

Fig. 22.8 Ulcer on the hand of patient with ulceroglandular tularemia. (Image courtesy of the Center of Disease Control and Prevention Public Health Image Library and Dr. Sellers of Emory University (ID #1344))

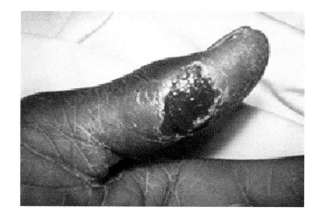

Fig. 22.9 An 8-year-old boy with inguinal lymphadenitis and associated tick-bite characteristic of ulceroglandular tularemia. (Used with permission from Citation: Kasper et al. [18])

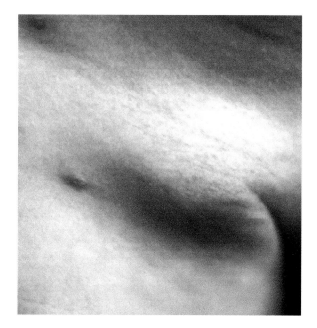

Atypical Presentation

Tularemia can present with lymphadenopathy alone without ulcerated lesion; this form is termed glandular tularemia. Those who present with other forms of tularemia may have other dermatologic findings such as erythema multiforme, urticaria, or erythema nodosum [22]. There is also an oculoglandular form of tularemia caused by direct inoculation which causes corneal ulcerations with associated chemosis, vasculitis, and lymphadenitis. Oropharyngeal disease may also occur with pharyngitis, cervical lymphadenopathy, and tonsillar exudates/

ulceration. The most difficult to recognize atypical form of tularemia is typhoidal which is a febrile disease without overt lymphadenopathy or mucocutaneous findings.

Associated Systemic Symptoms

All forms of tularemia usually start with sudden onset of fever, chills, and general malaise several days after initial exposure. There is a classically associated pulse-temperature dissociation (Faget's sign/sphygothermic dissociation) where patients have lower than expected heart rate for degree of fever.

Time Course of Disease (Incubation Period after Exposure to Infectious Agent or Drug Exposure)

A small papule develops at the inoculation site (bite site or other site of exposure) at the same time as systemic symptoms usually 3–5 days after exposure. The papule develops into a pustule and ruptures becoming painful ulcer over next few days. Ulcer and lymphadenopathy can persist for months even with proper therapy.

Common Mimics and Differential Diagnosis

Symptoms are frequently nonspecific and similar to many viral infections. The ulcer is similar in appearance to cutaneous anthrax; however, it is generally more painful, and eschar is less common. The regional lymphadenopathy may be similar to plague.

Key Physical Exam Findings and Diagnostic Features

The initial diagnosis is clinical and should be considered in a patient with character-istic lesions/symptoms and possible exposure. *F. tularensis* can be identified via culture of swabs or scrapings of skin lesions but will take days and may be missed if lab personnel are not notified of the suspicion for tularemia. Certain laboratories may have special stains or PCR to identify the bacteria from culture earlier. There are also serologic tests available but are usually not positive until weeks after expo-sure making them relatively useless to guide clinical management.

Patients with tularemia frequently develop a typically diffuse secondary skin eruption that may mimic other conditions. This rash has been described as maculo-papular, vesiculopapular, erythema multiforme, and erythema nodosum (particu-larly in pneumonic tularemia).

Management

Streptomycin 1 g IM BID for 10 days is the preferred treatment regimen for simple tularemia. Alternatives include gentamicin, doxycycline, chloramphenicol, and ciprofloxacin. Postexposure prophylaxis for high-risk exposure includes either oral ciprofloxacin 500 mg or doxycycline 100 mg bid for 14 days.

Standard isolation precautions are sufficient for potential cases due to the lack of human-to-human transmission. However, the laboratory that may be processing any infected specimens should be notified to ensure proper handling.

Complications

Untreated *F. tularensis* can spread to regional lymph nodes and disseminate throughout the body. Lymph node suppuration is the most common complication. Other serious complications include sepsis, renal failure, rhabdomyolysis, hepatitis, and meningitis. A prolonged convalescent phase is frequently described with persistent symptoms potentially lasting months.

> **Bottom Line: Tularemia Clinical Pearls**
> - Consider tularemia in anyone presenting with lymphadenopathy, skin findings, and systemic symptoms in endemic areas or with potential exposure/multiple concomitant infections in a community.
> - Tularemia may present with conjunctival injection and/or oropharyngeal erythema and exudates if mucosal surfaces are exposed to aerosolized particles or contaminated food or water.
> - Contact your local health officials if suspicion for tularemia exists to facilitate appropriate testing.

Smallpox

Background

The World Health Organization declared eradication of the variola virus, which causes smallpox, in 1980. However, stores of the virus remain in labs in the United States and Russia for research purposes which leaves concerns about outbreaks of the disease should it be intentionally or accidentally released. Such a release has the potential to be devastating as the majority of the world's population is no longer vaccinated [23]. Smallpox is very contagious via respiratory droplet and can be spread easily via contaminated bedding or clothing which has allowed for the use of smallpox as a biological weapon throughout history [19].

Classic Clinical Presentation

Variola major (ordinary smallpox), which accounted for nearly 90% of smallpox cases, presents with a prodromal phase of fever, headache, and malaise. The rash then appears gradually with small macules that enlarge to papules, vesicles, and pustules up to 4–6 mm in diameter over the course of 4–7 days. Lesions remain for about 5–8 days prior to becoming umbilicated and crusting over. Lesions appear first on the face/extremities and move to the trunk. Lesions exist in the same stage of development throughout (see Figs. 22.10 and 22.11) [23].

Atypical Presentation

There are several other less common forms of smallpox:

Hemorrhagic smallpox: rare form which leads to widespread skin and mucous membrane hemorrhage, high fatality rate, often within 5–6 days [24]. This form may be confused with meningococcemia or DIC [19].

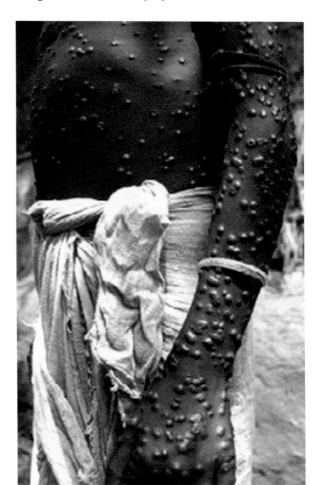

Fig. 22.10 Typical lesions of variola major (smallpox). (Image courtesy of the Center of Disease Control and Prevention Public Health Image Library and Jean Roy (ID #10661))

Fig. 22.11 Lesions of active smallpox infection with crusting [25]

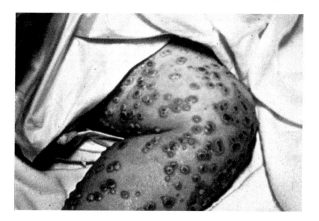

Flat-type (malignant) smallpox: rare form characterized by severe and sudden onset of constitutional symptoms. Lesions tend to develop more slowly and remain flat and soft instead of progressing to pustules. Most cases are fatal [26]. If patient survives they often have large sloughing of epidermis instead of scabbing [19].

Variola sine eruptione: occurs in previously vaccinated individuals. Patients usually are asymptomatic or have brief flu-like symptoms [23]. Rash usually evolves more quickly and resolves more rapidly. Also known as "modified-type smallpox."

Variola minor: milder form with smaller lesions than variola major [17]. Fatality rate < 1% [19].

Associated Systemic Symptoms

Abrupt onset of high-grade fever, headache, and backache usually lasts for 2–3 days and serves as prodrome to the rash itself. Patients may have a second febrile period associated with a secondary bacterial infection [23].

Time Course of Disease

Patients have onset of febrile prodrome and systemic symptoms approximately 10–14 days after inhalation of the virus. Prodrome lasts 2–3 days with onset of enanthema of mucous membranes approximately 24 h prior to onset of rash. Rash starts maculopapular and progresses to vesicles and papules over next 2–3 weeks.

Common Mimics and Differential Diagnosis

Variola can be mistaken for any other cause of papulovesicular rash including chickenpox/herpes zoster, monkeypox, drug eruptions, insect bites, measles, herpes simplex, or molluscum contagiosum (especially in immunocompromised patients) [23].

Table 22.2 Comparison of smallpox and chickenpox

	Smallpox	Chickenpox
Incubation period	10–14 days	14–16 days
Prodromal phase	2–4 days of fever, headache, malaise, transient rash	0–2 days of possible fever, headache, malaise (usually mild)
Rash distribution	Face/extremities (including palms/soles) → trunk	Trunk→ extremities (rarely palms/soles)
Rash appearance	Large, round pustules in *same stage of development*	Vesicles in *various stages of development*

Table 22.3 CDC algorithm for smallpox risk assessment

Major criteria:	Level of risk	Criteria	Response
1. Prodrome 1–4 days before rash with fever AND at least one of the following:Headache, backache, chills, vomiting, abdominal pain, prostration 2. Classic smallpox lesions. 3. Lesions in same stage of development on any one part of body.	High	Meets all 3 major criteria	Urgent ID or Derm consult, CDC notification, initiate treatment
Minor criteria: 1. Centrifugal distribution of rash 2. First lesions on face, oral mucosa, or forearms. 3. Toxic appearance 4. Slow rash evolution	Moderate	Febrile prodrome +1 major OR Febrile prodrome with at least 4 minor criteria	Urgent ID or Derm consult, diagnostic testing to rule out other causes including varicella
5. Lesions on palms/soles	Low	No febrile prodrome OR < 4 minor criteria	Varicella testing as needed

Most commonly confused is chickenpox especially in adults who may present with more severe cases of chickenpox [24]. See Table 22.2 for a comparison of the two conditions.

Key Physical Exam Findings and Diagnostic Features

The CDC has created the following algorithm/criteria to identify high-risk cases for smallpox based on the characteristics of classic smallpox (see Table 22.3). Assignment of risk based on this algorithm will help guide the appropriate level of public health response.

Management

Suspected cases should be isolated with airborne and contact precautions in a negative pressure room. Risk should be assessed via algorithm discussed above and then appropriate authorities notified should suspicion remain. Public health officials will help guide further management including length of quarantine and possible treatment with antiviral agents. Those early in the course of disease will be vaccinated to prevent progression. Otherwise treatment is generally supportive with IV fluids similar to other septic patients. Antibiotics may be given for possible bacterial superinfection of lesions. Close contacts and hospital workers should be immediately identified and vaccinated to prevent further spread. Vaccination is generally very effective at preventing major infection when given within 2–3 days of exposure. Infected persons are generally contagious from onset of enanthema through first week of rash [23].

Complications

Survivors of smallpox generally have scarring or "pockmarks." Other less common complications include blindness from viral keratitis or secondary infection, arthritis, or encephalitis [23]. Death from smallpox is usually a result from a toxemia leading to coagulopathy, hypotension, and multiorgan failure. The mechanism of these complications is not completely understood [24]. Smallpox has a fatality rate of approximately 30% [17].

> **Bottom Line: Smallpox Clinical Pearls**
> - Classic lesions: progressing lesions (papule>vesicle>pustule>crust) in the same stage of development spreading from face/extremities to trunk.
> - Smallpox is highly contagious so early recognition is crucial to prevent spread.
> - Potential contacts should be immediately vaccinated to prevent/attenuate infection.
> - Despite the eradication of smallpox, it is important for emergency providers to keep this disease on their differential to prevent a devastating outbreak in the event of its accidental or intentional release.

References

1. Sternbach G. The history of anthrax. J Emerg Med. 2003;24(4):463–7.
2. Bush LM, Perez MT. The Anthrax attacks 10 years later. Ann Intern Med. 2012;156:41–4.
3. Brachman PS. Bioterrorism: an update with a focus on anthrax. Am J Epidemiol. 2002;155:981–7.
4. Inglesby TV, O'Toole T, Henderson DA, Bartlett JG, Ascher MS, Eitzen E, et al. Anthrax as a biological weapon, 2002: updated recommendations for management. JAMA. 2002;287:2236–52.
5. Doganay M, Metan G, Alp E. A review of cutaneous anthrax and its outcome. J Infect Public Health. 2010;3:98–105.
6. Cinquetti G, Banal F, Dupuy AL, et al. Three related cases of cutaneous anthrax in France: clinical and laboratory aspects. Medicine. 2009;88(6):371–5.

7. Carucci JA, McGovern TW, Norton SA, et al. Cutaneous anthrax management algorithm. J Am Acad Dermatol. 2002;47:766–9.
8. Adalja AA, Toner E, Inglesby TV. Clinical management of potential bioterrorism-related conditions. N Engl J Med. 2015;372:954–62.
9. Swartz MN. Recognition and Management of Anthrax: an update. N Engl J Med. 2001;345(22):1621–6.
10. Inglesby TV, Henderson DA, Bartlett JG, Ascher MS, Eitzen E, Friedlander AM, et al. Anthrax as a biological weapon. JAMA. 1999;281:1735–45.
11. Hendricks KA, Wright ME, Shadomy SV, et al. Centers for Disease Control and Prevention Expert Panel Meetings on Prevention and Treatment of Anthrax in Adults. Emerging Infectious Diseases. 2014;20(2):e130687
12. Dixon TC, Meselson M, Guillemin J, Hanna PC. Anthrax. N Engl J Med. 1999;341:815–26.
13. Inglesby TV, Dennis DT, Henderson DA, et al. Plague as a biological weapon: medical and public health management. Working Group on Civilian Biodefense. JAMA. 2000 May 3;283(17):2281–90.
14. Prentice MB, Rahalison L. Plague. Lancet. 2007;369:1196.
15. CDC. Prevention of plague: recommendations of the Advisory Committee on Immunization Practices (ACIP). MMWR. 1996;45(RR-14):1–15.
16. CDC. Human plague – four States, 2006. MMWR. 2006;55(34):940–3.
17. Aquino LI, Wu JJ. Cutaneous manifestation of category A bioweapons. J Am Acad Dermatol. 2011;65:1213.e1–15.
18. Kasper D, Fauci A, Hauser S, Longo D, Jameson J, Loscalzo J. Harrison's principles of internal medicine, 19e; 2015 Available at: http://accessmedicine.mhmedical.com/content.aspx?sectionid=79736559&bookid=1130&Resultclick=2. Accessed: 20 Nov 2017.
19. Kman NE, Nelson RN. Infectious agents of bioterrorism: a review for emergency physicians. Emerg Med Clin North Am. 2008;26(2):517–47.
20. Hornick R. Tularemia revisited. N Engl J Med. 2001;345:1637–9.
21. Dennis DT, Inglesby TV, Henderson DA, et al. Tularemia as a biological weapon: medical and public health management. JAMA. 2001;285:2763–73.
22. Senel E, Satilmis O, Acar B. Dermatologic manifestations of tularemia: a study of cases in the mid-Anatolian region of Turkey. Int J Dermatol. 2015;54:e33–7.
23. Breman JG, Diagnosis HDA. Management of Smallpox. N Engl J Med. 2002;346(17):1300.
24. Moore ZS, Seward JF, Lane JM. Smallpox. Lancet. 2006;367:425–35.
25. Centers for Disease Control and Prevention. Smallpox: for clinicians. https://www.cdc.gov/smallpox/clinicians/index.html. Accessed 10 Aug 2017.
26. Cunha BA. Anthrax, tularemia, plague, ebola or smallpox as agents of bioterrorism: recognition in the emergency room. Clin Microbiol Infect. 2002;8:489–503.

Other Potentially Life-Threatening Conditions with Mucocutaneous Findings (Leptospirosis, Typhoid Fever, Dengue, Diphtheria, Murine Typhus)

Brett Lee and Emily Rose

Leptospirosis

Background

Leptospirosis is a potentially fatal zoonotic infection seen in both temperate and tropical regions exposed to heavy rainfall and flooding. Rodents are the most important reservoir for transmission. Commonly carried by the brown rat (*Rattus norvegicus*), the virus is excreted through urine of the rat or other infected animal and contracted by contact with mucosal surfaces or skin breaks [1]. It is most commonly seen in tropical areas subject to poverty, large rainfall, and flooding; however, cases do occur within the United States, particularly the South Pacific coastal states and Hawaii [2]. The organism can infect many types of mammals which can be either asymptomatic or fatal. Spontaneous abortion is a common complication in animals and frequently described in cattle, swine, sheep, and goats. Risk factors for acquiring leptospirosis infection include activities with exposure to infected animals or water. Farmers and animal caretakers are at particular risk. Sporadic outbreaks commonly occur and have been described in athletes participating in triathlons who swam in infected water [3–6].

B. Lee
Department of Emergency Medicine, Los Angeles County + University of Southern California Medical Center, Los Angeles, CA, USA

E. Rose (✉)
Department of Emergency Medicine, Keck School of Medicine of the University of Southern California, Los Angeles County + USC Medical Center, Los Angeles, CA, USA
e-mail: emilyros@usc.edu

© Springer International Publishing AG, part of Springer Nature 2018
E. Rose (ed.), *Life-Threatening Rashes*, https://doi.org/10.1007/978-3-319-75623-3_23

Clinical Presentation

Symptoms are largely nonspecific, and patients often present with flu-like illness including fever, myalgias, and headache. However, there are several distinguishing features that herald a diagnosis of leptospirosis (see Table 23.1). Ocular findings are quite common and may be present in up to 90% of cases. In particular, conjunctival suffusion, a dilatation of conjunctival vessels, is a common presentation in leptospirosis but rarely seen in other infectious diseases (see Fig. 23.1). Other ocular findings may include subconjunctival hemorrhage, icterus (seen in severe disease), and hypopyon [7].

Rash is less common and may lead one to consider other diagnoses such as dengue, hantavirus, chikungunya, and others; however, other cutaneous findings such as jaundice with intense pruritus (secondary to liver and renal failure) as well as petechiae or ecchymosis from hemorrhagic complications may be present [7].

Table 23.1 Classic features of leptospirosis

Typical presentation
Flu-like illness
Conjunctival suffusion[a]
Myalgias (especially calf pain)
Headache with retro-orbital pain

[a]Distinguishing clinical feature

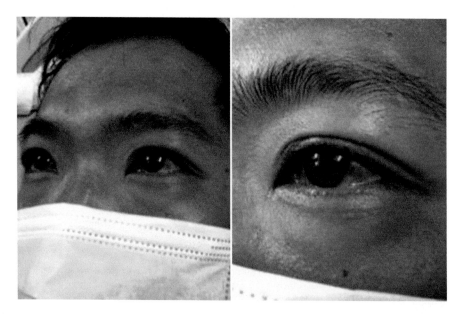

Fig. 23.1 Conjunctival suffusion with subconjunctival hemorrhage in a patient with leptospirosis. (From Lin et al. [57]. (Link to image: (may be better quality via the link) https://www.ncbi.nlm. nih.gov/core/lw/2.0/html/tileshop_pmc/tileshop_pmc_inline.html?title=Click%20on%20 image%20to%20zoom&p=PMC3&id=3269263_tropmed-86-187-g003.jpg)

Atypical Presentation

There have been documented cases of a pretibial rash with leptospiral infection; however, this is uncommon, as the majority of leptospiral diseases are without cutaneous findings. Other atypical findings include pharyngeal injection, maculopapular skin rashes, and cutaneous hyperesthesias [8, 9].

Associated Symptoms

Systemic symptoms are common, predominantly fever, myalgias, and headache. The headache is frequently described as a throbbing, bitemporal, frontal headache often accompanied by retro-orbital pain and photophobia. Myalgias with back and calf tenderness are commonly described. Cough, nausea, vomiting, diarrhea, and abdominal pain are also not infrequent [9].

Disease Progression

With leptospirosis, the disease course may vary significantly from patient to patient. Following exposure, the average incubation period is 10 days (see Fig. 23.2). In typical cases, patients then proceed to a biphasic illness. In the first phase, patients experience rapid onset of fever, rigors, myalgias, and headache that lasts 4–9 days. Patients then experience an afebrile phase for up to 3 days, followed by a recurrence of fever and possible complications such as meningitis and uveitis [9].

Common Mimics and Differential Diagnosis

Differential diagnosis includes malaria, dengue, chikungunya, typhus, rickettsial disease, and hantavirus. See Table 23.2 for distinguishing features of the differential diagnoses.

Complications

Severe leptospiral infections can lead to significant and potentially lethal complications (see Table 23.3). Weil's syndrome is characterized by liver and renal failure usually in association with altered level of consciousness, hemorrhage, and anemia. Advanced age and jaundice are associated with a higher mortality rate. Severe infections may also be complicated by progression to ARDS and circulatory collapse [9, 10].

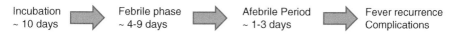

Incubation   Febrile phase   Afebrile Period   Fever recurrence
~ 10 days   ~ 4-9 days   ~ 1-3 days   Complications

Fig. 23.2 Leptospirosis disease timeline

Table 23.2 Differential diagnoses for leptospirosis

Differential diagnoses	
Malaria	Cyclical fevers Severe headache Rash is uncommon
Dengue	High fevers Headache with retro-orbital pain Conjunctival injection Maculopapular rash Palmar desquamation Petechiae/ecchymosis and positive tourniquet test
Chikungunya	High fever Maculopapular rash Myalgias, arthralgias
Typhoid fever	Fever with relative bradycardia Rose spot rash GI symptoms
Rocky Mountain spotted fever	Fever Headache Arthralgias, myalgias Maculopapular rash, petechiae, purpura that moves centripetally. Can affect palms and soles Predominantly eastern United States
Murine typhus	Fever Maculopapular rash that starts centrally and classically spares palms and soles
Hantavirus	Fever Headache GI symptoms Rash is uncommon Non-cardiogenic pulmonary edema

Table 23.3 Complications of leptospirosis

Complications
Weil's syndrome: hepatic and renal failure
Hemorrhagic complications: epistaxis, GI bleed, pulmonary hemorrhage, hemolytic anemia
Myocarditis
Neurologic: broad neurologic symptoms, aseptic meningitis, transverse myelitis
ARDS
Circulatory collapse

Hemorrhagic complications may also occur, secondary to coagulopathy and thrombocytopenia. Pulmonary hemorrhage is one of the most severe complications with a demonstrated fatality rate over 50%. GI bleeding, severe epistaxis, and hemolytic anemia are other hemorrhagic complications that may be present [1, 11].

Myocarditis, although rare, is another well documented complication of leptospirosis [9].

Patients may also experience a myriad of neurologic complications including aseptic meningitis (relatively common) and transverse myelitis [9].

Management

Diagnosis

Definitive diagnosis is made from PCR, antibody titers, or culture. However, as these diagnostic measures take time, empiric treatment should be initiated if there is a high clinical suspicion of the disease [12].

Treatment

While the majority of leptospirosis cases are mild and will resolve without intervention, early antibiotic therapy may prevent disease progression (see Table 23.4). Outpatient therapy is indicated for mild disease and consists of either doxycycline or azithromycin, with azithromycin being the preferred treatment for pregnant women and children. If rickettsial infection is a possible diagnosis, doxycycline should be given (see Chap. 16 for further discussion on rickettsial infections). Patients with evidence of complications, hemodynamic instability, or severe dehydration should be admitted for supportive care, targeted treatment of the specific complication and intravenous antibiotics [1, 13]. Inpatient treatment includes IV penicillin, ampicillin, ceftriaxone, or cefotaxime. A Jarisch-Herxheimer reaction may occur following treatment, which should be managed supportively [14].

Table 23.4   Treatment of leptospirosis

Treatment regimens	
Outpatient	Doxycycline 100 mg orally twice daily for 7 days
	Azithromycin 500 mg orally daily for 3 days
	Amoxicillin 50 mg/kg in 3 equally divided oral doses for 7 days
Inpatient	IV penicillin 1.5 million units every 6 h for 7 days
	Doxycycline 100 mg IV twice daily for 7 days
	Ceftriaxone 1–2 g IV once daily for 7 days
	Efotaxime 1 g IV every 6 h for 7 days

Bottom Line: Leptospirosis Clinical Pearls
- Leptospirosis can range from mild flu-like illness to multi-organ dysfunction.
- Patients typically present with flu-like illness, headache, and myalgias, predominantly in the back and calves.
- *Ocular findings are a key diagnostic clue to leptospirosis.*
- Conjunctival suffusion is the most common ocular finding in leptospirosis.
- Other ocular findings include subconjunctival hemorrhage, scleral icterus, and scattered petechiae.

- Diagnosis should be made clinically and is confirmed with serology, PCR, and culture.
- Outpatient treatment includes doxycycline, azithromycin, or amoxicillin.
- Inpatient regimens include IV penicillin, doxycycline, ceftriaxone, and cefotaxime.
- Complications may affect nearly any organ system and include hemorrhagic complications, liver failure, myocarditis, neurologic manifestations, ARDS, and renal failure.

Typhoid Fever

Background

Typhoid fever is a febrile illness common among travelers endemic to Asia, Africa, Latin America, and the Caribbean. It is caused by *Salmonella enterica* serotypes (Typhi and Paratyphi) and is commonly spread through urine and feces. Humans are the only reservoir and it is endemic in areas with poor sanitation [15].

Clinical Presentation and Disease Progression

Typhoid fever is a febrile illness that often develops mucocutaneous findings. Classically, typhoid fever is known for its "rose-spot" rash, which is characterized as a blanching salmon-colored maculopapular rash that appears across the trunk in groupings of 5–15 papules (Fig. 23.3). These lesions may extend across the back and to proximal extremities as well [16].

Atypical Presentation

One notable atypical finding that appears to be specific to typhoid fever is "furry tongue" (see Fig. 23.4). There are well-documented cases of white-yellow-coated tongues following infection with a reported specificity up to 94% [17, 18].

Associated Symptoms

In addition to fever and rash, patients commonly present with abdominal pain. This abdominal pain may be associated with either constipation or diarrhea which occur with similar frequency. In addition, relative bradycardia (Faget's sign/sphygmothermic dissociation) is a well-described phenomenon as are headache, sleep disturbance, cough, arthralgias, and myalgias (see Table 23.5) [19].

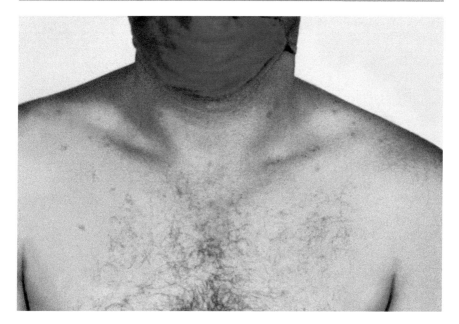

Fig. 23.3 Patient with a rose-colored rash on chest and shoulders with acute typhoid fever. (Photo courtesy: https://phil.cdc.gov/details.aspx?pid=2215)

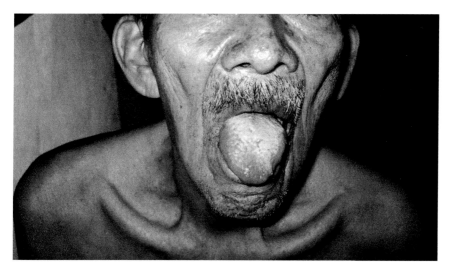

Fig. 23.4 Coated tongue in a patient with typhoid fever. (From Bal and Czarnowski [18]. Open access https://www.ncbi.nlm.nih.gov/pmc/articles/PMC374215/bin/21FF1.jpg)

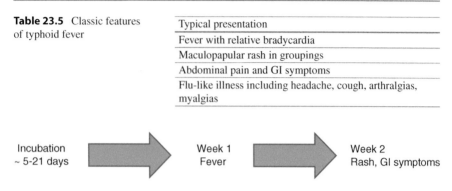

Table 23.5 Classic features of typhoid fever

Typical presentation
Fever with relative bradycardia
Maculopapular rash in groupings
Abdominal pain and GI symptoms
Flu-like illness including headache, cough, arthralgias, myalgias

Incubation
~ 5-21 days → Week 1
Fever → Week 2
Rash, GI symptoms

Fig. 23.5 Typhoid fever disease timeline

Time Course

Classically, typhoid fever presents in stages (see Fig. 23.5). The incubation period lasts roughly 5–21 days after ingestion of the microorganism. In the first week of clinical symptoms, patients often develop fever which classically rises in a stepwise fashion and, if left untreated, may persist for weeks. In the second week of infection, the classic "rose-spot" rash appears with lesions usually lasting 3–5 days before remitting. Patients commonly complain of abdominal pain at this time and may suffer from a myriad of GI symptoms. In the third week, patients may develop complications of ongoing illness as discussed below [15].

Common Mimics and Differential Diagnosis

Findings in typhoid fever are largely nonspecific, and therefore a wide differential needs to be maintained. The differential diagnosis includes malaria, tuberculosis, brucellosis, tularemia, leptospirosis, rickettsial infections, dengue fever, hepatitis, and infectious mononucleosis.

Complications

Left untreated, typhoid fever can lead to a number of significant complications, which commonly present as GI complaints in the later weeks of infection (see Table 23.6). These include small bowel ulceration, intestinal perforation, and subsequent septic shock. Other complications are also possible, including psychosis, neurologic deficits, and "typhoid encephalopathy" which can be described as altered level of consciousness or delirium. The bacteria can also seed nearly every other organ system so there may potentially be cardiac, respiratory, genitourinary, musculoskeletal, and central nervous system abnormalities. Finally, patients if untreated, may become chronic carriers causing autoinoculation and or transmission to other contacts [19–21].

Table 23.6 Complications of typhoid fever

Complications
GI: Ulceration, perforation, peritonitis
Neurologic: Encephalopathy, psychosis, neurologic deficits
Sepsis
Nearly any other organ system may be affected, but the above complications are the most common

Table 23.7 Treatment of typhoid fever

Treatment
Select treatment based on severity of disease and local susceptibilities
Inpatient regimen: IV ceftriaxone or fluoroquinolones
Outpatient regimen: PO azithromycin or fluoroquinolones
In severe cases, add IV dexamethasone 3 mg/kg followed by repeat doses at 1 mg/kg every 6 h

Management

Diagnosis

The diagnosis of typhoid fever should largely be clinical with high suspicion in patients exposed to endemic areas. Diagnosis can be confirmed with cultures from blood, stool, urine, rose spots, and bone marrow; however, these diagnostic methods are imperfect. Serology is of limited utility as a positive result may indicate a prior infection rather than an ongoing one. Other developing modalities include ELISA and PCR [22].

Treatment

Historically, chloramphenicol or amoxicillin were the drugs of choice for treatment of typhoid fever; however, drug resistance has become a significant problem (see Table 23.7). Treatment should be directed by local resistance patterns and severity of illness. In severe disease with systemic signs, IV ceftriaxone or fluoroquinolones should be initiated if there is local susceptibility. Glucocorticoid therapy has been shown to reduce severity of illness and mortality in patients with severe disease based on a randomized, double-blind placebo-controlled trial out of Indonesia with a relatively low side effect profile. Therefore, if patients develop delirium, coma, shock, or DIC, glucocorticoid therapy should be considered with dexamethasone loading at 3 mg/kg IV followed by 1 mg/kg IV every 6 h for eight doses. Steroid treatment beyond this is contraindicated as it may increase relapse rate [23–26].

In uncomplicated disease, oral agent therapy with ciprofloxacin 500–750 mg PO BID for 14 days should be initiated. In quinolone-resistant regions, azithromycin 1 g PO may be taken daily for 5 days [23].

Bottom Line: Typhoid Fever Clinical Pearls
- Typhus is endemic to Mexico, Peru, Indonesia, and the Indian subcontinent.
- Classic presentation includes high fevers, abdominal discomfort, and a maculopapular rash that appears in clusters across the torso.
- Significant complications may occur from untreated typhoid fever particularly throughout the GI tract, but any organ may be affected.
- Diagnosis is clinical and treatment initiated empirically in suspected cases, while confirmatory tests are pending.
- Treatment choice should be based on severity of disease and local susceptibilities.

Dengue Fever

Background

Dengue fever, caused by several serotypes of Flaviviridae, is one of the most common etiologies of arthropod-borne viral disease in the world. While often asymptomatic and self-limited, dengue fever can vary significantly in severity and is a significant public health concern in developing nations [27].

Clinical Presentation

Dengue fever classically presents with high fever, headache, abdominal pain, myalgias, and arthralgias as well as mucocutaneous findings (see Tables 23.8 and 23.9). During the febrile portion of the illness, conjunctival injection and oropharynx hyperemia are commonly present (see Fig. 23.6). Facial flushing or erythematous mottling may occur at the beginning of fever or just before, usually resolving within 2 days after onset of symptoms (Fig. 23.7). Rash can occur in up to 50% of patients, occurring either early or late. The rash is typically described as maculopapular and can occur diffusely across face, throat, abdomen, and extremities. Patients may endorse pruritus as well. With defervescence, a late cutaneous eruption develops, characterized by confluent and erythematous islands, which are often pruritic in nature (Figs. 23.8 and 23.9). The rash often resolves within 2–3 days but may last up to as many as 5 days. In addition, as the disease resolves, pruritic desquamation of the palms and soles may occur. Other cutaneous manifestations occur secondarily to hemorrhagic complications, as discussed below, and include petechiae, purpura, and ecchymosis (see Fig. 23.10) [28].

Table 23.8 Mucocutaneous findings in dengue

Mucocutaneous findings
Conjunctival injection
Oropharynx hyperemia
Facial flushing
Maculopapular rash across face, throat, abdomen, and extremities
Confluent erythematous islands
Desquamation of palms and soles
Petechiae, purpura, ecchymosis

Table 23.9 Typical presentation of dengue

Typical presentation
Flu-like illness including fevers, myalgias, arthralgias
Mucocutaneous findings as above
Headache with retro-orbital pain
Nausea and vomiting
Relative bradycardia
Less common findings: anorexia, altered taste sensation, sore throat

Associated Symptoms

As above, patients may experience a myriad of symptoms consistent with viral illness. Patients commonly complain of frontal headache with retro-orbital pain, myalgias, arthralgias, nausea, and vomiting. During the febrile phase of the illness, patients commonly have a relative bradycardia to the degree of fever. Less common associated symptoms include anorexia, altered taste sensation, and mild sore throat. Other symptoms may occur secondarily to complications and will be discussed below [28].

Physical Exam

Patients may have conjunctival injection and pharyngeal erythema. Given propensity for hemorrhagic complications, patients commonly develop petechiae, purpura, and ecchymosis. Additionally, lymphadenopathy, hepatomegaly, facial plethora, or signs of overload secondarily to vascular leak may be present [28].

Time Course of Disease

Dengue virus is typically transmitted by the *Aedes* mosquito and is typically found in densely forested areas. The viral incubation period is 3–14 days after inoculation. Dengue fever is divided into three phases: the febrile phase, the critical phase, and the convalescent phase [28].

Fig. 23.6 Scleral injection in a patient with dengue fever. (From Thomas et al. [58] (open access))

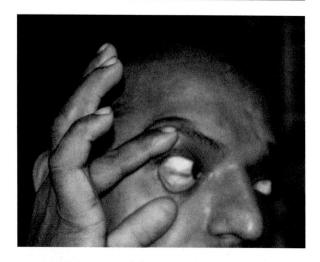

Fig. 23.7 Erythematous blanching rash of a patient with dengue infection. (From Thomas et al. [58] (open access))

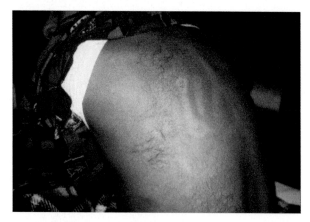

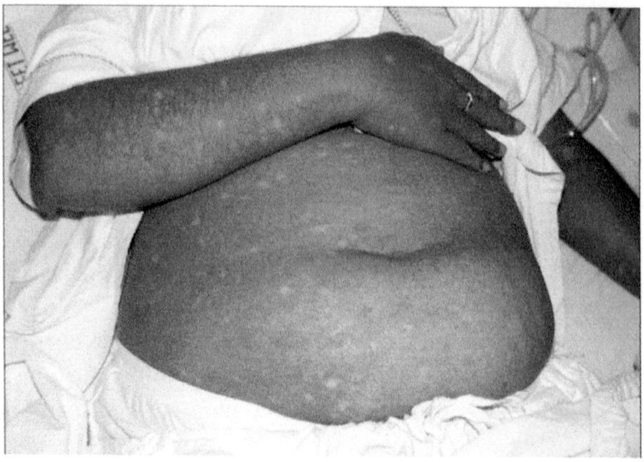

Fig. 23.8 Confluent erythematous rash with islands of sparing in a patient with dengue fever. (From Thomas et al. [58] (open access))

Fig. 23.9 Early erythematous mottling and secondary maculopapular rash. (Used with permission from Kenzaka and Kumabe [59])

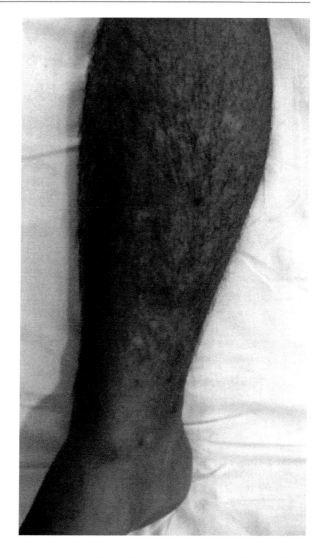

In the febrile phase, patients experience fever that waxes and wanes, lasting from 2 to 7 days, as well as many of the symptoms above [28].

The critical phase occurs around the time of defervescence, often 3–7 days after fever onset. This phase usually lasts 24–48 h and may be complicated by systemic vascular leak syndrome. This syndrome is characterized by plasma leak, bleeding, shock, and organ dysfunction [29].

The convalescent phase, often occurring 1–2 days after defervescence, is characterized by resolution of plasma leakage and hemorrhage. A pruritic confluent erythematous rash often is present during this phase as seen above [28].

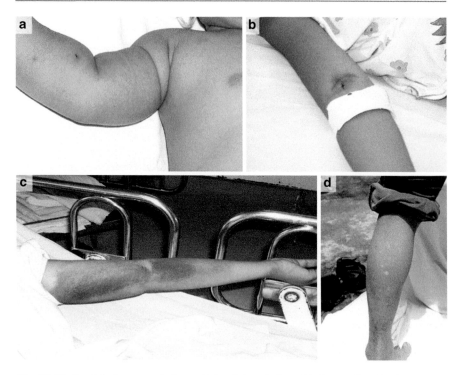

Fig. 23.10 Panel A shows a typical petechial rash in an infant with dengue. Panel B shows minor bleeding around injection sites, a very common feature in dengue. Panel C shows a hematoma in a patient with severe dengue. Panel D shows characteristic diffuse macular rash that appears after recovery from the acute illness in an adult patient with dengue (typically 3-6 days after fever onset). Note the "islands of white" of normal skin surround by an erythematous rash Simmons et al. [60]

Common Mimics and Differential Diagnosis

Differential diagnosis should include malaria, dengue, chikungunya, typhus, rickettsial disease, and hantavirus. See Table 23.2 for distinguishing features of the differential diagnoses.

Complications

The complications of dengue are many and involve multiple organ systems with potential organ failure. Table 23.10 outlines many of the common complications [28–33].

Management

Diagnosis
Early diagnosis of dengue fever is usually clinical and should be suspected in patients with the signs and symptoms above and exposure to endemic regions. Although neither sensitive nor specific, providers may perform a tourniquet test to

Table 23.10 Complications of dengue

Complications	
Systemic vascular leak syndrome	Third spacing
	Liver injury and failure
	Acute kidney injury
Hemorrhagic	Easy bleeding
	Petechiae and purpura
	DIC
Neurologic	Encephalopathy
	Seizures
	Neuropathies (including pure motor weakness)
	Guillain-Barre
	Transverse myelitis
Cardiovascular	Myocarditis
	Arrhythmia
	Heart failure

help in diagnosis (Figs. 23.11 and 23.12). In this test, a blood pressure cuff is inflated midway between systolic and diastolic pressures and left for 5 min. A positive test is characterized by ten or more new petechiae in 1 square inch. Diagnosis may be confirmed by detection of viral components in serum or PCR, although these methods are labor intensive and costly. Serology is also available but is of lower specificity. Viral culture is also available but of limited utility given time needed for test to result [34–36].

Management

Management is largely supportive because there is no antiviral therapy for dengue fever. Outpatient management may be appropriate in patients without systemic complications or comorbid conditions such as pregnancy, infancy, advanced age, renal failure, underlying hemolytic disease, or poor social support/access to follow-up care [37].

Inpatient management should be considered for any patient with comorbid conditions or for those with signs of severe infection. Signs of severe infection include abdominal pain, persistent nausea and vomiting, fluid accumulation (ascites, pleural effusion), mucosal bleeding, lethargy or altered mental status, hepatomegaly, increased hematocrit with rapid decrease in platelet count, and signs of shock or end-organ dysfunction. Aggressive IV fluid supplementation is warranted in those with signs of dehydration. Fevers, myalgias, and arthralgias can be managed with acetaminophen. NSAIDs and aspirin should be avoided, given the potential hemorrhagic complications. During the disease course, hemoglobin and platelets should be monitored. Transfusion with packed red blood cells is indicated for worsening anemia and suspected bleeding. Platelet transfusion is indicated for severe thrombocytopenia (<10,000/mm^3) but should not be pursued prophylactically. Vitamin K may be indicated if the prothrombin time is prolonged which may occur as a result of liver dysfunction or DIC [37–39].

Fig. 23.11 Positive
tourniquet test in dengue.
(Used with permission
from Kenzaka and Kumabe
[59])

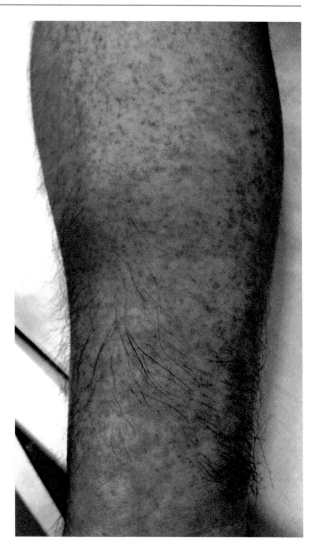

Fig. 23.12 Positive
tourniquet test in dengue.
(Source: https://www.cdc.
gov/dengue/training/cme/
ccm/images/tourniquet_
test1.png)

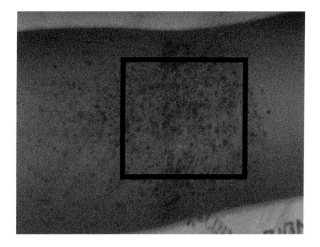

Bottom Line: Dengue Fever Clinical Pearls
- Dengue is endemic to tropical regions and transmitted by the *Aedes* mosquito.
- The disease presents in three phases: The febrile phase, the critical phase, and the convalescent phase.
- Symptoms may vary significantly; patients commonly present with fever, headache, retro-orbital pain, GI symptoms, and rash.
- The initial rash is maculopapular and may last several days.
- A secondary rash may present in the convalescent phase, which is erythematous, occurs in clusters, and is often pruritic.
- There are a wide range of complications that can occur from dengue fever, including vascular leak, hemorrhagic sequelae, and multi-organ dysfunction.
- Diagnosis is largely clinical and confirmed with titers and PCR.
- Treatment is largely supportive with IV fluids and antipyretics, particularly acetaminophen.
- Aspirin and NSAIDs should be avoided due to potential hemorrhagic complications.
- Transfusion and vitamin K may be required for hemorrhagic complications.

Diphtheria

Background

Caused by the gram-positive rod *Corynebacterium diphtheriae*, diphtheria is a disease that can cause a myriad of symptoms, ranging from asymptomatic infection to respiratory distress. It is often associated with mucocutaneous symptoms. Diphtheria was a significant cause of morbidity and mortality in the pre-vaccine era; however, since the advent of the diphtheria vaccine, the disease has largely been eliminated in developed countries but may sporadically occur [40].

Clinical Presentation

Patients infected with *C. diphtheria* usually present in one of two fashions: respiratory diphtheria or cutaneous diphtheria. Respiratory diphtheria is often caused by toxigenic strains, whereas cutaneous diphtheria may be caused by both toxigenic and non-toxigenic strains.

Respiratory diphtheria often presents with sore throat, malaise, cervical lymphadenopathy, and low-grade fever. Early in the disease course, only pharyngeal erythema may be present, which then progresses to isolated areas of gray and white exudate (see Figs. 23.13 and 23.14; Table 23.11). Although known as the hallmark of this disease, pseudomembranes form in only one third of cases. Pseudomembranes

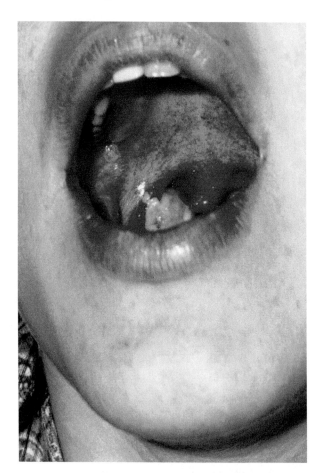

Fig. 23.13 Early diphtheria in a 26-year-old female. Note the membrane on the right tonsil. (Used with permission from Kadirova et al. [61])

Fig. 23.14 Diphtheritic membrane extending from the uvula to the pharyngeal wall with associated neck edema in a 47-year-old female. (Used with permission from Kadirova et al. [61])

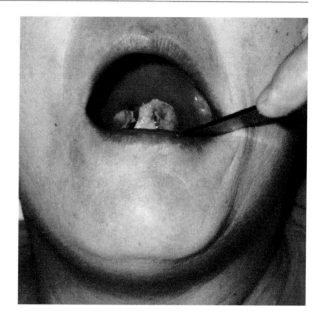

Table 23.11 Mucocutaneous findings in diphtheria

Classic presentations	
Respiratory diphtheria	Pharyngeal erythema
	Gray-white exudate
	Pseudomembrane
	note that these findings can occur anywhere along respiratory tract
Cutaneous diphtheria	Blisters or pustules that progress to shallow ulcers
	Gray membranes
	Hemorrhagic or violaceous base
	Painful lesion that becomes anesthetic
	Heals poorly

are easily friable gray tissue adhering to underlying tissue, composed of necrotic fibrin, leukocytes, epithelial cells, and organisms. These membranes can spread anywhere along the respiratory tract; however, the majority of cases are found along tonsils and oropharynx. Extensive spreading of these membranes can lead to respiratory compromise which will be discussed below [41].

Cutaneous diphtheria is often the more benign of the two conditions as systemic toxicity is rare. Early, patients may experience a small blister or pustule, often over a site of minor skin trauma, with straw-colored fluid that ruptures early forming a punched-out ulcer. These shallow ulcers usually become chronic, poorly healing lesions (taking from 6 weeks to up to a year to heal) that become covered by gray membrane. While initially painful during the first 2 weeks, these lesions often become anesthetic and develop a hemorrhagic or purple base (see Fig. 23.15). In addition, this variant of the disease tends to predominately affect the impoverished and intravenous drug users. Patients with cutaneous diphtheria rarely develop the respiratory variant of the disease but commonly serve as a reservoir of infection for others [42–44].

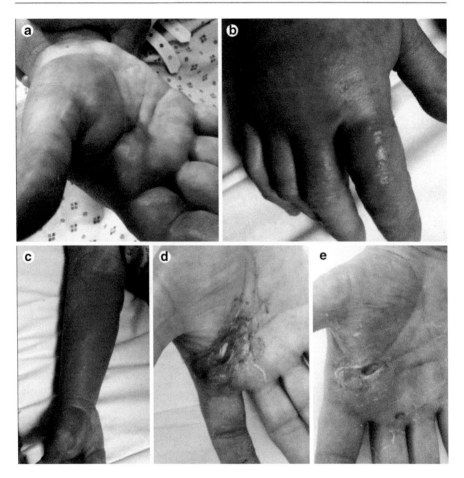

Fig. 23.15 Clinical presentation and progression of *Corynebacterium ulcerans* cutaneous diphtheria. (**a**) Palmar aspect of the hand at time of presentation. (**b**) Dorsal aspect of the hand at the
time of presentation. (**c**) Ipsilateral forearm with spreading inflammatory response at time of presentation. (**d**) Palmar aspect of hand after surgical debridement of synovial sheath necrotic tissue
at 7 days after presentation. (**e**) Palmar aspect of hand at 28 days after presentation and debridement. (Used with permission from Moore et al. [42])

Cutaneous Diphtheria

Associated Symptoms

Respiratory diphtheria often presents similar to streptococcal pharyngitis with sore
throat, malaise, lymphadenopathy, and low-grade fever; however, patients may also
experience cough as areas of the respiratory tract become involved. Symptoms may
become significantly more severe in cases of systemic toxicity as discussed below.
Symptoms are not solely limited to cutaneous and respiratory systems, however,
and further manifestations will be discussed below [45, 46].

Fig. 23.16 The "bull neck" of diphtheria infection. (Source: https://www.cdc.gov/diphtheria/images/symptoms.jpg)

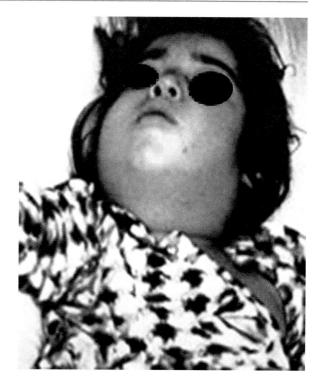

Physical Exam

As above, findings consistent with diphtheria are posterior oropharynx erythema and pseudomembrane formation. In cases of nasal diphtheria, the clinician may find serosanguineous to purulent nasal discharge. In laryngeal diphtheria, hoarseness and cough may be present. In severe cases, the pseudomembranes may be extensive causing massive swelling of the tonsils, uvula, cervical lymph nodes, submandibular region, and neck. This presentation is colloquially known as the "bull neck" of diphtheria, and such swelling may cause stridor and respiratory distress (see Fig. 23.16) [41].

Time Course of Disease

Humans are the only known reservoir of disease, with spread primarily occurring via respiratory secretions or direct contact with mucocutaneous manifestations. Symptoms often appear 2–5 days postexposure. After symptoms begin, in untreated patients, the disease often lasts up to 2 weeks but can last up to 6 weeks. In appropriately treated patients, the infection is often cleared within 4 days [41, 47].

Common Mimics and Differential Diagnosis

Differential diagnosis should include infectious mononucleosis, group A streptococcal pharyngitis, epiglottitis, viral pharyngitis, acute necrotizing ulcerative gingivitis, oral candidiasis, and viral pharyngitis.

Complications

See Table 23.12 for a summary of complications associated with diphtheria. The primary and most feared complication is severe membranous pharyngitis which can lead to thickening of the neck, narrowing of the airway, and resultant respiratory distress. Airway management is of the utmost importance in the emergent management of these patients [41].

Another well-described complication of diphtheria is myocarditis, which is more common in severe infections. Cardiac manifestations of diphtheria have been noted in up to 10 to 25 percent of patients with diphtheria, often occurring 1–2 weeks after symptom onset. Patients may experience heart blocks, arrhythmia, heart failure, and, in severe cases, circulatory collapse. These potential complications mandate cardiac monitoring in patients with potential systemic disease [41, 48].

Neurologic toxicity is another well-known complication of severe diphtheria infection. As with cardiac complications, neurologic symptoms are more common with worsening systemic illness. Manifestations of neurologic involvement often include paralysis of the soft palate and posterior pharyngeal wall. These neuropathies can progress to cranial neuropathies and peripheral neuritis ranging from mild weakness to total paralysis [49].

Management

Diagnosis
A diagnosis of diphtheria should first be suspected clinically in the unvaccinated or exposed population in the setting of above findings, particularly with friable pseudomembrane formation. Culture from respiratory tract or cutaneous lesions is

Table 23.12 Complications of diphtheria

Complications	
Respiratory	Airway narrowing
	Respiratory failure
Cardiovascular	Myocarditis
	Heart blocks
	Arrhythmia
	Heart failure
Neurologic	Cranial nerve palsies
	Soft palate and posterior pharynx paralysis
	Peripheral neuropathies

required for definitive diagnosis; however, a presumptive diagnosis can be made in the setting of gram-positive rods on gram stain with the above findings. PCR and toxin assay are also available to help distinguish whether a toxigenic form of diphtheria is causing the patient symptoms [50].

Treatment

The most important aspect of treatment of treatment in diphtheria is airway management given risk for obstruction. Patients should also be monitored for dysrhythmias and hypotension secondary to cardiac involvement with supportive management as needed [41].

In cases of early suspected or confirmed respiratory diphtheria, antitoxin should be administered. Of note, antitoxin is only effective before the toxin enters the cell. In addition, there is a 5–20% risk of hypersensitivity or serum sickness; therefore, ideally a scratch test can be performed before IV administration, and epinephrine should be readily available in cases of anaphylaxis [51].

Antibiotic therapy also plays a role in the treatment of diphtheria, with the antibiotics of choice being erythromycin or penicillin. Benefits of antibiotic therapy are threefold: killing of bacteria preventing further toxin formation, slowing spread of local infection, and reducing of transmission. Treatment with these antibiotic regimens is for 2 weeks followed by a repeat culture to ensure eradication [47, 51]. See Table 23.13 for antibiotic treatment regimens.

Table 23.13 Antibiotic treatment regimens for diphtheria

Treatment	
Erythromycin	500 mg four times daily for 2 weeks
Penicillin	PO intolerant Penicillin G IM injections 600,000 units every 12 h PO tolerant: Oral penicillin V 250 mg four times daily for 2 weeks

Bottom Line: Diphtheria Clinical Pearls
- Diphtheria is a potentially life-threatening illness of two variations: Respiratory and cutaneous.
- Respiratory diphtheria classically causes pseudomembrane formation which may be diffuse and can lead to airway obstruction.
- Cutaneous findings are generally nonspecific, characterized by grayish non-healing ulcers.
- Diphtheria may affect multiple organ systems with cardiac and neurologic manifestations being the most common in severe systemic illness.
- Diagnosis is initially clinical and confirmed with cultures and PCR.
- Treatment includes antibiotics and antitoxin (if early in the disease course).

Murine Typhus

Background

Murine or endemic typhus is a flea-borne infectious disease caused by *Rickettsia typhi*. The infection is often mild and self-limited and likely frequently remained undiagnosed as a nonspecific febrile illness with rash. As with other rickettsial disease, infection induces a widespread vasculitis [51, 52].

Murine typhus is primarily transmitted via the rat flea, particularly in the developing world and in locations with large rat populations. However, any type of flea may carry and transmit the disease. In suburban United States, cats, opossums, mice, and shrews may host infected fleas. Humans are infected via infected flea bite. Most cases of murine typhus in the United States are reported in people from California, Hawaii, and Texas [51, 52].

Classic Clinical Presentation

Murine typhus is typically a mild illness of nonspecific viral-type symptoms (see Table 23.14). Typically, the onset of illness is abrupt with fever, headache, chills, and myalgias. A rash is present in 20–50 percent of patients. The classic rash is a fine, maculopapular rash that begins on the abdomen and spreads centripetally to the extremities (see Fig. 23.17). Classically, the palms, soles, and face are spared. The rash is frequently faint and less apparent in dark-skinned individuals [51, 53].

Atypical Presentation

Children are more likely to additionally have abdominal pain, vomiting, and diarrhea [54]. In approximately 10 percent of patients, the rash may be petechial. In contrast to the typical mild disease course, severe complications may potentially occur, particularly in patients with glucose-6-phosphate dehydrogenase deficiency (G6PD) and the elderly (see Complications below).

Table 23.14 Classic murine typhus presentation

Classic presentation
Flu-like illness
Fevers
Headache
Myalgias
Fine maculopapular rash
Spreads from trunk to extremities
No palms or soles involvement

Fig. 23.17 Diffuse murine typhus rash consisting of multiple erythematous macules. (Source: Gorchynski et al. [53] *(open access)*)

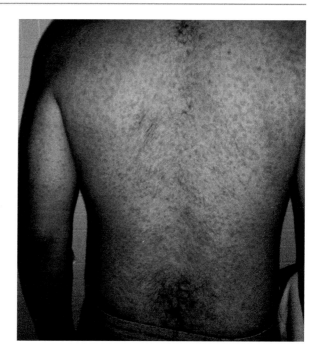

Time Course of Disease

After inoculation, there is a 7–14-day incubation period prior to symptom onset. Low-grade fever generally occurs within the first 1–2 days and resolves within 2 days. Rash onset classically occurs 5 days after onset of symptoms and usually resolves spontaneously within 4 days. Total resolution of symptoms generally occurs within 14 days (see Fig. 23.18) [55].

Common Mimics and Differential Diagnosis

There is a wide differential diagnosis to the nonspecific symptoms of murine typhus. Important diagnoses to consider include viral infections, rubella, measles (see Chap. 6), mononucleosis, and classically tropical infections such as dengue and Zika.

Key Physical Exam Findings and Diagnostic Features

Diagnosis typically occurs with initial clinical suspicion in a patient with fever, headache, rash, and possible exposure to infected fleas. Similar to other rickettsial infections, there is no reliable diagnostic test early in the disease course. Serologic confirmation may occur with an indirect fluorescent antibody testing which is

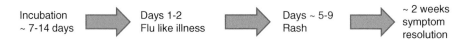

Fig. 23.18 Murine typhus disease timeline

Table 23.15 Treatment regimens for murine typhus

Treatment	
Adults	Doxycycline 100 mg twice daily[a]
Children	Doxycycline 4 mg/kg/day divided into two doses every 12 h[b]

[a]Treatment duration is controversial and not clearly outlined
[b]Tetracyclines and chloramphenicol can be used as alternatives, but are generally less effective

typically only available at a health department laboratory. Other laboratory findings are nonspecific and also nondiagnostic. Thrombocytopenia occurs in approximately half of all patients with murine typhus [51, 55].

Management

Treatment of murine typhus rapidly improves clinical symptoms and decreases complication rates; therefore, empiric treatment should be initiated in those with a high enough index of suspicion (see Table 23.15). While tetracyclines and chloramphenicol are effective treatments, doxycycline is the antibiotic of choice for rickettsial infections (see Chap. 16), and adults should receive 100 mg twice daily. In children, doxycycline is still the recommended agent of choice regardless of age. The recommended dosing of doxycycline in children is 4 mg/kg daily divided into two doses to be received every 12 h. Of note, fluoroquinolones and chloramphenicol may also be used but appear to be less efficacious. In addition, fluoroquinolones should not be used in children under the age of 18 years. While duration of therapy is controversial, some sources recommend treatment until 3 days after defervescence, and evidence of clinical improvement is documented. In addition, it should be noted that most individuals will recover from illness within 2 weeks without treatment [51, 52, 56].

Complications

While complications are rare, nearly any organ system may be affected by murine typhus. Notable complications include renal dysfunction, pulmonary edema, respiratory failure, aseptic meningitis, splenomegaly, and rarely septic shock and multi-organ system failure. Severe disease is more likely to occur in patients with G6PD deficiency and advanced age [52].

Bottom Line: Murine Typhus Clinical Pearls
- Murine typhus is a flea-borne illness that causes an abrupt onset of symptoms including fever, headache, and myalgias.
- It is often generally a mild, self-limited disease.
- A faint maculopapular rash begins on the trunk and spreads peripherally, sparing the palms and soles.
- Patients with G6PD deficiency and advanced age are at risk for life-threatening complications.
- Treatment is with doxycycline.

References

1. Haake DA, Levett PN. Leptospirosis in humans. Curr Top Microbiol Immunol. 2015;387:65–97.
2. Jesus MS, Silva LA, Lima KM, Fernandes OC. Cases distribution of leptospirosis in City of Manaus, State of Amazonas, Brazil, 2000-2010. Rev Soc Bras Med Trop. 2012;45(6):713–6.
3. Morgan J, Bornstein SL, Karpati AM, et al. Outbreak of leptospirosis among triathlon participants and community residents in Springfield, Illinois, 1998. Clin Infect Dis. 2002;34(12):1593–9.
4. Stone SC, Mcnutt E. Update: outbreak of acute febrile illness among athletes participating in Eco-Challenge-Sabah 2000 – Borneo, Malaysia, 2000. Ann Emerg Med. 2001;38(1):83–4.
5. Radl C, Müller M, Revilla-fernandez S, et al. Outbreak of leptospirosis among triathlon participants in Langau, Austria, 2010. Wien Klin Wochenschr. 2011;123(23–24):751–5.
6. Brockmann S, Piechotowski I, Bock-hensley O, et al. Outbreak of leptospirosis among triathlon participants in Germany, 2006. BMC Infect Dis. 2010;10:91.
7. Rathinam SR. Ocular manifestations of leptospirosis. J Postgrad Med. 2005;51(3):189–94.
8. Gochenour WS, Smadel JE, Jackson EB, Evans LB, Yager RH. Leptospiral etiology of Fort Bragg fever. Public Health Rep. 1952;67(8):811–3.
9. Sanford JP. Leptospirosis – time for a booster. N Engl J Med. 1984;310(8):524–5.
10. Gulati S, Gulati A. Pulmonary manifestations of leptospirosis. Lung India. 2012;29(4):347–53.
11. Gouveia EL, Metcalfe J, De carvalho AL, et al. Leptospirosis-associated severe pulmonary hemorrhagic syndrome, Salvador, Brazil. Emerging Infect Dis. 2008;14(3):505–8.
12. Limmathurotsakul D, Turner EL, Wuthiekanun V, et al. Fool's gold: why imperfect reference tests are undermining the evaluation of novel diagnostics: a reevaluation of 5 diagnostic tests for leptospirosis. Clin Infect Dis. 2012;55(3):322–31.
13. Suputtamongkol Y, Niwattayakul K, Suttinont C, et al. An open, randomized, controlled trial of penicillin, doxycycline, and cefotaxime for patients with severe leptospirosis. Clin Infect Dis. 2004;39(10):1417–24.
14. Guerrier G, D'ortenzio E. The Jarisch-Herxheimer reaction in leptospirosis: a systematic review. PLoS One. 2013;8(3):e59266.
15. Parry CM, Hien TT, Dougan G, White NJ, Farrar JJ. Typhoid fever. N Engl J Med. 2002;347(22):1770–82.
16. Hoffman SL, Punjabi NH, Kumala S, et al. Reduction of mortality in chloramphenicol-treated severe typhoid fever by high-dose dexamethasone. N Engl J Med. 1984;310(2):82–8.
17. Haq SA, Alam MN, Hossain SM, Ahmed T, Tahir M. Value of clinical features in the diagnosis of enteric fever. Bangladesh Med Res Counc Bull. 1997;23(2):42–6.
18. Bal SK, Czarnowski C. A man with fever, cough, diarrhea and a coated tongue. CMAJ. 2004;170(7):1095.
19. Gupta SP, Gupta MS, Bhardwaj S, Chugh TD. Current clinical patterns of typhoid fever: a prospective study. J Trop Med Hyg. 1985;88(6):377–81.

20. Ali G, Rashid S, Kamli MA, Shah PA, Allaqaband GQ. Spectrum of neuropsychiatric complications in 791 cases of typhoid fever. Tropical Med Int Health. 1997;2(4):314–8.
21. Huang DB, Dupont HL. Problem pathogens: extra-intestinal complications of Salmonella enterica serotype Typhi infection. Lancet Infect Dis. 2005;5(6):341–8.
22. Hoffman SL, Punjabi NH, Rockhill RC, Sutomo A, Rivai AR, Pulungsih SP. Duodenal string-capsule culture compared with bone-marrow, blood, and rectal-swab cultures for diagnosing typhoid and paratyphoid fever. J Infect Dis. 1984;149(2):157–61.
23. Thaver D, Zaidi AK, Critchley J, Madni SA, Bhutta ZA. Fluoroquinolones for treating typhoid and paratyphoid fever (enteric fever). Cochrane Database Syst Rev. 2005;(2):CD004530.
24. Kalra SP, Naithani N, Mehta SR, Swamy AJ. Current trends in the management of typhoid fever. Med J Armed Forces India. 2003;59(2):130–5.
25. Butler T, Islam A, Kabir I, Jones PK. Patterns of morbidity and mortality in typhoid fever dependent on age and gender: review of 552 hospitalized patients with diarrhea. Rev Infect Dis. 1991;13(1):85–90.
26. Cooles P. Adjuvant steroids and relapse of typhoid fever. J Trop Med Hyg. 1986;89(5):229–31.
27. Guzman MG, Harris E. Dengue. Lancet. 2015;385(9966):453–65.
28. Gubler DJ. Dengue and dengue hemorrhagic fever. Clin Microbiol Rev. 1998;11(3):480–96.
29. Kalayanarooj S, Vaughn DW, Nimmannitya S, et al. Early clinical and laboratory indicators of acute dengue illness. J Infect Dis. 1997;176(2):313–21.
30. Chhour YM, Ruble G, Hong R, et al. Hospital-based diagnosis of hemorrhagic fever, encephalitis, and hepatitis in Cambodian children. Emerging Infect Dis. 2002;8(5):485–9.
31. Solomon T, Dung NM, Vaughn DW, et al. Neurological manifestations of dengue infection. Lancet. 2000;355(9209):1053–9.
32. Carod-artal FJ, Wichmann O, Farrar J, Gascón J. Neurological complications of dengue virus infection. Lancet Neurol. 2013;12(9):906–19.
33. Neeraja M, Iakshmi V, Teja VD, et al. Unusual and rare manifestations of dengue during a dengue outbreak in a tertiary care hospital in South India. Arch Virol. 2014;159(7):1567–73.
34. Cao XT, Ngo TN, Wills B, et al. Evaluation of the World Health Organization standard tourniquet test and a modified tourniquet test in the diagnosis of dengue infection in Viet Nam. Tropical Med Int Health. 2002;7(2):125–32.
35. Guzman MG, Jaenisch T, Gaczkowski R, et al. Multi-country evaluation of the sensitivity and specificity of two commercially-available NS1 ELISA assays for dengue diagnosis. PLoS Negl Trop Dis. 2010;4(8):e811.
36. Hunsperger EA, Muñoz-jordán J, Beltran M, et al. Performance of dengue diagnostic tests in a single-specimen diagnostic algorithm. J Infect Dis. 2016;214(6):836–44.
37. Rajapakse S, Rodrigo C, Rajapakse A. Treatment of dengue fever. Infect Drug Resist. 2012;5:103–12.
38. Thomas L, Kaidomar S, Kerob-bauchet B, et al. Prospective observational study of low thresholds for platelet transfusion in adult dengue patients. Transfusion. 2009;49(7):1400–11.
39. Khan assir MZ, Kamran U, Ahmad HI, et al. Effectiveness of platelet transfusion in dengue fever: a randomized controlled trial. Transfus Med Hemother. 2013;40(5):362–8.
40. English PC. Diphtheria and theories of infectious disease: centennial appreciation of the critical role of diphtheria in the history of medicine. Pediatrics. 1985;76(1):1–9.
41. Naiditch MJ, Bower AG. Diphtheria; a study of 1,433 cases observed during a ten-year period at the Los Angeles County hospital. Am J Med. 1954;17(2):229–45.
42. Moore LSP, Leslie A, Meltzer M, Sandison A, Efstratiou A, Sriskandan S. Corynebacterium ulcerans cutaneous diphtheria. Lancet Infect Dis. 2015;15(9):1100–7.
43. Höfler W. Cutaneous diphtheria. Int J Dermatol. 1991;30(12):845–7.
44. Zeegelaar JE, Faber WR. Imported tropical infectious ulcers in travelers. Am J Clin Dermatol. 2008;9(4):219–32.
45. Murphy JR. Corynebacterium Diphtheriae. In: Baron S, editor. Medical microbiology. 4th ed. Galveston: University of Texas Medical Branch at Galveston; 1996. Chapter 32. Available from: https://www.ncbi.nlm.nih.gov/books/NBK7971/.

46. Walters RF. Diphtheria presenting in the accident and emergency department. Arch Emerg Med. 1987;4(1):47–51.
47. Kneen R, Pham NG, Solomon T, et al. Penicillin vs. erythromycin in the treatment of diphtheria. Clin Infect Dis. 1998;27(4):845–50.
48. Kneen R, Nguyen MD, Solomon T, et al. Clinical features and predictors of diphtheritic cardiomyopathy in Vietnamese children. Clin Infect Dis. 2004;39(11):1591–8.
49. Sanghi V. Neurologic manifestations of diphtheria and pertussis. Handb Clin Neurol. 2014;121:1355–9.
50. Efstratiou A, Engler KH, Mazurova IK, Glushkevich T, Vuopio-varkila J, Popovic T. Current approaches to the laboratory diagnosis of diphtheria. J Infect Dis. 2000;181(Suppl 1):S138–45.
51. American Academy of Pediatrics. Diphtheria. In: Kimberlin DW, Brady MT, Jackson MA, Long SS, editors. Red book: 2015 Report of the Committee on infectious diseases. 30th ed. Elk Grove Village: American Academy of Pediatrics; 2015. p. 307–11, 770–771.
52. Civen R, Ngo V. Murine typhus: an unrecognized suburban vector-borne disease. Clin Infect Dis. 2008;46(6):913–8.
53. Gorchynski JA, Langhorn C, Simmons M, Roberts D. What's hot, with spots and red all over? Murine typhus. West J Emerg Med. 2009;10(3):207.
54. Tsioutis C, Zafeiri M, Avramopoulos A, Prousali E, Miligkos M, Karageorgos SA. Clinical and laboratory characteristics, epidemiology, and outcomes of murine typhus: a systematic review. Acta Trop. 2017;166:16–24.
55. Peniche lara G, Dzul-rosado KR, Zavala velázquez JE, Zavala-castro J. Murine typhus: clinical and epidemiological aspects. Colomb Med. 2012;43(2):175–80.
56. Fergie JE, Purcell K, Wanat D. Murine typhus in South Texas children. Pediatr Infect Dis J. 2000;19(6):535–8.
57. Lin CY, Nan-Chang C, Lee CM. Leptospirosis after Typhoon *Americal*. J Trop Med Hyg. 2012;86(2):187–8.
58. Thomas EA, Mary J, Kanish B. Mucocutaneous manifestations of dengue fever. Indian J Dermatol. 2010;55(1):79–85.
59. Kenzaka T, Kumabe A. Skin rash from dengue fever. BMJ Case Rep. 2013;2013:bcr2013201598. https://doi.org/10.1136/bcr-2013-201598.
60. Simmons CP, Farra JJ, van Vinh Chau N, Wills B. Dengue. N Engl J Med. 2012;366:1423–32.
61. Kadirova R, Kartoglu HU, Strebel PM. Clinical characteristics and management of 676 hospitalized cases, Kyrgyz Republic, 1995. J Infect Dis. 2000;181(Suppl 1):S110–5.

Index

© Springer International Publishing AG, part of Springer Nature 2018
E. Rose (ed.), *Life-Threatening Rashes*, https://doi.org/10.1007/978-3-319-75623-3

Erythematous rash, 94
Erythroderma, 106–108
    atypical presentation, 269
    causes of, 267
    clinical presentation, 267–269
    complications, 274
    CTCL, 265
    diagnosis features, 270–272
    differential diagnosis, 270, 271
    exfoliative skin scaling, 265, 266
    incidence, 265
    initial management, 272, 273
    systemic symptoms, 269
    physical examination, 270, 271
    time course of disease, 270
    treatment modalities, 272, 273
Exfoliation, 274
Exfoliative toxins A (ETA), 127
Exfoliative toxins B (ETB), 127
Exotoxins, 104

F
Febrile phase, 331
Fixed drug eruptions, 67
Flaccid bullae, 128
Flat-type (malignant) smallpox, 315
Flaviviridae, 328
Food allergy, 19
Forchheimer spots, 87, 117, 118
Frambesiform secondary syphilis, 195
Francisella tularensis, 310
Fresh frozen plasma (FFP), 137

G
Gastrointestinal complications, 50
Gastrointestinal symptoms, 169
Gentamicin, 163
Glucagon infusion, 16
Glucocorticoids, 31, 32, 327
Granulocyte colony stimulating factor
    (G–CSF), 49
Group A *Streptococcus* (GAS), 103,
    117, 123
Guillain-Barré syndrome (GBS), 237
Gummatous syphilis, 191
GVHD, 45

H
Hematologic abnormalities, 283
Hematoxylin, 69
Hemophagocytic syndrome, 283

Hemorrhagic fever, 292
Hemorrhagic smallpox, 314
Henoch-Schönlein purpura (HSP), 68
    atypical presentation, 242, 245, 248
    clinical presentation, 241, 242, 245
    complications, 254
    diagnosis and management, 252, 253
    differential diagnosis, 251, 252
    pathogenesis, 241
    physical examination, 252
    systemic symptoms, 249
    time course of disease, 250, 251
Hepatosplenomegaly, 192, 234
Herpes simplex virus (HSV), 55, 58, 68,
    69, 72
Herpes zoster, *see* Varicella-zoster
    virus (VZV)
Human granulocytic anaplasmosis
    (HGA), 228
Human immunodeficiency virus (HIV),
    167–177
    crusted scabies
        atypical presentation, 173
        clinical presentation, 173
        complications, 175
        differential diagnosis, 174
        physical examination, 174
        symptoms, 173
        time course of disease, 174
        treatment, 175
        widespread proliferation, 173
    dermatologic conditions, 168
    eosinophilic folliculitis
        atypical presentation, 171
        clinical presentation, 170, 171
        complications, 172
        differential diagnosis, 171, 172
        incidence, 170
        management, 172
        physical examination, 172
        symptoms, 171
    herpes zoster, 180
    Kaposi sarcoma, 178
        atypical presentation, 176
        clinical presentation, 176
        complications, 177
        differential diagnosis, 177
        incidence, 176
        management, 177
        physical examination, 177
        signs and symptoms, 176
        time course of disease, 177
    molluscum contagiosum, 178, 179
    primary infection

Printed by Printforce, the Netherlands